A Colour Atlas of

Gynaecological Surgery

Volume 1: Vaginal operations

David H. Lees
FRCS(ED), FRCOG
Consultant Obstetrician and Gynaecologist,
Jessop Hospital for Women, Sheffield
Honorary Clinical Lecturer,
University of Sheffield

Albert Singer
Ph.D, D.Phil (OXON), MRCOG
Senior Lecturer in Obstetrics and Gynaecology,
University of Sheffield
Honorary Consultant Obstetrician and Gynaecologist,
Jessop Hospital for Women, Sheffield

Wolfe Medical Publications Ltd

Published by Wolfe Medical Publications Ltd,
London, England
Printed by Smeets-Weert, Holland
ISBN 0 7234 0723 1

Introduction

There is probably no substitute for the type of personal tuition provided by teacher and pupil working together in the operating theatre as surgeon and assistant, with knowledge and experience being passed on directly. There is, however, the disadvantage that such a relationship is not available to everyone and is, at best, transient. In addition the learner is frequently not at a stage in his career when he can take full advantage of what is available. The majority, therefore, have to look elsewhere for such instruction.

Textbooks of operative surgery provide the principal source of information, but these are only as good as their illustrations. The occasional colour plate does not instruct and there is something unreal about the well-executed drawings prepared by a medical artist to the specification of the author. The one worthwhile teaching aid is the simple line diagram or sketch, which demands considerable skill and ingenuity and allows the student to see and follow what is required. But to carry that information in one's mind and apply it in practice is another matter. In surgery, with all its accompanying distractions, the real life structures are frighteningly different from those which the simple diagrams have led one to expect, and these same structures obstinately refuse to adopt the position and behaviour expected of them.

Cine films are excellent but the cost of their production in time and money is high, besides which they are clumsy to use. This series of atlases offers what we consider to be the next best thing: a series of step-by-step colour photographs accompanied by an appropriate written commentary. This form of presentation follows almost exactly the colour slide plus commentary method most often used to teach surgery. Using slides, of course, it is necessary to have projection apparatus and access to a library or bank of suitable material. The method adopted in this series – of using high quality colour reproduction processes – retains the advantages of the slide and commentary method while avoiding its drawbacks.

The present series of atlases sets out to provide detailed instruction in the techniques of standard gynaecological operations. Its methodology is straightforward. The technique of each operation is clearly shown, step-by-step, using life-size photographs in natural colour, and with liberal use of indicators and accompanying diagrams. Where a step is repetitive or there is a natural sequence of steps, grouping has sometimes been used, but the natural size of the structures is maintained.

The accompanying commentary is concise and is printed on the same page as the photograph or photographs to which it refers. Every effort has been made to include only necessary material, but in situations where experience and special training have provided additional information and knowledge, that has been included.

The illustrations are selected and the accompanying commentaries so arranged as to carry the reader forward in a logical progression of thought and action in which he becomes involved. Occupied with one step he is at the same time anticipating the next, and in due course confirms his foresight as logical and correct. The photographs are those of a real patient having a real operation and the picture seen is exactly what the reader will see in the operation theatre when he does it himself. Interest is concentrated on the one step of the operation being taken at that time.

In any form of medical teaching there is the inevitable problem of pitching instruction at the level required by the audience and the presumption that the reader has insight into the specialist knowledge of the author is just as irritating as being patronised. We do not think there is a problem in this context because an atlas is by definition a guide and therefore for general use. It is just as likely to be consulted by a junior house surgeon about to assist at his first hysterectomy as by a senior colleague seeking an alternative method of dealing with a particular problem. That, at least, is the spirit in which it has been written.

Certain assumptions have had to be made to avoid verbosity, tediousness and sheer bulk of paper. It is hoped that the reader will be kind enough to attribute any omissions and shortcomings to the acceptance of such a policy. No one should be embarking on any of the procedures described without training in surgical principles, nor should he attempt them without knowledge of abdominal and pelvic anatomy and physiology.

Several areas have purposely been avoided in preparing the Atlas. There is no attempt to advise on the indications for operative treatment and only in the most general terms are the uses of a particular operation discussed. Individual surgeons develop their own ideas on pre- and post-operative care and have their personal predilections regarding forms of anaesthesia, fluid replacement and the use of antibiotics.

Even on the purely technical aspects the temptation to advise on the choice of instruments and surgical materials is largely resisted and it is assumed that the reader is capable of placing secure knots and ligatures. Each volume of the Atlas contains a photograph of the instruments used by the authors and some of these are shown individually. Most readers will have their own favourites but the information may be useful to younger colleagues. We do not consider the choice of suture material to be of over-riding importance. The senior author has used PGA suture material since its inception and although generally preferring it to catgut does not consider it perfect. It has disadvantages and can be very sore on the surgeon's hands but it does have advantages in that it is particularly suitable for vaginal work and for closing the abdomen.

There are, of course, several methods of performing the various operations but those described here have consistently given the authors the best results. It need hardly be reiterated that the observance of basic surgical principles is probably more important than anything else.

The Atlas is produced in six volumes, each of which relates approximately to a regional subspecialty. This is done primarily to keep the size of the volumes convenient for use but also to allow publication to proceed progressively.

From what has been written it might appear that the authors think of gynaecologists as necessarily male. The suggestion is rejected: the old-fashioned usage of the inclusive masculine gender is merely retained for simplicity and neatness. Anyone questioning the sincerity of this explanation would have to be reminded that every gynaecologist must, in the very nature of things, be a feminist.

Introduction to Volume 1

In presenting Volume 1 of this series of Atlases some short explanation of policy is appropriate. The various volumes were planned to be in all essentials self-sufficient and it therefore became important that subject matter be carefully apportioned to its correct place. One would not expect undue difficulty in relation to the volume on vaginal surgery because it would include only those operations done *per vaginam*. The vaginal surgery of malignancy and infertility would be retained for their own particular sections and some operations loosely thought of as vaginal really come under the heading of 'Surgery of the Vulva'. It is difficult to know whether to include the operations for stress incontinence; in that matter we have gone for a straight compromise by describing a Sling procedure which is mainly a vaginal operation and reserving for Volume 2 the Marshall–Marchetti–Krantz operation which is essentially an abdominal procedure.

There is a further difficulty when it comes to listing the operations described. A time-honoured classification exists which would be convenient to follow but it is unrealistic in that it does not include several operations which a practical gynaecologist needs to perform.

For example, much of vaginal surgery is concerned with prolapse and the usual course has been to describe a case of anterior colporrhaphy and posterior colpoperineorrhaphy as the basic procedure. Subsequently, there are built on that, the necessary variations to suit other aspects of prolapse. We could not remember when last we used this set operation, and a long waiting list provided no prolapse patient whose needs would have been served by it. It would obviously be wrong to describe an operation which has no application in reality, although the fact remains that anterior and posterior vaginal wall repair, singly or together, are necessarily embodied in practically every vaginal procedure.

The problem has been met by including a full description of both exercises with the Manchester repair. The recognised procedures for prolapse such as vaginal hysterectomy with repair and the Manchester repair, are of course fully described. We have added several operations so frequently required as to qualify as standard and which require special techniques. Post-hysterectomy prolapse, constricted vagina, enterocele and the tedious problem of major rectocele are given full coverage because the practical gynaecologist repeatedly meets them. We have felt much lighter in spirit since discarding the traditional list of contents and substituting a more honest, if less tidy, catalogue.

There is the debatable place of vesico-vaginal fistula in an Atlas such as this. Closure of a vesico-vaginal fistula is not a standard operation in the Western world, being only occasionally required; in the developing countries it is a commonly performed procedure. As far as actual management is concerned, the really important requirements are to define the fistula with accuracy and plan the operation to suit the particular problem, bearing in mind that the lesion may prove to be anything from reasonably simple to hideously complex.

The actual technique for the commonly encountered types is described and the emphasis has been on a diagrammatic rather than photographic representation. We hope we have been logical in choosing such an approach to what can be a very inexact condition.

Acknowledgements

This six volume colour atlas of Gynaecological Surgery was produced at the Jessop Hospital for Women, Sheffield as part of a postgraduate project to teach operative surgery by edited colour slides. We are indebted to all who took part in the exercise, but there are some whom we would particularly like to mention.

Mr Alan Tunstill, Head, Department of Medical Illustration, Sheffield Area Health Authority (Teaching), organised the whole of the actual photography. Mr Stephen Hirst took nearly all the photographs, and the high standard of work is obvious. Mrs Dorothy Huntingdon was responsible for the remainder; her photography too was excellent.

Professor I. D. Cooke generously gave full access to clinical material in his unit. All our other consultant colleagues were helpful when their cases were of interest to the project and acknowledgement is made in the text where appropriate.

The anaesthetists at all levels were very co-operative. Dr A. G. D. Nicholas, Dr D. K. Powell and Professor J. A. Thornton were the consultants involved. Of the numerous senior registrars and registrars we remember particularly Drs Bailey, Birks, Burt, Clark, Dye, Mullins, Saunders and Stacey.

Miss J. Hughes-Nurse, Mr I. V. Scott, Miss P. Buck and Dr H. David were the senior registrars and lecturers in obstetrics and gynaecology during the time and greatly assisted by keeping us informed of suitable cases and in the organising of operations. Drs Katherine Jones, E. Lachman, Janet Patrick, K. Edmonds, A. Bar-am and C. Rankin were involved in the management of the cases and assisted at operations.

Miss M. Crowley, nursing officer in charge of the Jessop Hospital operating theatres saw that we had every facility, and Sisters J. Taylor, M. Henderson, E. Duffield, M. Waller and A. Broadly each acted as theatre sister or 'scrub' nurse at the individual operations. Mr Leslie Gilbert and Mr Gordon Dalton, the operating room assistants were valuable members of the team. We particularly wish to thank the whole theatre staff for their courtesy and efficiency.

The line and colour diagrams featured in chapters 5, 11 and 12 were drawn by Miss Sue Hunter of Sheffield.

A large amount of secretarial work was involved. We are grateful to Mrs Jennifer Haydn-Smith and Mrs Valerie Prior of the University Department who dealt with most of it. Mrs Talya Singer has been responsible for typing the manuscript and has given much genial/general help and constructive advice throughout.

The photographs in this book were taken on Kodachrome 25 colour reversal film. The camera was a 35 mm Nikkormat FTN fitted with a 105 mm f2.5 Nikkor auto lens. A PK-3 extension ring was used for close ups and a 55 mm f3.5 Micro-Nikkor auto lens for general views. Illumination was provided by a Sunpak auto zoom 4000 electronic flash unit, set on full power. An exposure setting of 1/60th of a second at f16 was used.

Contents

To our wives

Anne & Talya

MINOR OPERATIONS

1: Dilatation and curettage

Dilatation of the cervix with curettage of the uterus is by far the commonest gynaecological operation. It is generally a diagnostic procedure but is sometimes used therapeutically. To allow an adequate examination of the uterus and appendages at the same time, a short general anaesthetic is administered, although local infiltration analgesia can be used in a frail patient. Suction curettage using a metal cannula of the Vabra type without anaesthesia can be carried out in the consulting room or clinic, but has limitations – in that an intra-uterine polyp will probably be missed and it is a theoretical possibility that the whole cavity of the endometrium may not be sampled by such a limited procedure.

Suction curettage is therefore adequate for symptomatic bleeding and as a check on endometrial histology but is not really adequate for cases of post-menopausal bleeding. A dilatation and curettage operation done under general anaesthesia is suitable for day-case management. It is not generally considered necessary to shave the patient when the D & C is a purely diagnostic procedure.

When done with care a D & C has several possible complications including perforation of the fundus uteri; when done roughly or carelessly the dangers make a formidable list. It is advisable therefore to adhere to and insist on a strict procedure or regime and one such is described here. In the event of the uterus being perforated the only situation demanding immediate surgical intervention is bleeding and this is only likely to occur where the uterus is or recently has been pregnant. Alterations in pulse rate (i.e. tachycardia) or the development of signs of peritonism, such as rebound tenderness or guarding, will indicate the need for laparotomy.

Many major and minor procedures are combined with curettage in gynaecological practice. Cervical erosions and polypi may be treated by diathermy and excision repectively and curettage is a necessary precursor to the prolapse repair operations and to abdominal hysterectomy where the endometrium has not been studied to exclude malignancy.

The term fractional curettage is used when an attempt is made to obtain separate specimens from the cervical canal and the cavity of the uterus or even from different parts of the cavity itself. Its application is in differential diagnosis and in estimating the extent of a malignancy, usually in the endocervix. The authors are not convinced that it is particularly accurate as a procedure. The method of using it is described in relation to uterine carcinoma in Volume 3.

The authors make no apology for the detailed description of D & C which follows. Experienced readers may think it tedious but they above all know how carelessly and even dangerously this common operation is sometimes done. They are aware also of the considerable amount of short-term and long-term disability that results. Neither can the medical-legal aspect be disregarded, especially in certain western countries.

Mishaps during investigative procedures are particularly unacceptable to the laity and litigation is always a possibility.

1

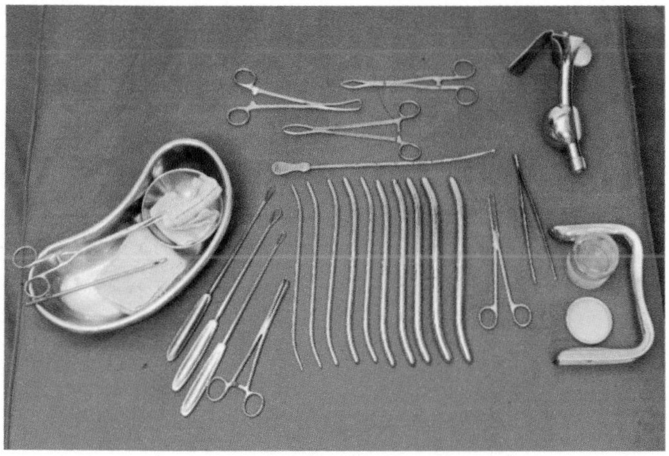

2

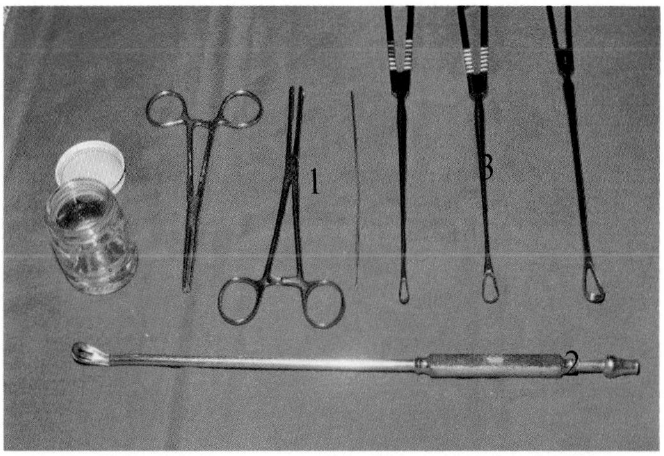

1 Instruments for dilatation and curettage (i)

A suitable set of instruments for D & C. The equipment shown is quite comprehensive and indicates that the procedure is looked on as a formal if minor operation to be done with full aseptic precautions. It should not be necessary to catheterise the patient if the bladder is emptied prior to the operation but a catheter and urine container are available in case there is doubt or difficulty. Decompression of the bladder allows a more accurate assessment of pelvic structures.

2 Items of particular value in dilatation and curettage

A pair of small Spencer Wells forceps are useful in stretching a cervix which is very tight and where the dilator will not enter. The closed blades are inserted into the cervical canal and then opened very slowly to give just enough stretch to allow dilatation to proceed (1).

A spoon-shaped flushing curette (2) but without any flushing attachment is particularly helpful in exploring the cavity of the uterus when evacuating it in an incomplete abortion case. The curette is gently inserted until its smooth distal end lies against the fundus of the uterus and it is then drawn down the uterine wall as a spoon to detach and remove retained products.

The ordinary sharp curettes are shown (3).

3

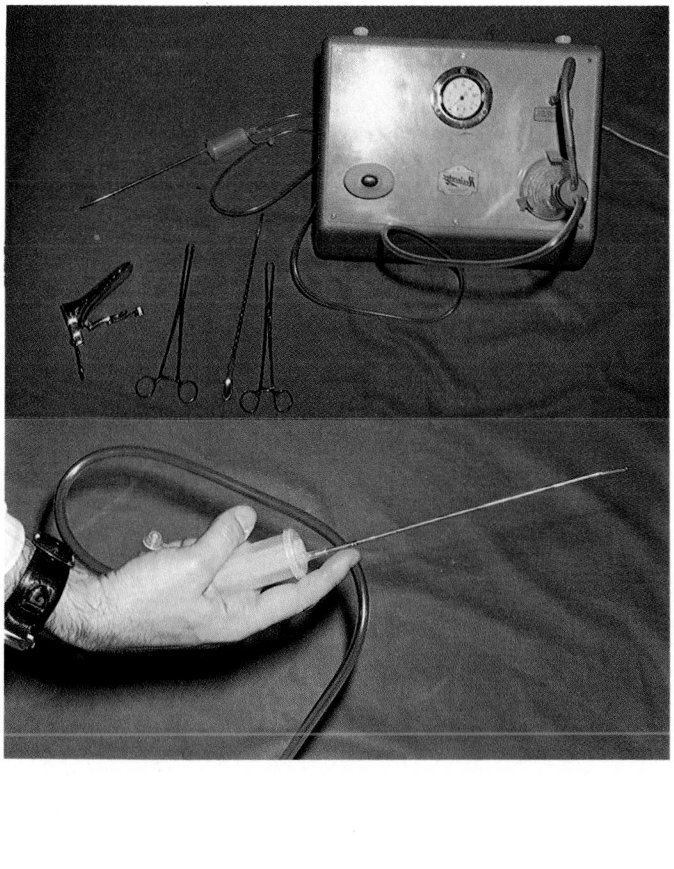

3 Instruments for dilatation and curettage (ii)

The Vabra suction curettage equipment. The curette itself is composed of a metal aspirator 240 mm long and 3 mm thick. A small slit measuring 1.5×16 mm is situated at the angled distal end. Proximally there are two small holes for pressure equalisation. The cannula is mounted on a plastic chamber with incorporated filter which collects the curettings. After use the combined cannula and lid are removed from the chamber which is then filled almost to capacity with 4 percent formaldehyde solution or some other fixative. The chamber is closed with a spare lid provided in the packing and the specimen sent in the polythene bag provided, for pathological examination. The procedure is preferably carried out in the outpatient department and some form of pre-medication may be given (diazepam or pentazocine). After preparation of the vulva and vagina by sterile swabbing a gynaecological examination is performed and a sound is then passed into the uterine cavity. The aspirator is then introduced into the uterine cavity without preceding dilatation of the cervical canal. A suction pressure of 600 mm Hg vacuum is used and is obtained from a central suction pump. The procedure may be carried out under a paracervical nerve block in which case Carbocaine 1 per cent solution is used and 10 ml are injected on each side of the cervix.

This figure shows the aspirator with the operator's finger over the pressure equalisation holes. Figure 3 shows the portable vacuum pressure apparatus connected to the aspirator. The limited number of instruments needed are displayed, i.e. vaginal speculum, uterine sound and holding forceps (single tooth).

4

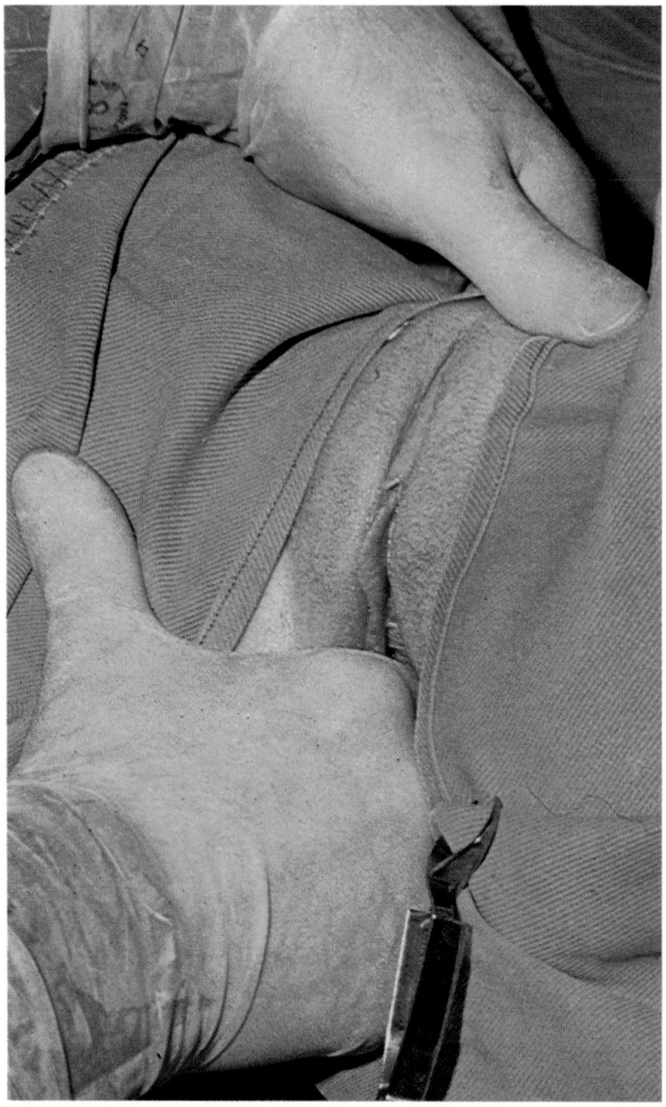

5

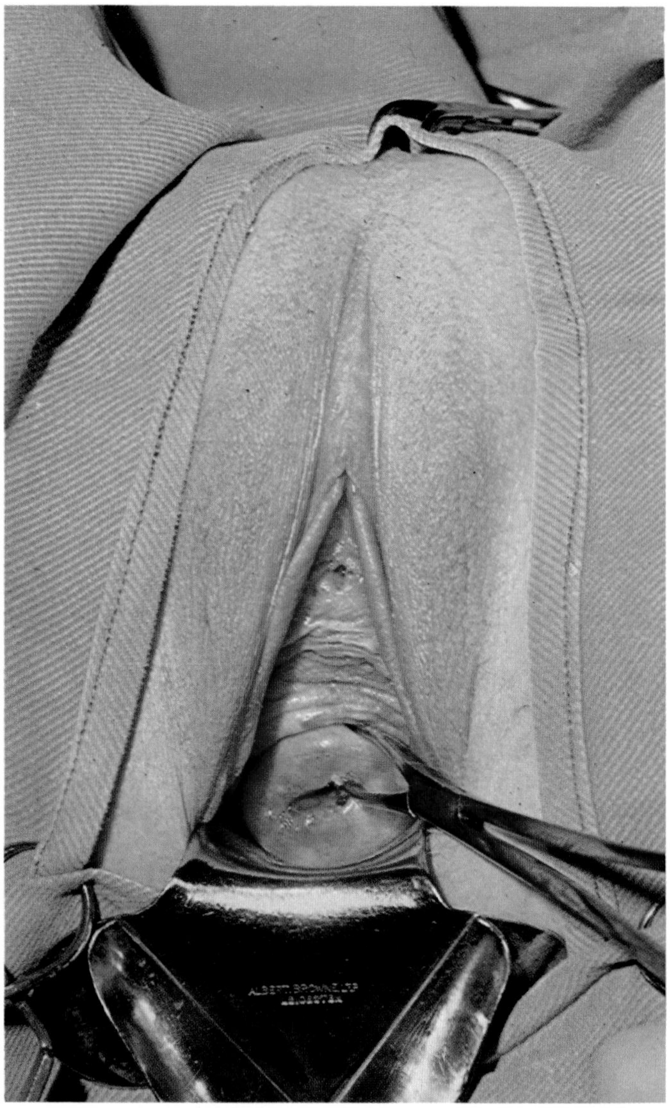

4 Bimanual examination

The patient is in the lithotomy position and the vagina and vulva have been swabbed with chlorhexidene solution (formula: see below*). The posterior vaginal wall is retracted with a Sims' speculum to expose the vagina and cervix and allow preparation. The drapes are then applied as shown. Bimanual examination at this stage is important for several reasons. Apart from obtaining essential information about the uterus it is necessary to know about the appendages and any abnormality in relation to them. The size, position, mobility and outline of the uterus should be established as all these have a bearing on the proposed operation. An indication of the axis or direction of the uterine cavity is an important safety factor in avoiding perforation by the uterine sound or a dilator.

* Chlorhexidine 0.5% in 70% spirit.

5 Securing the cervix

The anterior lip of the cervix is grasped at its mid-point by Littlewood's forceps. These forceps are less traumatic to the cervix than a volsellum. This serves to steady and fix the whole uterus during both dilatation and curettage. If necessary two pairs of forceps can be placed side by side to give a firmer hold.

6

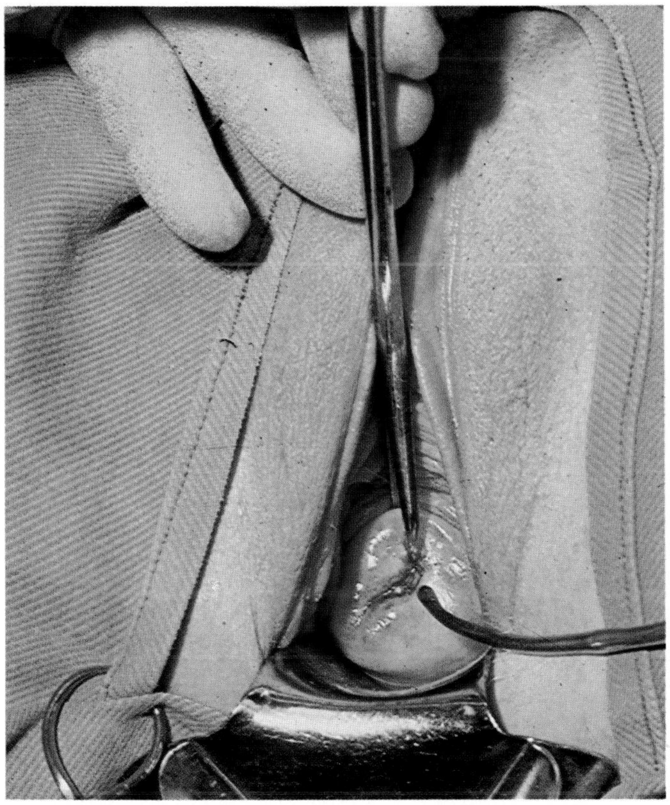

7

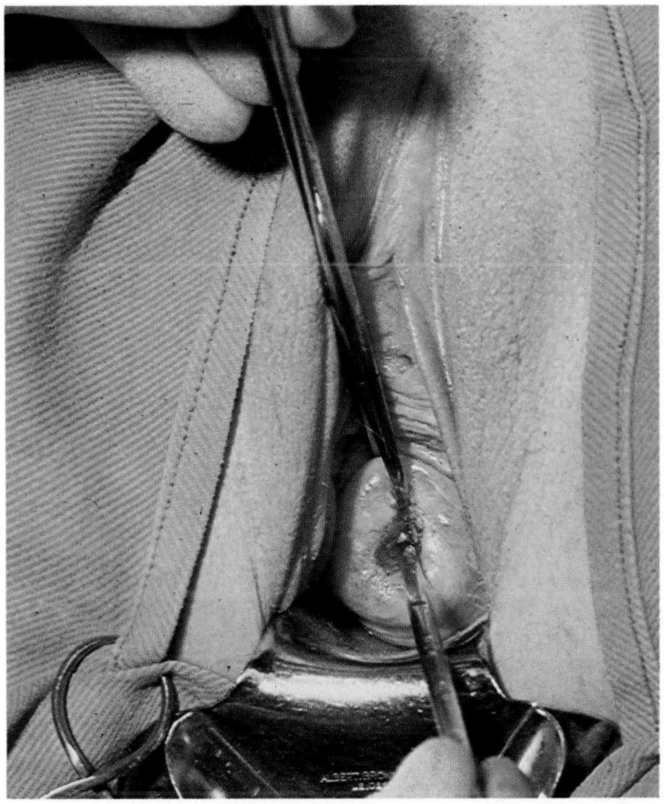

8

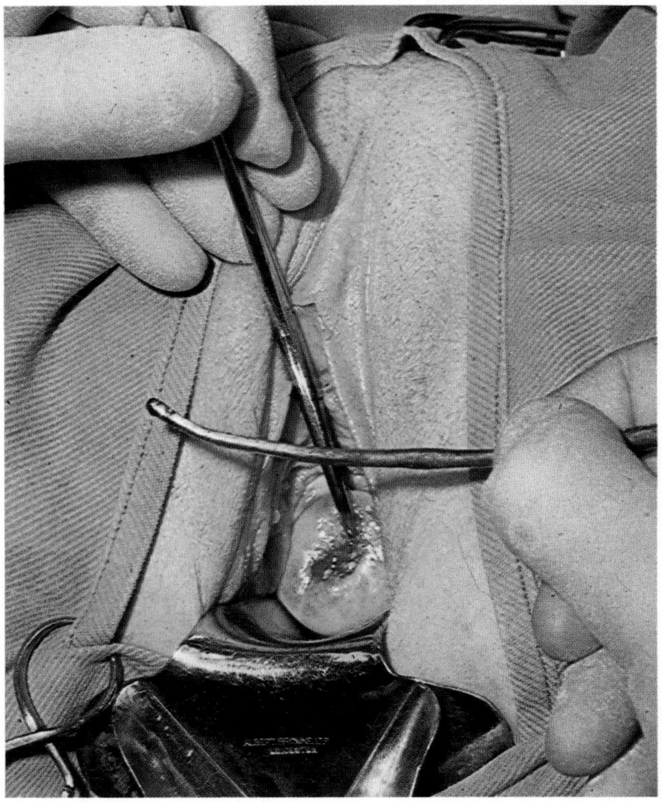

6 and 7 Exploring uterine cavity with sound

The uterine sound is introduced through the undilated cervix with its curve or concavity in line with what was estimated as the axis of the uterine cavity. It is held lightly like a pen and introduced gently towards the fundus of the uterus. The main purpose is to estimate the length of the uterine cavity and exclude major abnormalities. If the cervix is too tight to admit the rather bulbous tip of the sound easily, it is advisable to use one of the smaller dilators to prepare access for it. This would particularly apply in a case of post-menopausal bleeding or where the cervix had been amputated or repaired. Dilators have a gradually increasing gauge from the tip proximally and easily enter the cervical canal. Figure **6** shows the sound being introduced at the external os and **7** shows the cavity being examined. A Spencer Wells forceps is ideal for stretching a cervix which stubbornly resists an increased size of dilator. It must be used with care lest the cervix be split; if that happens it should be sutured immediately.

8 Measurement of uterine cavity

The depth to which the sound has been inserted to reach the fundus is shown on the scale which is imprinted on it but it is usual to fix the position on the sound at the external os with the forefinger and read it off again when the sound has been withdrawn from the uterus.

9
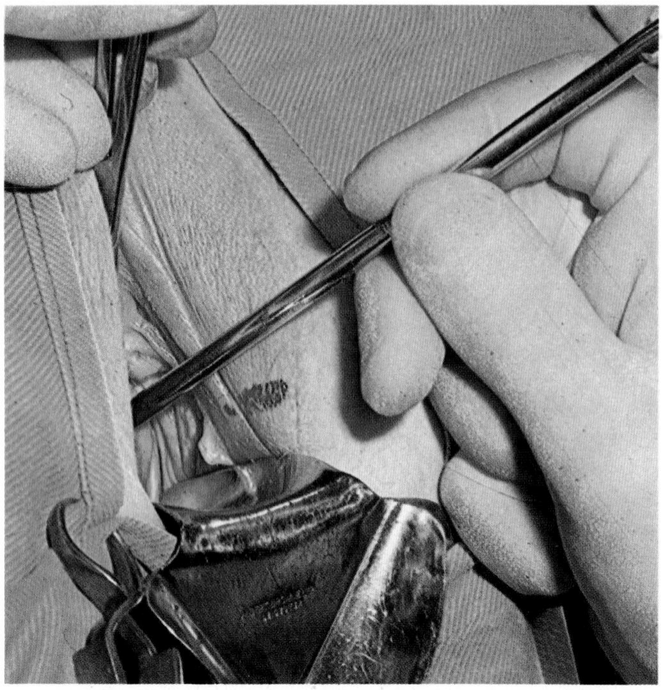

9 and 10 Dilatation of cervix

Starting with the smaller sized dilators these are used in turn to dilate the canal to the requisite amount. The point of each is lubricated and as with the sound the dilator is held in the fingers like a pen so that control is delicate and undue force is not used. As explained above, if the cervix is very resistant a pair of small Spencer Wells forceps introduced into the cervical canal and opened out gently and slowly will solve the difficulty.

It is in overcoming the resistance of a tight cervix that the uterus tends to be injured and it occurs in the following manner. The surgeon is pressing firmly on the dilator to overcome cervical spasm or narrowing. Suddenly that is achieved, the dilator is unchecked and is driven right through the fundus of the uterus. This hazard can be obviated by ensuring that the ring and little fingers of the right hand holding the dilator are flexed and so held that they and the ulnar border of the hand form a buffer which will meet and impinge on the vulva and pelvic floor before the advancing tip of the dilator reaches the fundus of the uterus. In **9** and **10** increasing sizes of dilators are being used and the method of flexing the hand as a safety measure is shown in both.

10
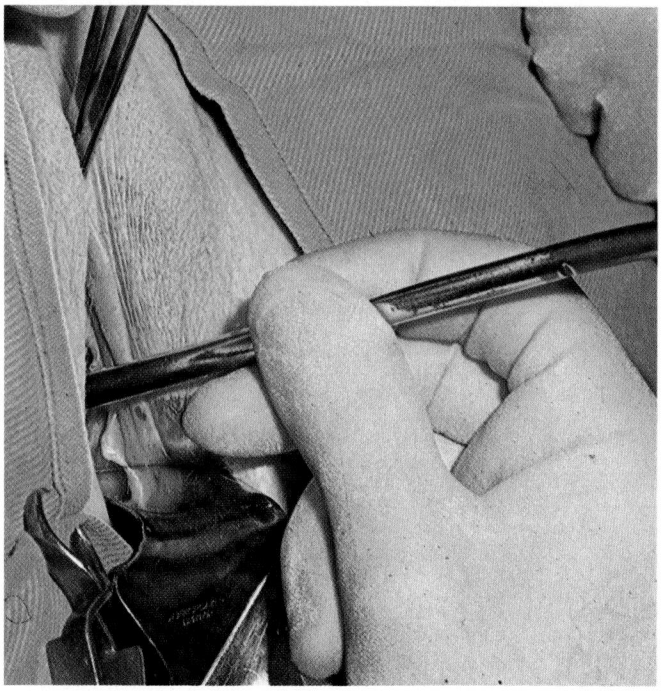

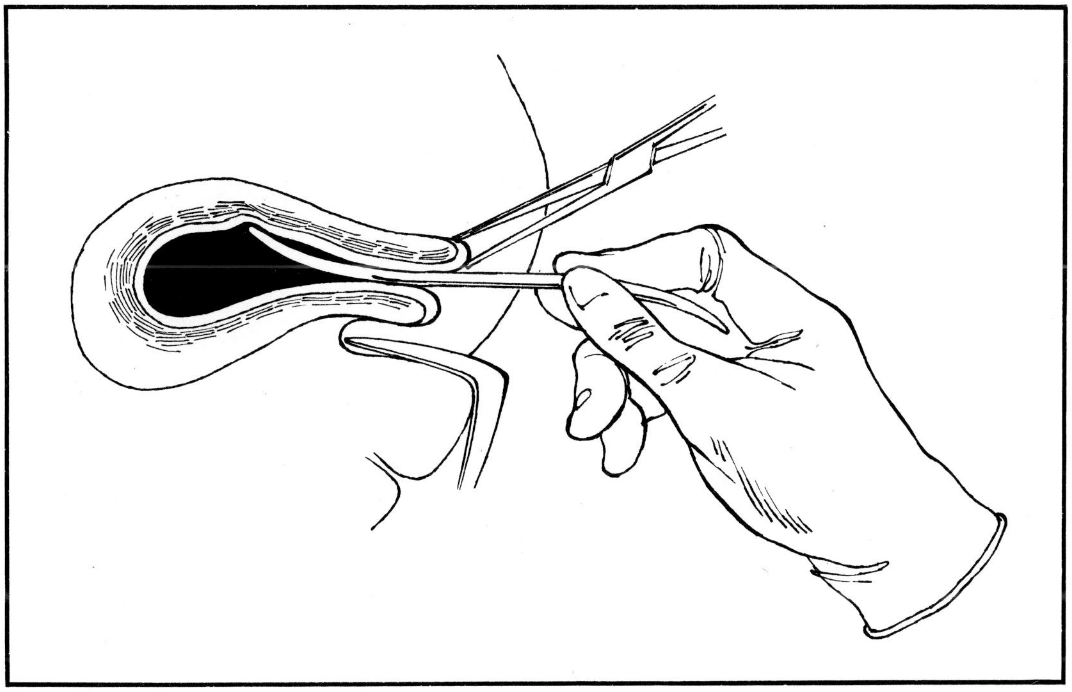

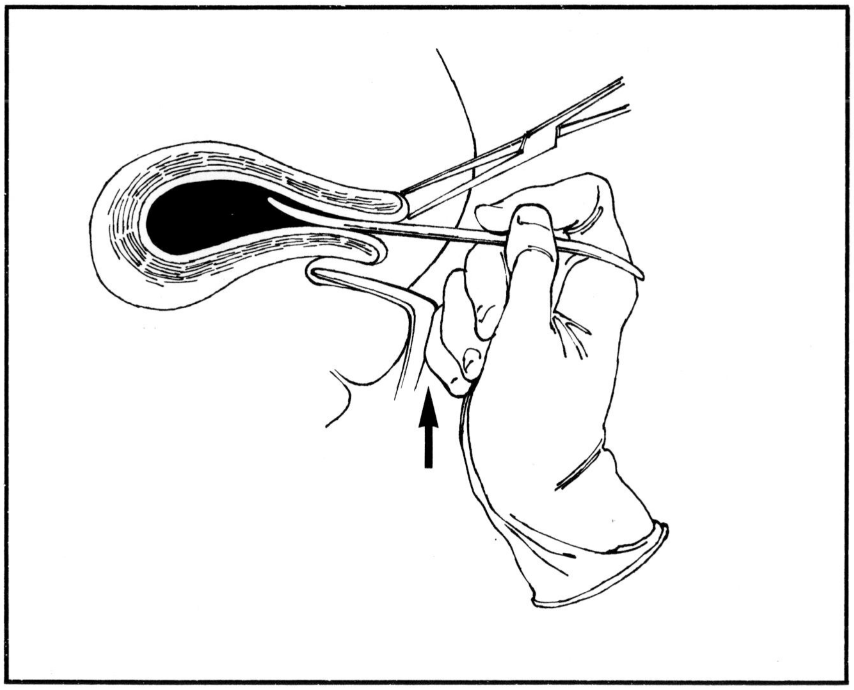

These diagrams illustrate the safety measures described in **9** and **10**.

In the first diagram the surgeon is holding the dilator in a potentially dangerous manner. Once he has overcome resistance at the internal cervical os, there is no barrier to impair the forward movement of the instrument. Perforation of the anterior wall of a retroposed uterus is possible.

In the second diagram the attitude of the hand holding the dilator prevents such an occurrence. Any excess and uncontrolled forward movement is obviated as indicated by the arrow which shows how the flexed hand forms a buffer to impinge on the perineum.

11

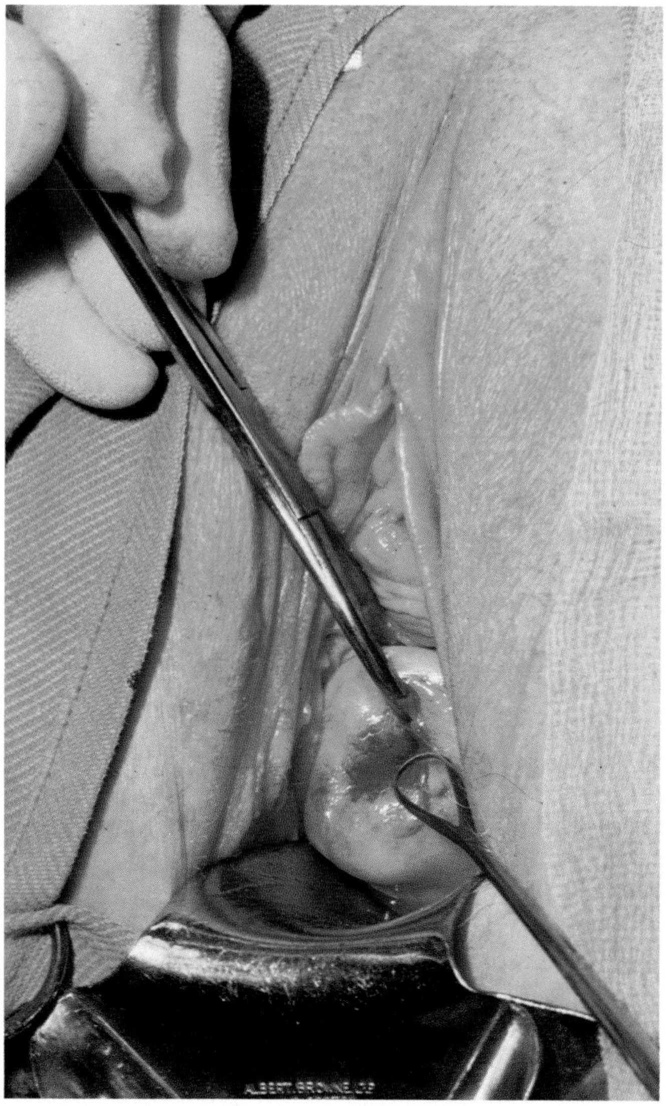

12

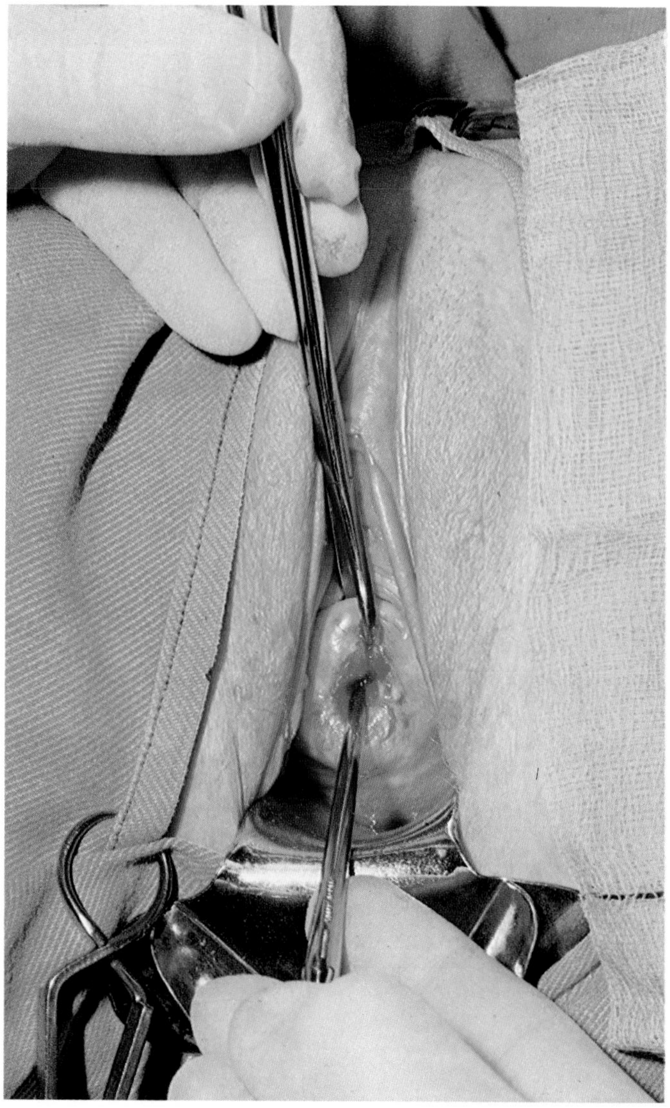

11 and 12 Curettage of uterus

The curette to be used is selected according to the circumstances. It is generally more satisfactory to use one with a broad end but if the cervix is non-elastic or resistant and there is fear of damaging it by further dilatation then a smaller sized curette should be chosen.

Held lightly between the thumb and forefinger of the right hand it is introduced into the uterine cavity in its known axis and as far as the fundus. It is definitively scraped down the anterior, posterior and each lateral wall of the uterus in turn to obtain sizeable specimens of endometrium for examination. The process is completed by curetting the fundus from side to side and making a further general curettage of the whole cavity. The curette is always held lightly between the finger and thumb or as one would hold a pen.

The curettings are transferred to a gauze swab placed lateral to the vulva either as they are obtained or by retrieval from the posterior vaginal fornix. While he is removing the endometrium the surgeon is looking out for any abnormality or roughness of the cavity wall such as might suggest a submucous fibroid or a large polyp. In **11** a medium sized sharp curette is about to be introduced into the cervical canal and in **12** curettage of the anterior wall is in progress.

13
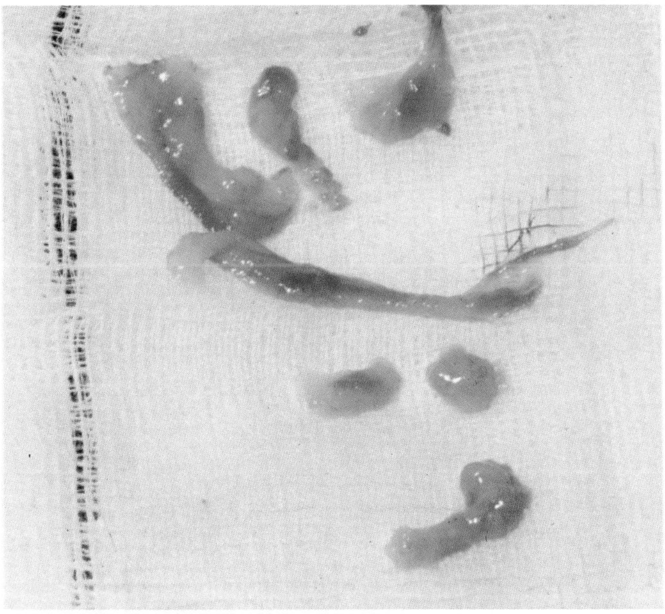

14
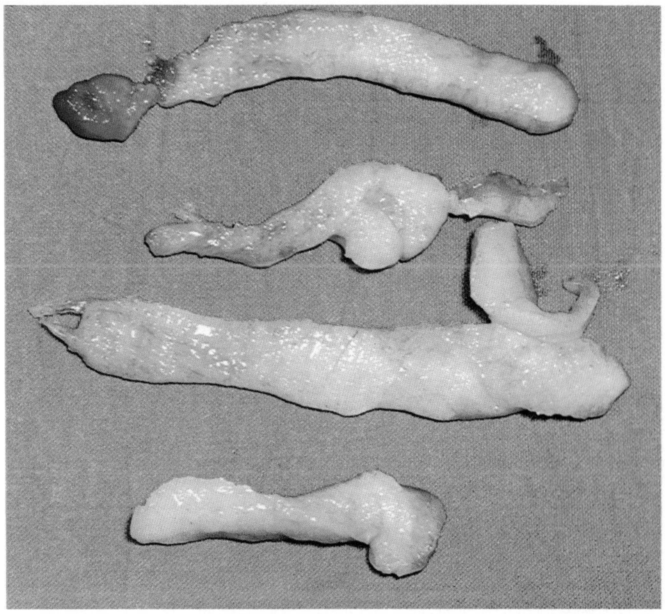

15
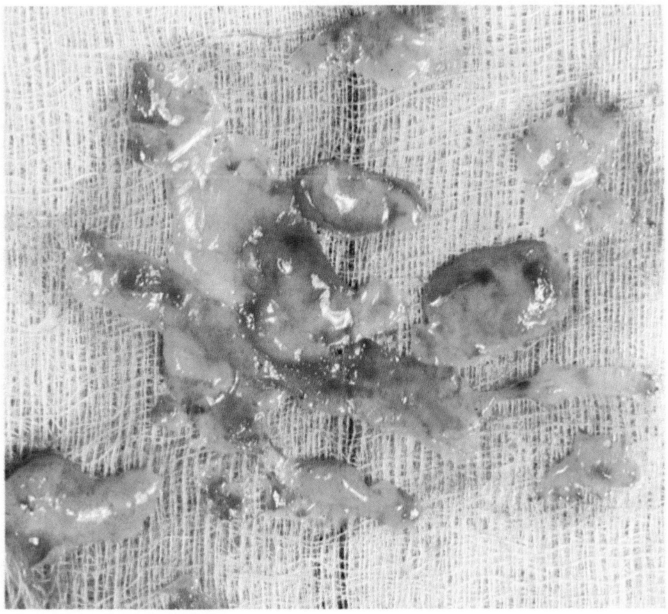

16
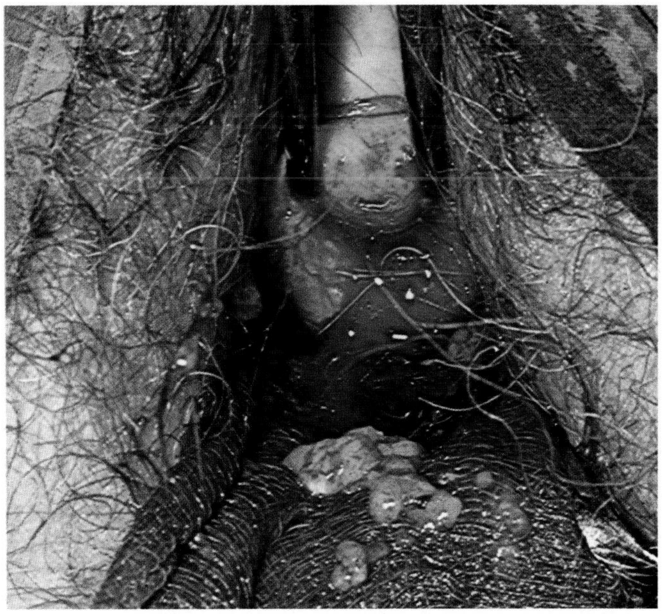

Figures **13** to **16** show the types of endometrium commonly obtained on curettage.

13 Normal curettings

These are usually minimal in amount and retrieved as thickened threads of tissue. When held to the light they are seen to have a smooth, moist and glistening surface.

14 Hyperplastic endometrium – benign

When the uterus is subjected to excessive amounts of oestrogenic hormone as occurs in cystic glandular hyperplasia or when an excessive amount of oestrogen is given in the post-menopausal state, the endometrium becomes very thickened. When held to the light it still retains its smooth, glistening surface, but has a rather pale, opaque appearance. A definite opinion as to the absence of neoplasia cannot be given until proper histological examination has been made. The absence of surface breakdown in this tissue specimen makes neoplastic change unlikely.

15 Endometrial polyp

This photograph shows typical endometrial polypi removed from a patient with intermenstrual bleeding. They have a smooth glistening exterior, but neoplasia cannot be excluded without histological examination.

16 Endometrial adenocarcinoma

The signs of endometrial carcinoma in a curettage specimen are usually those of profuse curettings associated with marked necrotic change. This is seen by the loss of the glistening sheen on the endometrial sample and the cheesy type appearance of this tissue. Histological confirmation must of course be obtained.

17

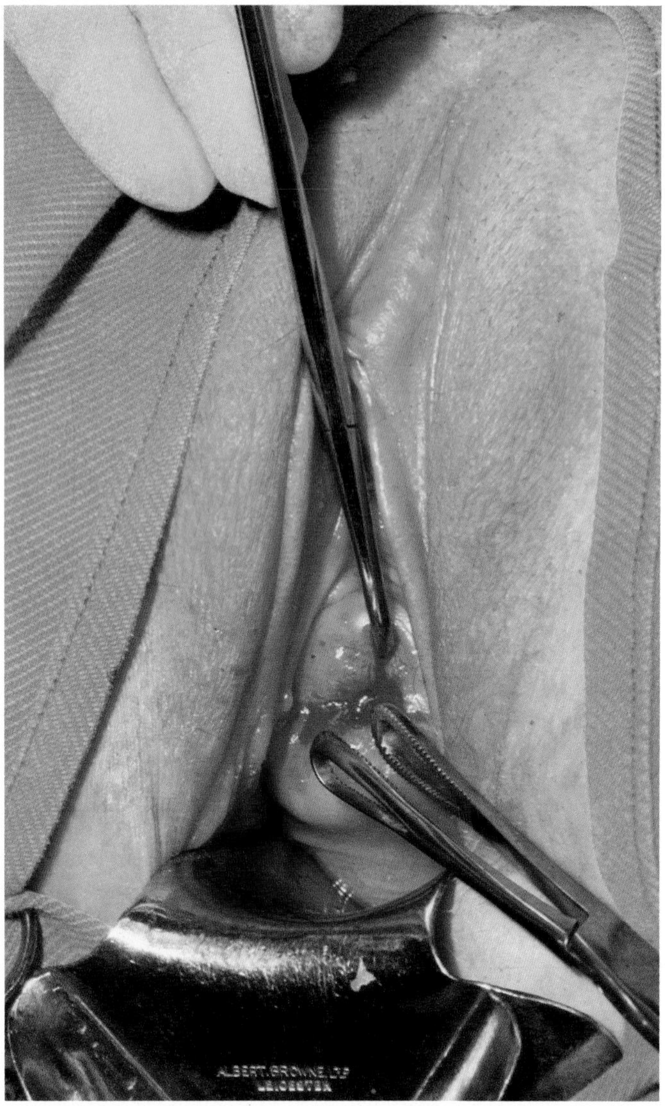

18

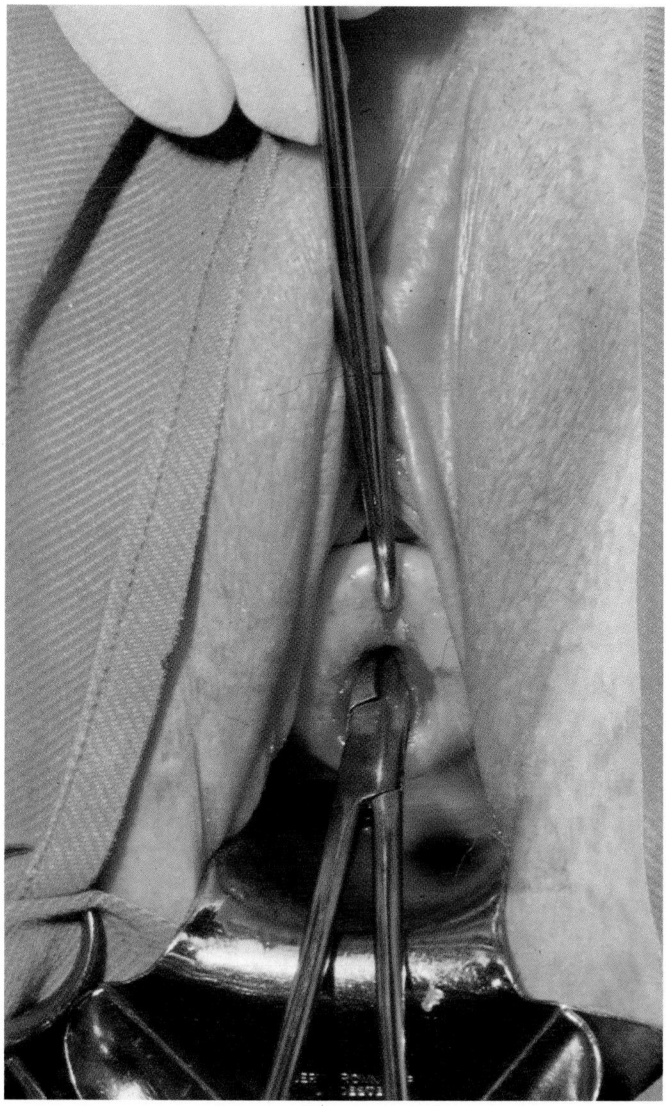

17 and 18 Exploration of uterine cavity with sponge forceps

In **17** the forceps are shown ready to be introduced. In **18** they are seen reaching the uterine cavity. The possibility of missing an intra-uterine polyp is reduced or obviated by exploring the cavity with these forceps. Introduced through the cervix into the cavity of the uterus, the blades are opened and the cavity is searched in all directions to exclude polypi which, if on a narrow stalk, can otherwise escape detection.

19

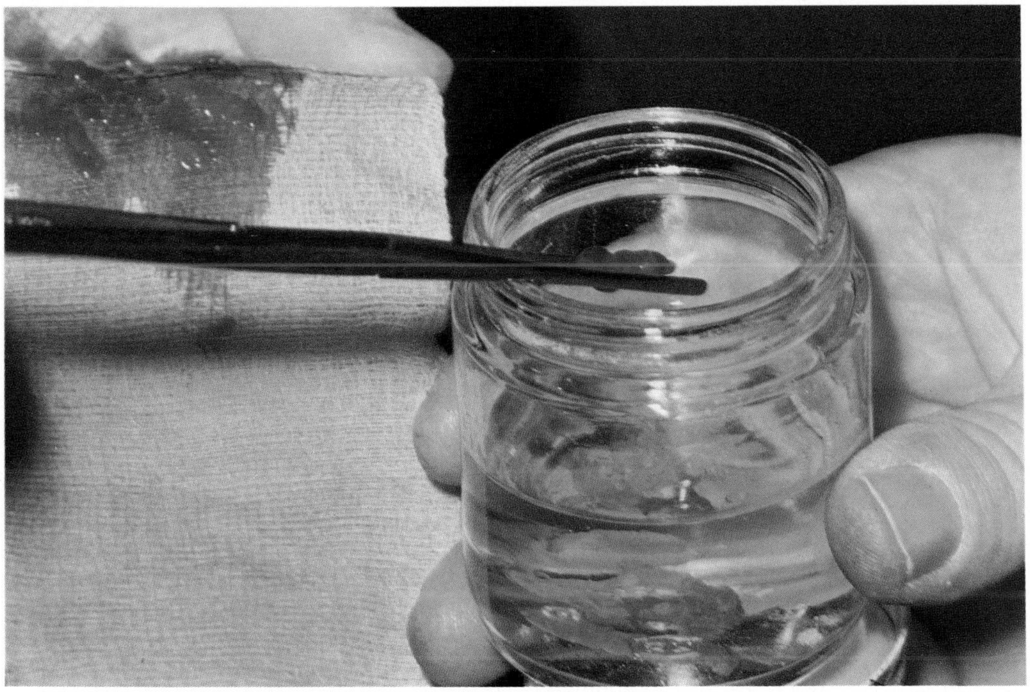

19 Collection and labelling of specimens

This is a most important and essential part of the operation. The curettings are transferred from the gauze swab with sinus forceps to a wide-mouthed jar containing Masson's solution* which has been labelled in preparation. The laboratory request form is completed at the end of the operation giving the necessary clinical information and the date of the last menstrual period of all patients in that group. As with the laboratory request form, the clinical notes should be completed without delay at the end of the operation. The virtual impossibility of remembering relevant information where even two operations are written up retrospectively has to be attempted to be believed.

* Formula: 1 per cent each of glacial acetic acid, picric acid and water in 60:40 per cent solution of methylated spirits and formaldehyde.

2: Diathermy coagulation of the cervix

The operation of diathermy coagulation of the cervix is used in circumstances where there are symptoms arising from an excessive amount of glandular secreting tissue present on the ectocervix. This common condition is usually referred to as an 'erosion'. This, however, is an incorrect term as there is no loss of superficial tissue. Illustrations **1** and **2** show the presence of excessive glandular epithelium.

It is important to remember that an artificial eversion of the endocervix occurs when a bivalve speculum is used. In figures **3** and **4** such an example is seen. In **3** the cervix is viewed with the speculum open and clearly displays the endocervix with glandular tissue present. When the speculum is withdrawn into the lower vagina and imitates the normal *in vivo* relationship of the upper vaginal and cervical tissues, the previously exposed glandular tissue is now seen to be withdrawn within the endocervix. Treatment of the cervix as seen in **3** would have been irrelevant to the patient's symptoms.

Excessive amounts of such glandular secretory tissue are found in the cervix in cases where there has been severe cervical trauma with delivery. It is also becoming more common to find it in women who are taking the oral contraceptive steroids. In the latter condition the endocervical columnar tissue is hyperplastic and hypertrophic as a result of progestogenic stimulation. When these lesions are present they tend to produce symptoms in the form of muco-purulent vaginal discharge, intermenstrual and post-coital bleeding, and as such require treatment.

The purpose of the treatment is to excise and destroy the more superficial secretory glands of the endocervix and ectocervix. This in turn allows healing to occur by the replacement of the secretory tissue by non-secretory squamous epithelium. Removal of the endocervical portion of the lesion is effected by a coning out type of procedure using the diathermy loop. The ectocervical part is treated by making deep linear cuts within it which radiate out from the external os. A diathermy needle or flat electrode is also used to incise and drain nabothian follicles which are small, cervical, glandular retention cysts. This procedure also destroys redundant tissue and aligns the incision.

Although apparently crude as a surgical procedure diathermy coagulation gives excellent results. It takes about six weeks for the cervix to heal over and there is increased discharge during the first three or four weeks of that time, but at the end of six weeks the cervix looks almost nulliparous. The cervical canal heals without stenosis, the 'erosion' is replaced by squamous epithelium and the result of the contraction following the radial incisions is to draw in and reform the cervix to a normal outline.

Before using diathermy coagulation of the cervix it is essential to be sure to have excluded the presence of cervical neoplasia by the use of exfoliative cytology. Curettage is a routine preliminary to the diathermy treatment; the cervix requires dilation in any case and this offers an opportunity to exclude intra-uterine cause for any of the symptoms.

The main disadvantages of the operation are that general anaesthesia is required and there is a small risk of secondary haemorrhage. This risk can be reduced by ensuring proper healing of the area with squamous epithelium by the application of an acid pH cream into the area immediately after diathermy. It has been shown that this influences the regenerating cells to produce a keratin type of epithelium. There is an increasing tendency, however, in recent times to use cryosurgery in the treatment of such cases and the advantages of such treatment are described under that heading.

Figures **1** to **4** are situated overleaf.

Suggested reading

1 'The Cervix', *eds.* Jordan, J. & Singer, A., p. 13–36. W. B. Saunders, London, 1976.
2 Reid, B. L., Singer, A. & Coppleson, M. (1967). 'The Process of Cervical Regeneration after Electrocauterization', *Aust. & N.Z. J. Obstet. & Gynaec.* **7** 125–133.

1
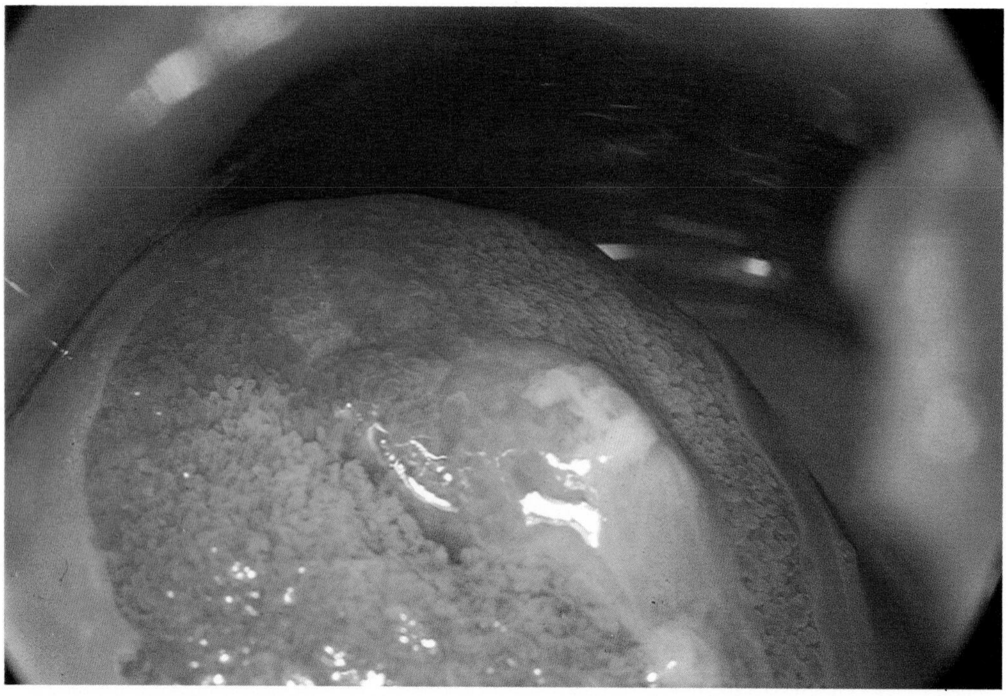

2
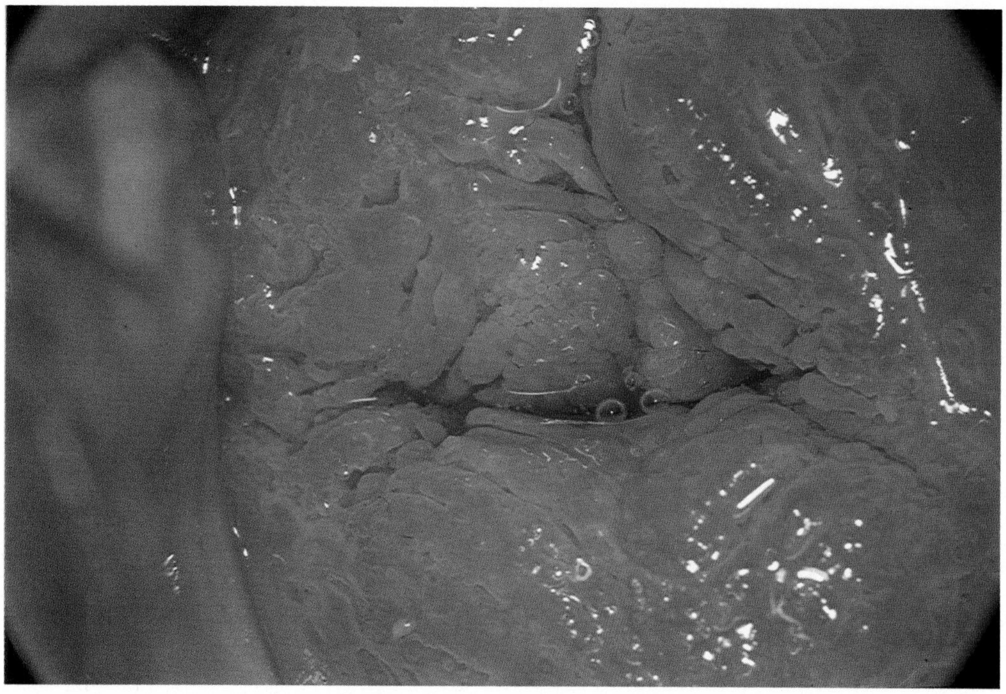

1 and 2 Cervices suitable for diathermy

As explained in the introduction above, the cervix here shows an excessive amount of glandular secretory tissue. This condition is usually referred to as an 'erosion'. This is incorrect as previously explained.

3

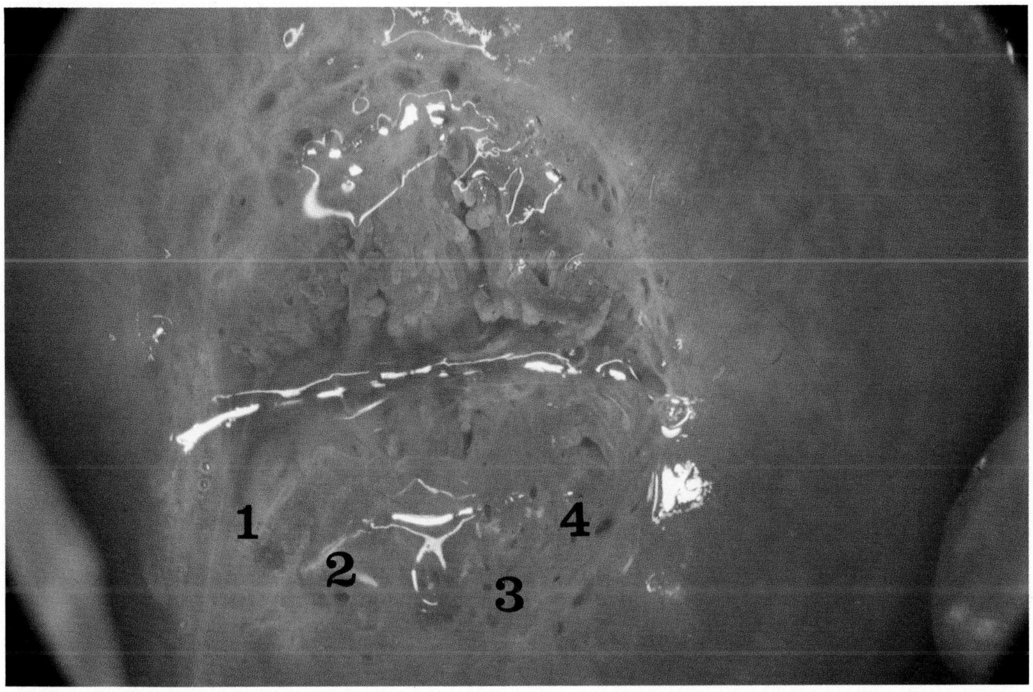

4

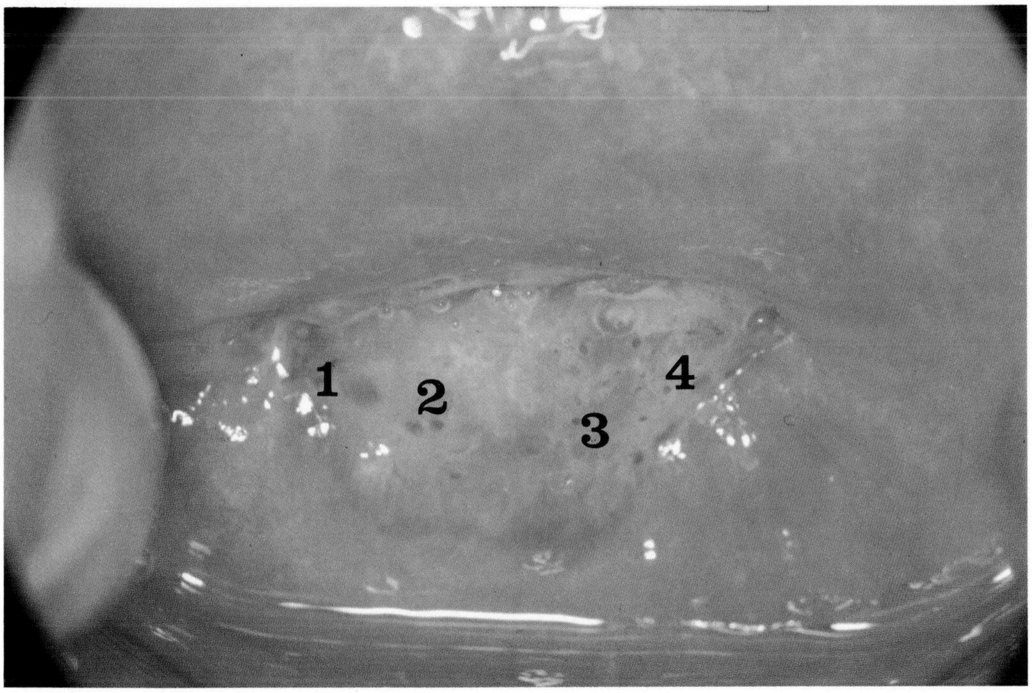

3 and 4 The true appearance of the cervical epithelium

The cervix as seen with a bivalve speculum fully opened displaying endocervical and ectocervical tissue. However, in the *in vivo* situation, only the ectocervical tissue is in contact with the vagina. Treatment of such an area not containing glandular tissue would be unnecessary. The cervix must be viewed with the speculum partly withdrawn into the vagina. This view, as seen in Figure **4**, imitates the natural *in vivo* position of the cervical epithelium. Points 1 to 4 show gland openings within the squamous epithelium.

5

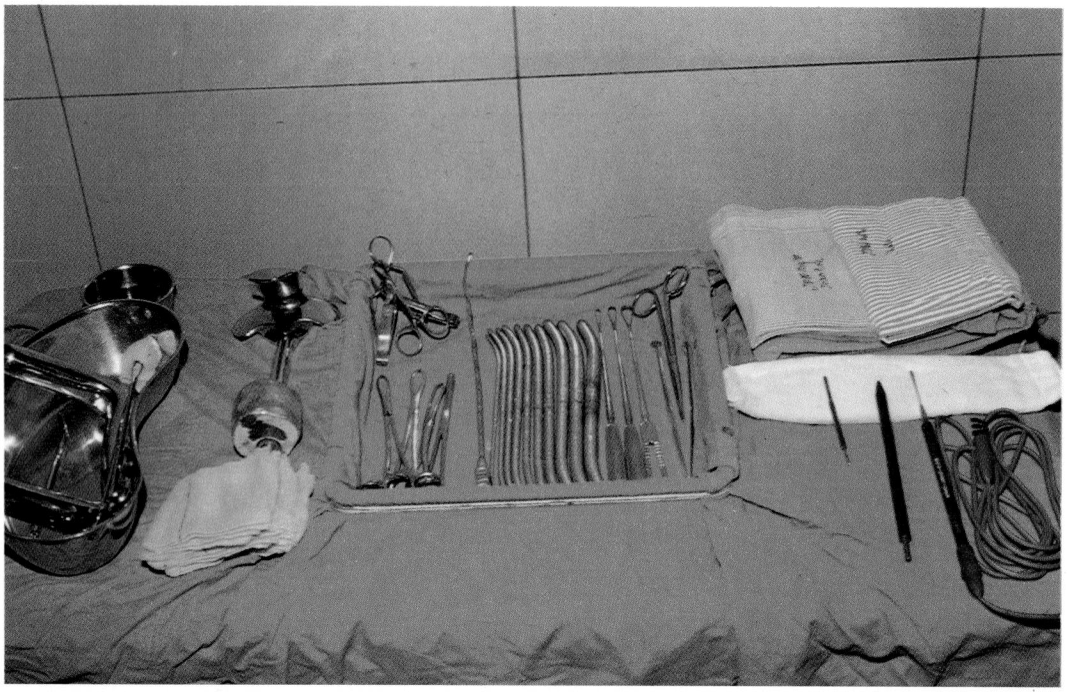

6

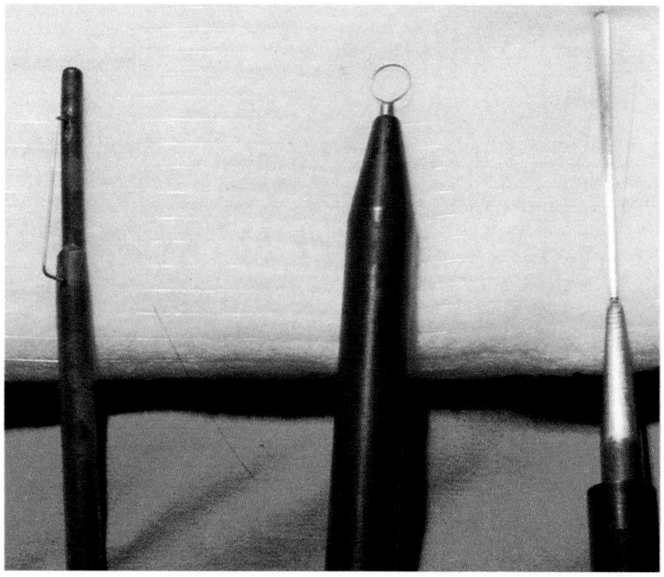

7

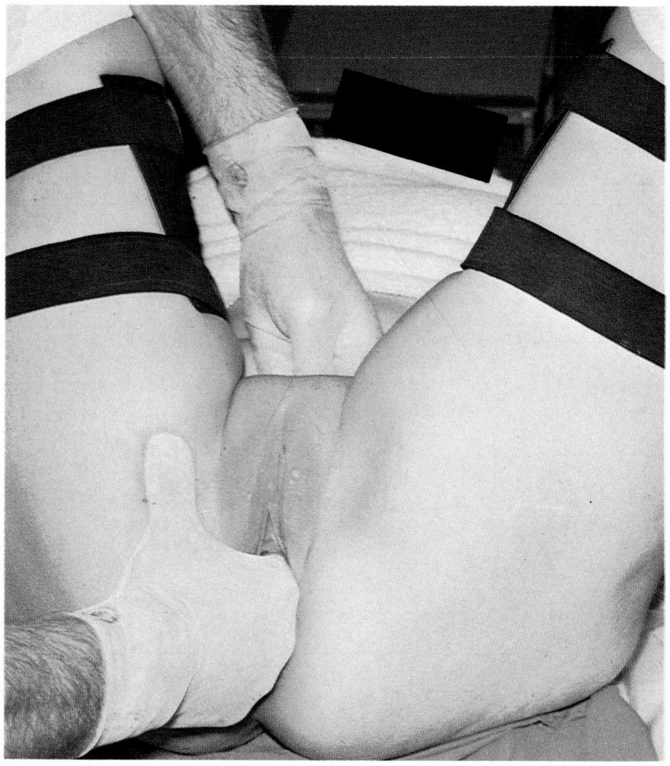

5 and 6 Instruments for diathermy to cervix

Since a uterine curettage is normally done with diathermy coagulation a basic dilatation and curettage set of instruments is required. The necessary diathermy leads, applicators and points are added. These instruments are shown in **5**. Figure **6** shows the type of diathermy points which are available and generally used. That on the left, when inserted into the cervical canal and rotated, will remove a narrow cone of tissue and this can be a useful method of starting the operation.

The loop is used to cone out the lower cervical canal by a series of downward strokes, each of which removes a strip of diathermised tissue. The loop shown here is of rather small diameter and a slightly larger one is generally more practical. The flattened cutting electrode on the right is used to make the radiating linear cuts and is superior to a needle in that it electro-coagulates a wider zone.

7 Preparation for treatment

The patient, in the lithotomy position, has the diffuse electrode applied in the form of two plates – one strapped to each side. This is preferred to a flat pad electrode under the sacrum where the swabbing solution may collect as a pool and cause a short-circuit burn. Note that the metal stirrups on the operating table are rubber insulated. A bimanual examination is made to establish the position and the size of the uterus and to exclude abnormal pelvic findings.

8
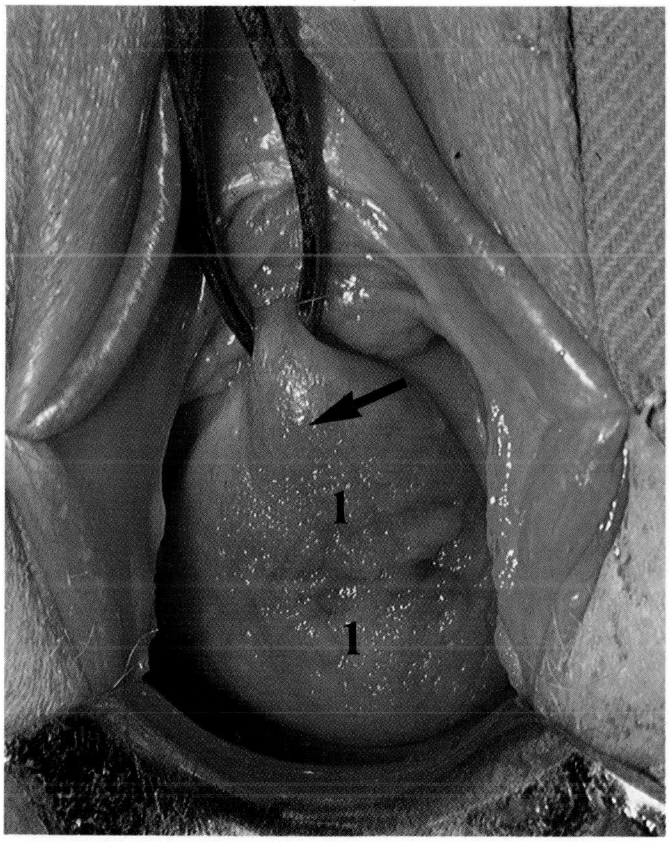

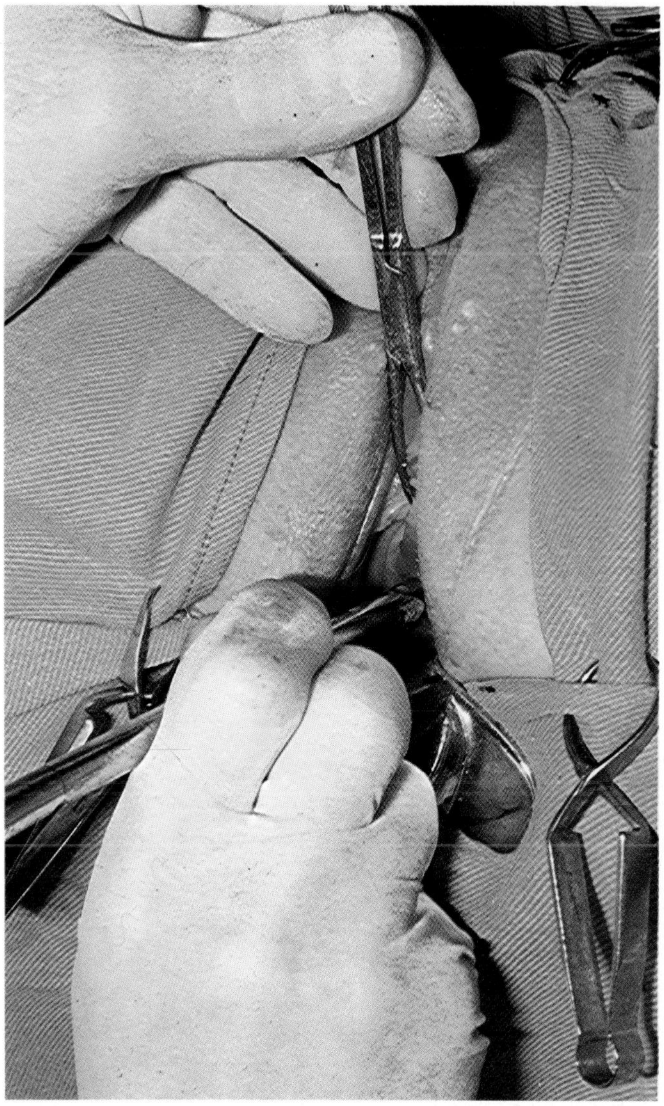
9

8 Appearance of cervix pre-operatively

The appearance is that of ectocervical and endocervical hypertrophic columnar epithelium (1); there are several nabothian follicles, one of which is arrowed.

The cervix is grasped with a Littlewood's forceps clear of the area to be treated. The labia have been stitched back in this case for demonstration purposes and this step is not normally required. The Auvard's speculum should give adequate vision and access.

10
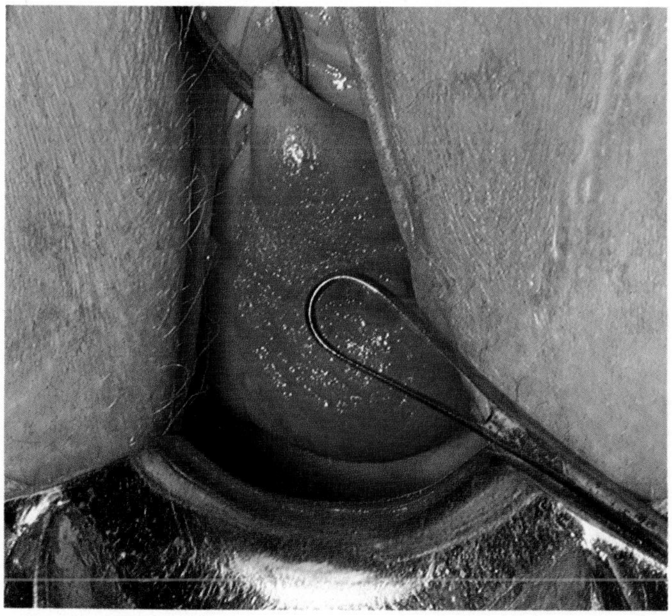

9 and 10 Dilatation and curettage (D & C) (i)

A D & C is performed and two stages in the process are shown. In **9** a medium-sized dilator is being used and the cervix is offering considerable resistance. Note how the right hand is holding the dilator so that when the resistance of the cervix is overcome the heel of the hand is almost immediately arrested on the perineum with no risk of fundal perforation. Dilatation should only be effected up to a Hegar 7. Any further dilatation is unnecessary and may damage the sphincteric mechanism of the internal os.

In **10** it can be seen that a moderately large sharp curette is about to be introduced into the uterus. It is generally safer to use the larger sizes since perforation is less likely and allows a suitable endometrial sample to be obtained.

11

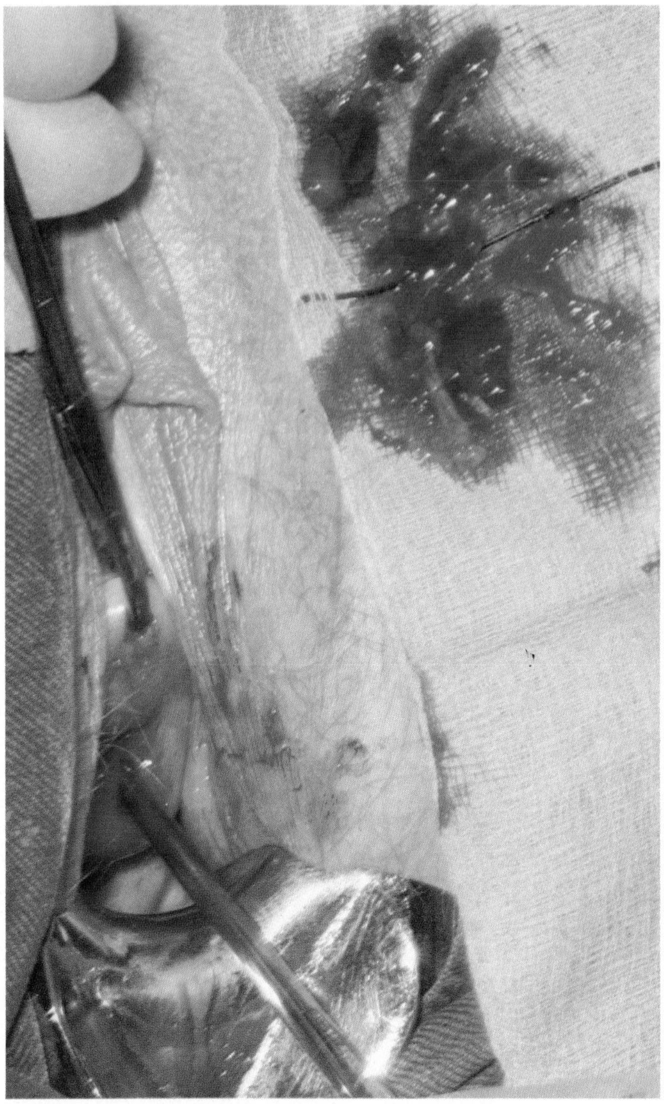

12

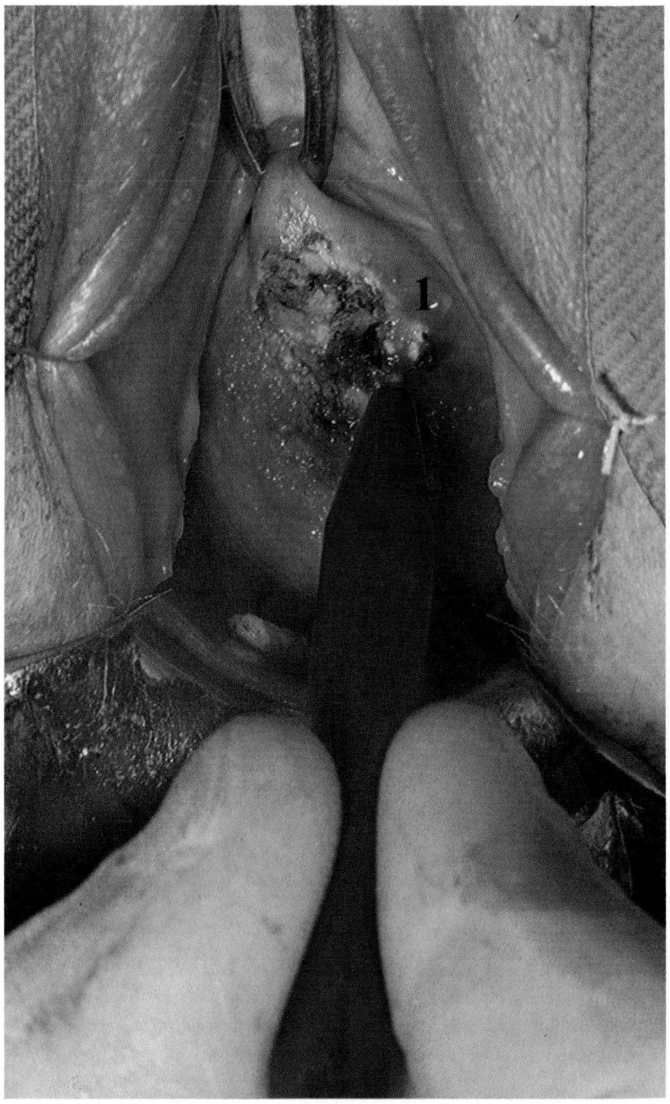

11 Dilatation and curettage (ii)

In **11** curettage continues and the curettings are being transferred to a gauze swab on the patient's thigh.

12 Diathermy conization (i)

The process of conization has been started on the anterior aspect of the lower cervical canal which has been dilated up to 20 mm. The loop diathermy is used for this stage and starts each stroke about the junction of the upper and middle thirds of the cervical canal. It is drawn down slowly with the current on and this removes a strip of tissue of whatever depth is required. A white or slightly charred vertical furrow results and the process is continued until these are joined up and deepened to the extent required. Polypoid projections are removed and occasional mucoid cysts are encountered and punctured. In the photographs the loop has made several strokes on the patient's right side and is actually cutting a strip towards the left. A small mucoid cyst is seen rupturing just ahead of the loop (1) and a strip of tissue which has been removed is seen lying on the blade of the Auvard's speculum. Treatment of the anterior part is nearly complete.

13

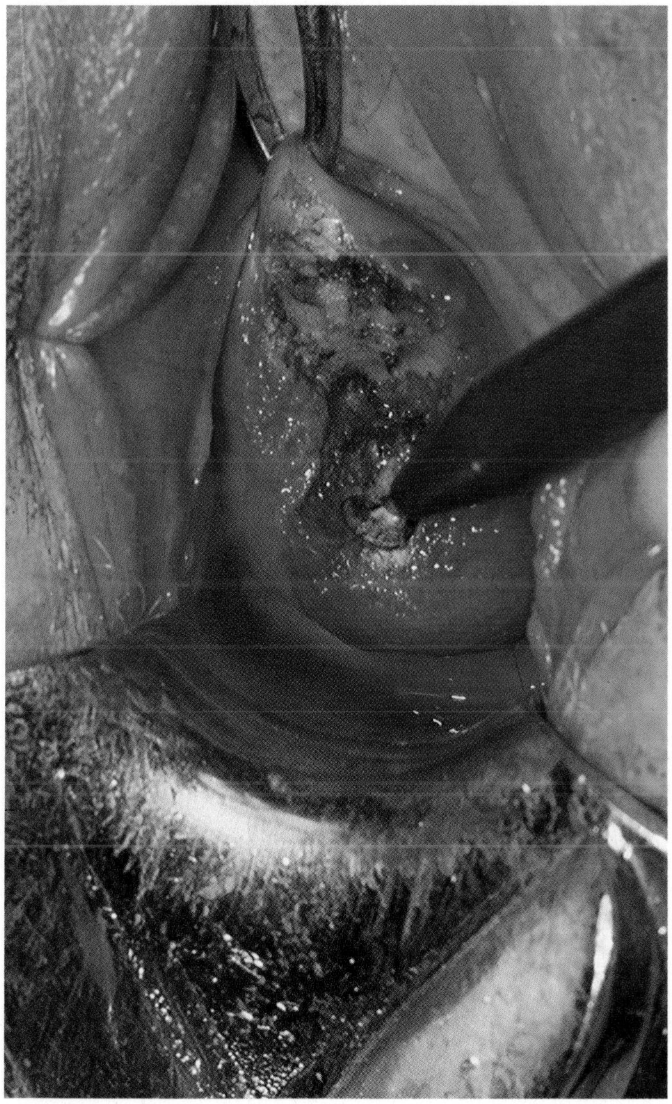

14

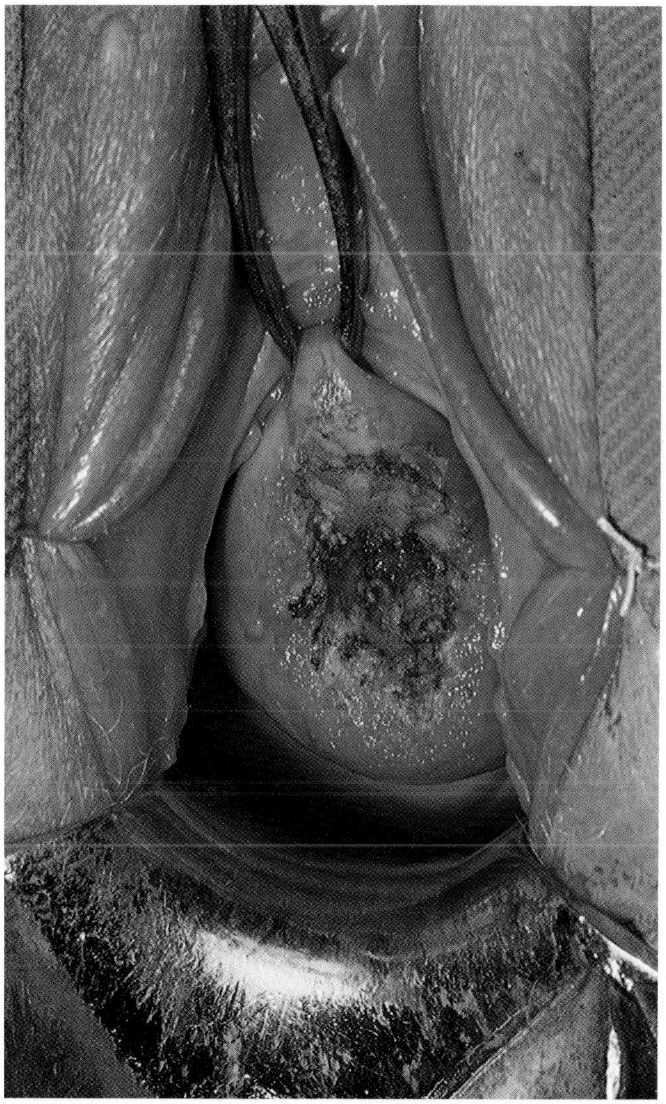

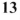

13 Diathermy conization (ii)

The same procedure is followed posteriorly and in this photograph the anterior aspect has been treated and the loop is cutting a strip posteriorly. It is necessary to deal with the endocervix in this way because of the depth of the glands: the loop is not used on the ectocervix where surface and linear diathermy are quite adequate.

14 Diathermy conization (iii)

The conization has been completed and the area of hypertrophic glandular tissue has been removed. The cervical canal is open to allow adequate drainage and the emergence of mucus from deeper glands is seen at the apex of the cone. It will be seen that the 'erosion' is largely a surface one and of no great depth laterally although there are some nabothian follicles near the muco-cutaneous junction.

15

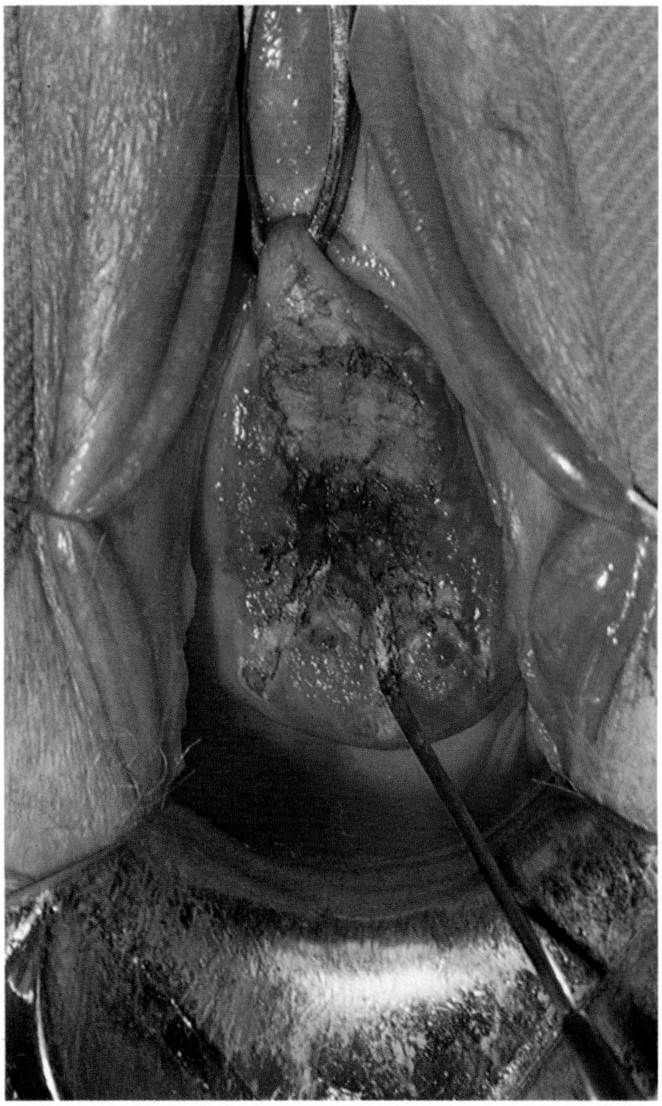

16

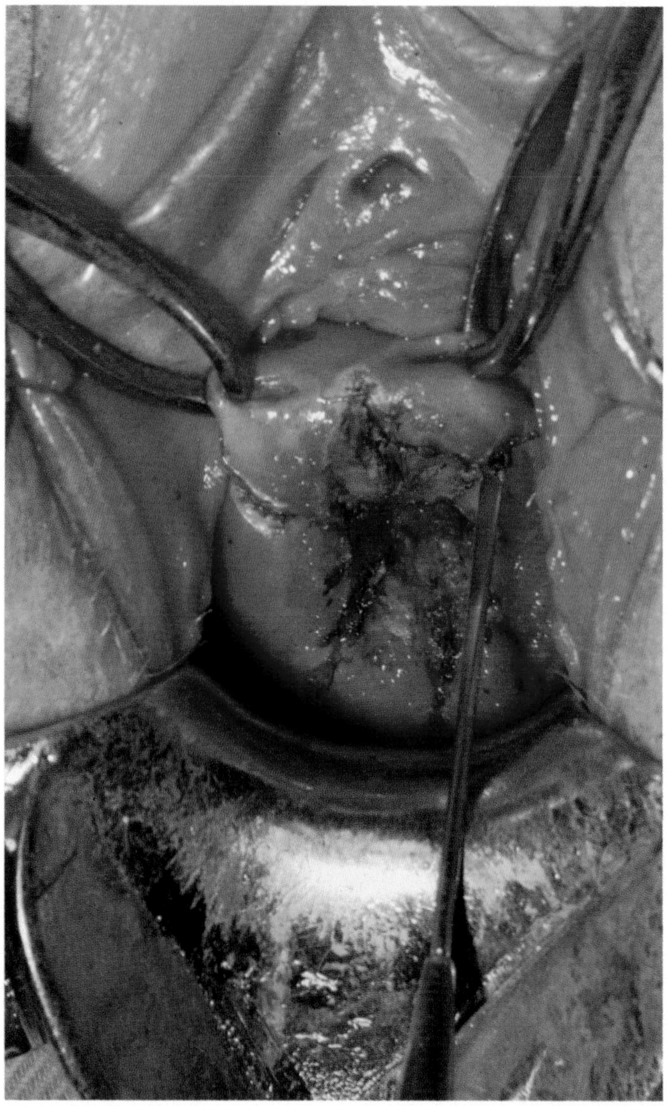

15 Linear cauterisation of cervix (i)

The flat cutting electrode is being used to make radial cuts from the edge of the external os outwards for about 2 cm and cutting to a depth of about 0.5 cm. Three or four such cuts are made on each lip of the cervix and since there is no bleeding it is immaterial whether one starts anteriorly or posteriorly. Nabothian follicles of varing sizes are encountered and one such can be seen opened in the 5 o'clock position.

16 Linear cauterisation of the cervix (ii)

The operation is continued on the anterior lip of the cervix in the same fashion. The cuts extend to the outer edge of the erosion and open up and drain small nabothian follicles. There is no bleeding.

17

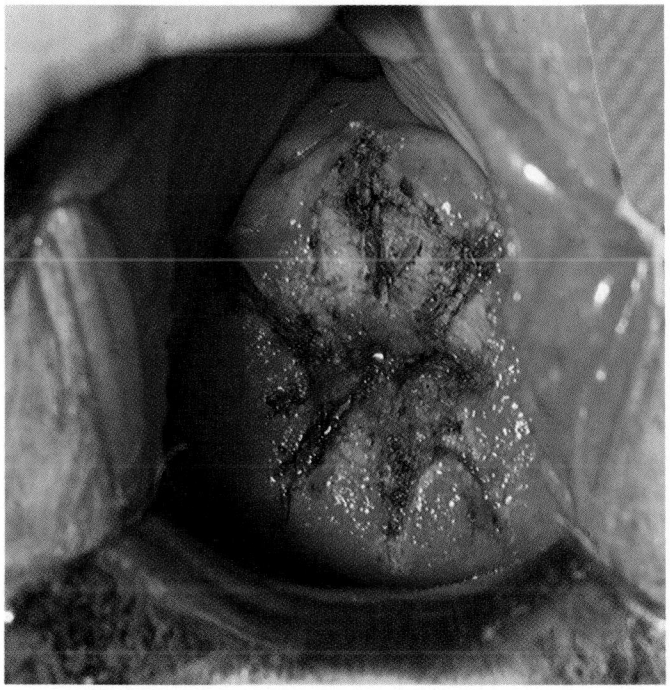

18

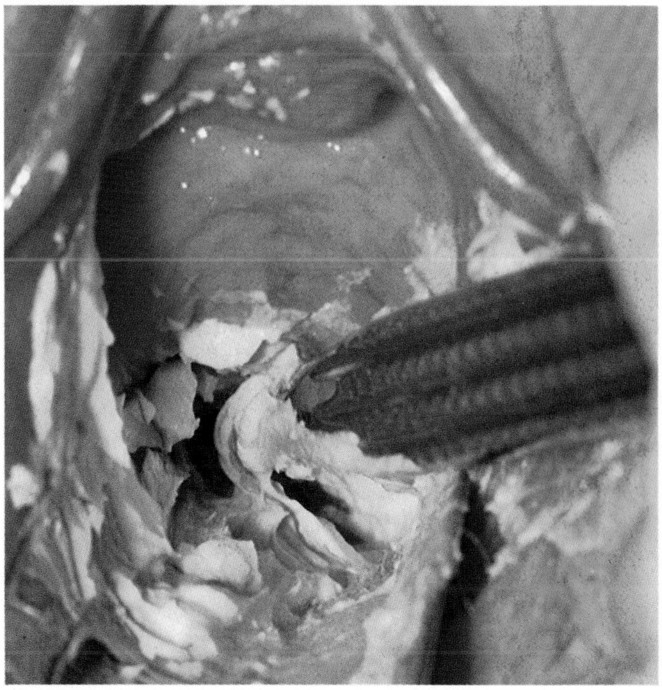

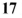

17 Appearances at completion of operation

The cervix is shown with the coned out lower cervical canal and the radiating linear cuts on the ectocervix. There is no need to apply the button electrode to the surface reddened areas between the cuts as this will only cause unnecessary sloughing of tissue and these areas will acquire a squamous epithelium if left alone.

18 Application of triple sulpha cream

Triple sulpha cream is applied immediately as shown here. This cream has an acidic pH which stimulates the development of squamous epithelium in the regeneration area. It has been found that the application of this cream intra-vaginally for 10 days results in a perfectly healed ectocervix.

19

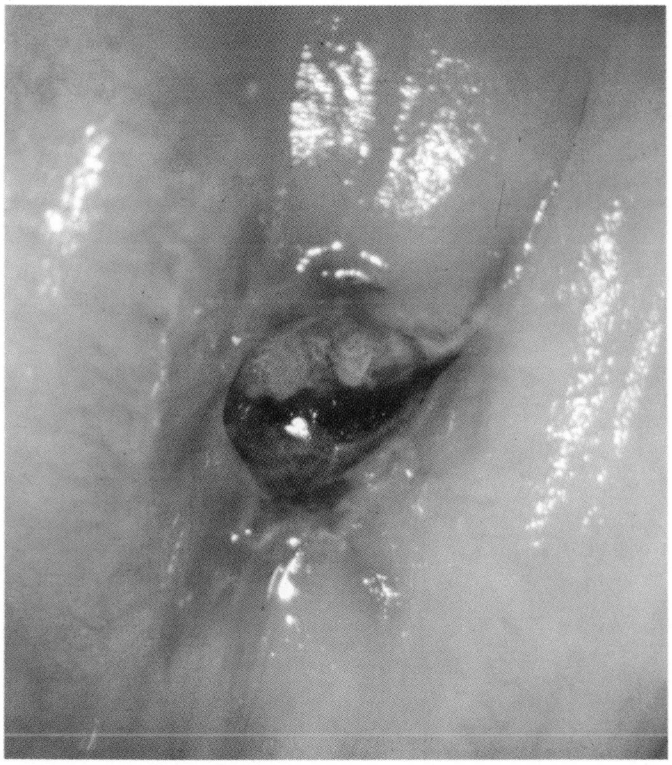

19 Appearance of cervix six weeks following treatment

The ectocervix previously occupied by an excessive amount of glandular secreting tissue (Figure **8**), has now been replaced by normal squamous epithelium. A small area of columnar epithelium still remains within the endocervix, thereby retaining one of the physiological functions of the cervix i.e. provide adequate mucus for sperm transport.

3: Cryosurgical treatment of cervical 'erosion'

Cryosurgery in gynaecology has developed enormously since Weitzner's freezing of a cervical 'erosion' using dry ice rods in 1940. Liquid nitrogen and freon were originally used but these rather expensive cryogens with their bulky delivery systems have been replaced by agents i.e. carbon dioxide and nitrous oxide, which are cheaper and can be stored indefinitely in small sealed containers. These gases are currently available in a variety of delivery units, most of which have a gun-type configuration with a variety of interchangeable probe tips (**1b**). Carbon dioxide and nitrous oxide are not only refrigent but are also used as the heating agent.

The principle of cryosurgery depends on the fact that the temperature at which ice forms in tissue is between 0°C and —10°C. The mechanism of cryosurgical cell death is uncertain but cellular dehydration is certainly of importance. Water removal increases cellular solute concentration which affects structural and enzyme systems in the cell. With water crystallisation the cell membrane is weakened, making rupture possible and resultant cell death.

Tissue destruction is more readily achieved by rapid freezing; thawing, and particularly the rate at which this occurs, also plays a role in determining cellular disintegration. Rapid freezing and slow thawing appears to be the most lethal freeze-thaw combination with repeated episodes of this being particularly injurious to the tissues.

The cervix, because of its anatomical location, accessibility and variety of benign and premalignant conditions, is ideally suited for cryosurgical therapy. Excessive amounts of glandular cervical epithelium, commonly called 'erosions', and giving rise to symptoms, may be treated very effectively with cryosurgery. Obviously cervical precancer or cancer must be excluded although certain of the former can be treated by this method (see Volume 3). Healing is complete in six to eight weeks and about 80 per cent of patients will be cured by one treatment. Ninety-five per cent are symptom free after a second therapy course. About 25 per cent of patients will complain of a mild vasomotor reaction during and after treatment but this can be alleviated by analgesics and rest. A watery and malodorous discharge will last for some 10 to 14 days; a mucoid discharge persists from two to four weeks afterwards.

Theoretical long-term sequelae such as infertility, delay in labour, or cervical incompetence, do not seem to be associated with cryosurgery. Very occasionally cervical stenosis may occur, but this can be overcome by simple outpatient or office cervical dilatation.

Suggested reading

1 Collins, R. J. & Pappas, H. J. (1972). 'Cryosurgery for benign cervicitis; follow-up of six years', *Amer. J. Obstet. Gynec.* **113** 744–750.

2 Townsend, D. E., Ostergard, D. & Lickrish, G. M. (1971). 'Cryosurgery for benign disease of the uterine cervix', *J. Obstet. Gynaec. Brit. Cwlth.* **78** 667–670.

3 Townsend, D. E. 'The management of cervical lesions by cryosurgery' in 'The Cervix', *eds.* Jordan, J. A. & Singer, A., p. 305–313. W. B. Saunders, London, 1976.

Office/outpatient cryosurgery

1a Cryosurgery source

The actual apparatus is simple in concept and compact, besides being easy to use. The various items are indicated in the figure and it need not be pointed out that the foot-switch would normally be on the floor and accessible to the surgeon's foot. A raising and tilting gynaecological-style chair as shown ensures the comfort of patient and doctor but is not essential. Any gynaecological table or chair with stirrups to provide for the lithotomy position is adequate.

1b Applicator tips

Detachable applicator tips for cryoprobe (model 40-D7: Spembly Ltd., England).

1a

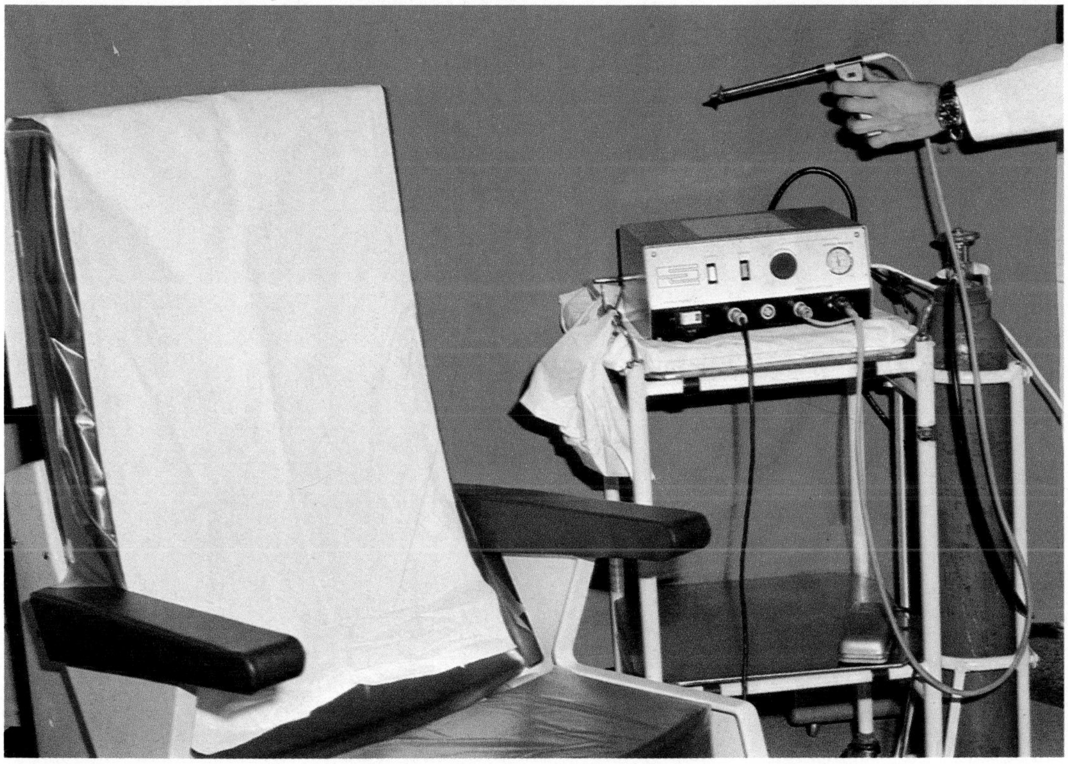

1b

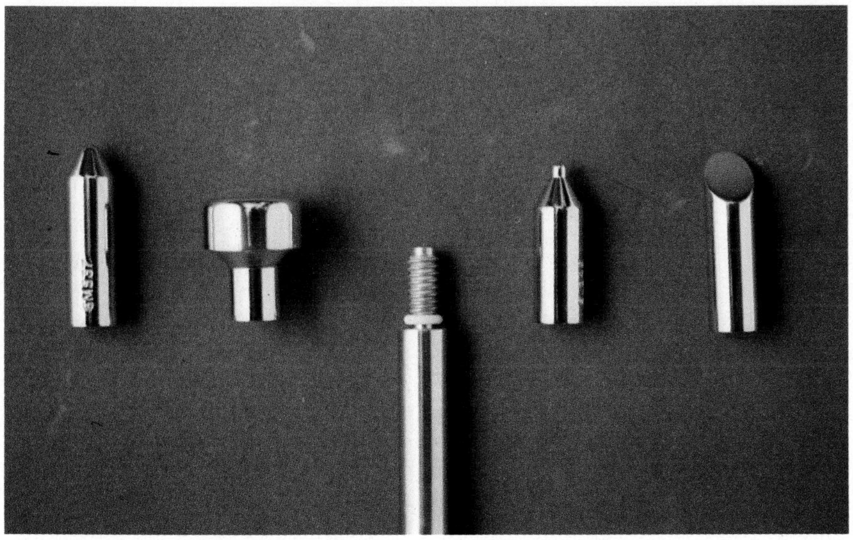

2

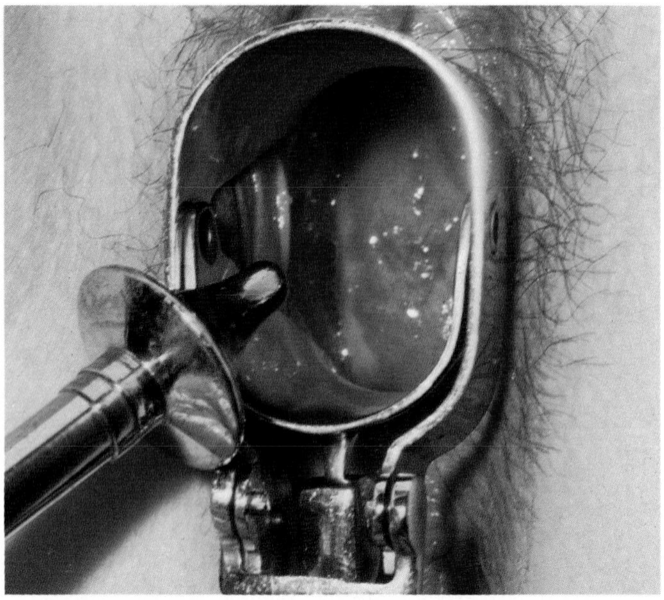

3

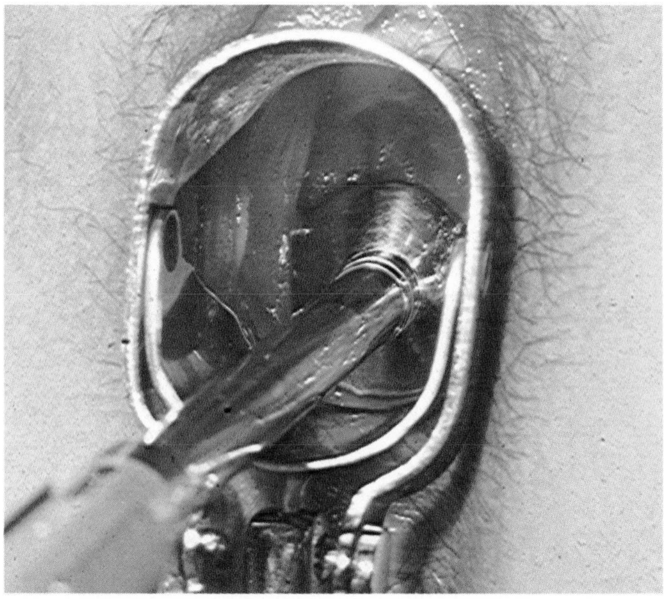

4

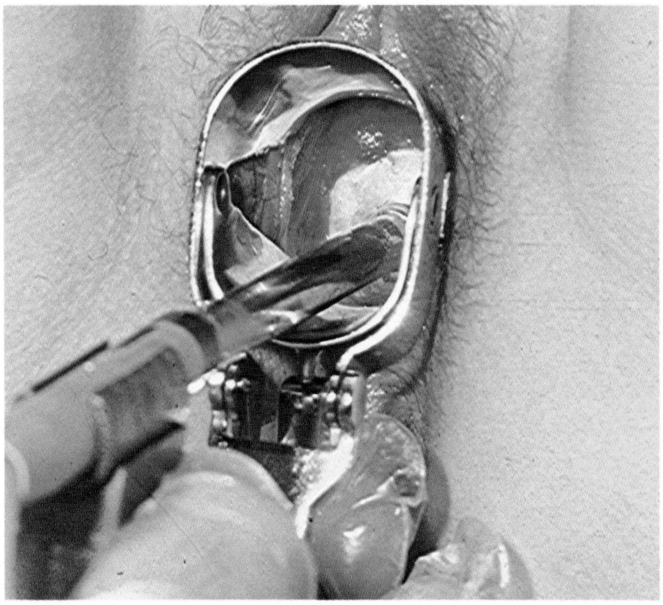

5

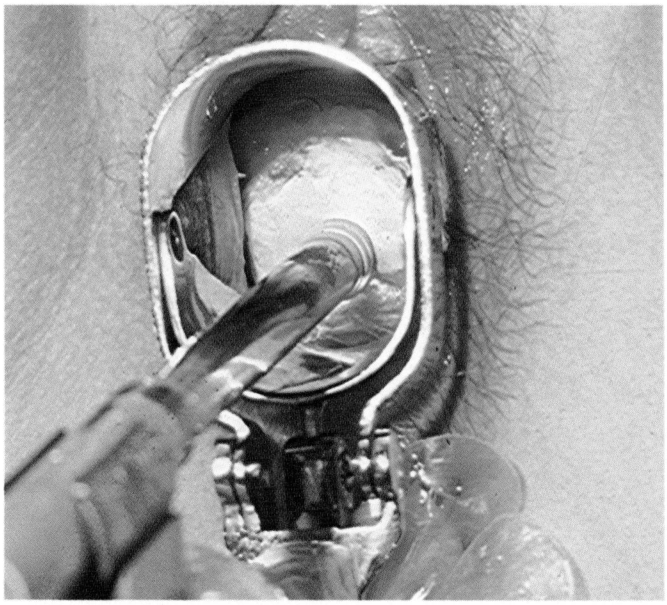

2 and 3 Application of cryosurgery button probe to cervix

A Cusco or duckbill speculum is ideal for this work and acts as a self-retaining retractor. The 'erosion' in this case is a large one and is uniformly involving the ectocervix. Its full extent can be seen on the right side and the external os is clearly visible towards the left side in **2**.

The button type probe is the standard one for cervical application and meets the requirements of practically all cases. The knob on the button enters the external os and the shoulder of the probe rests against the ectocervix over the actual 'erosion' as seen in **3**. In the case of a really large 'erosion' like this one there may be a peripheral ring of 'erosion' not covered by the button but it is narrow enough to be included in the ice ball which will be formed by the treatment. Before commencing cryotherapy it is important to remove all mucous and cellular debris from the cervix and vagina by washing with cotton ball swabs soaked in 3 per cent acetic acid solution or other mucolytic agents. Some authors recommend the application of a thin layer of lubricating jelly to the probe surface to expedite heat transfer.

4 and 5 Treatment in progress

In **4** the freezing process has been set in motion by depressing the foot-switch and within seconds a white frozen circular area spreads outwards from the point of application. The button is held against the cervix and as freezing is established it becomes firmly adhered to it. It is important to see that the rim of the button does not lie in contact with any loose fold of upper vaginal wall skin otherwise it too will adhere and if not realised will cause an area of sloughing later.

Figure **5** illustrates this point. The vaginal skin in the 5 o'clock position has adhered on a short and narrow attachment as the probe sagged against the posterior wall. The situation was immediately rectified by releasing the foot-switch for a few seconds, when the re-heat travelling distally on the probe released the skin and allowed the cryosurgical treatment to continue safely. One has to be on the look-out for this happening – indeed it is about the only complication of this exceedingly simple technique.

6

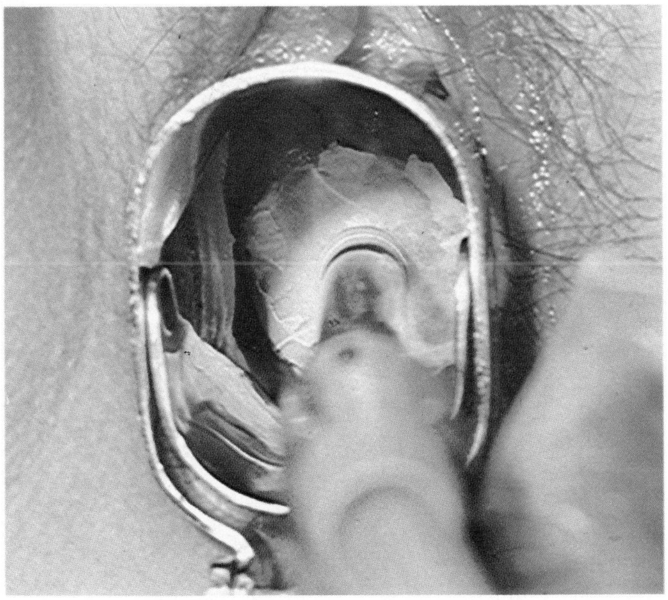

7

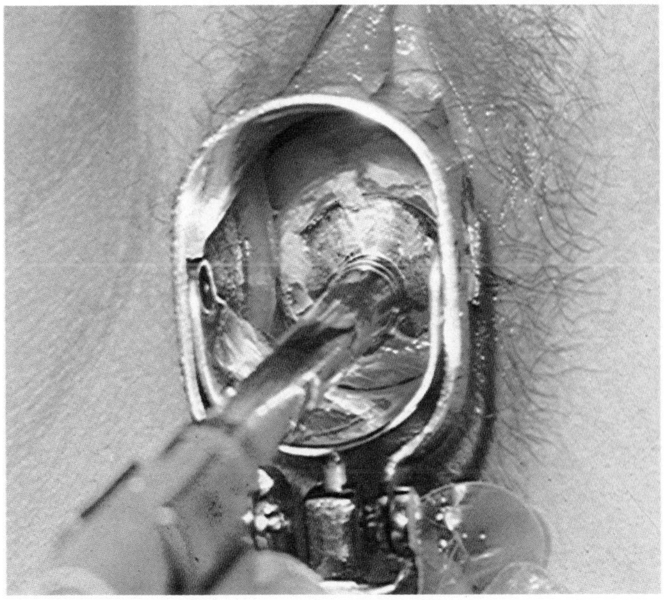

8

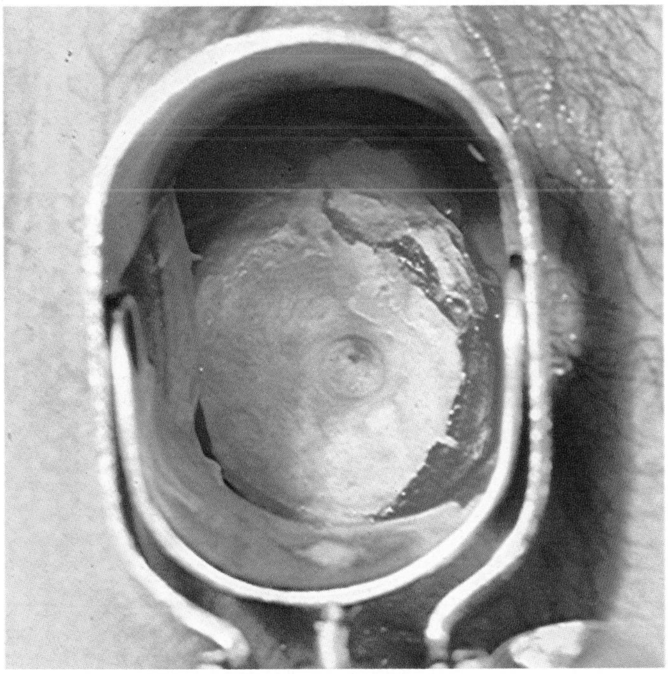

9

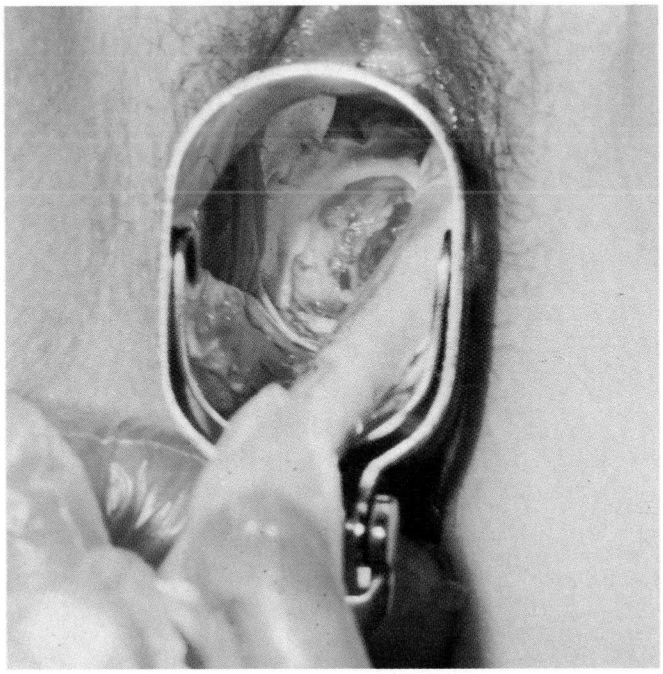

6 and 7 Completion of treatment

It is almost standard procedure to freeze the tissue to a depth of 3 mm, and this is achieved by keeping the probe in position and the foot-switch depressed for 3 minutes. An ice ball of about 2.5 cm diameter develops (**6**). When the cryosurgical equipment is switched off it takes a few seconds for the probe to re-heat and release itself from the cervix and this stage is in progress in **7**. The whitened frozen shaft of the probe de-ices distally and the camera has just caught this stage of commencing separation. It is important to ensure that at least 3 mm of normal epithelium has been included by the ice ball. Any areas that do not appear to have been adequately treated should be retreated at this time. If this is necessary then it is important that the ice balls overlap.

8 and 9 Appearance of cervix following treatment

The area of the erosion is seen as a white flattened and frozen surface, with the depression centrally at the external os. It will be seen that the effects of the freezing have extended beyond the rim of the probe and there is a crescentic vascular area on the left side which has only been partially frozen and is already 'blushing-up' with blood. Figure **9** shows the application of triple sulpha cream to the treated cervix; it is inserted in a measured quantity by a vaginal applicator. This ensures an acid pH during the stage of healing and greatly assists and accelerates the process.

10
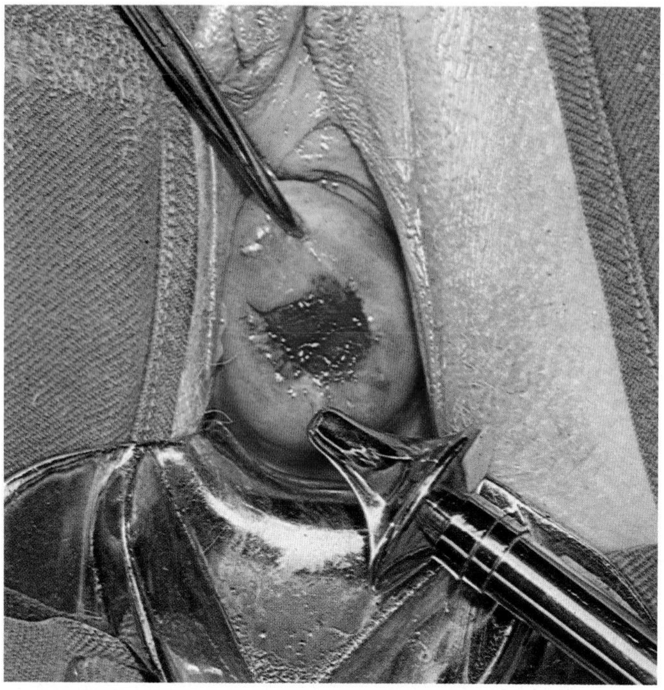

11
 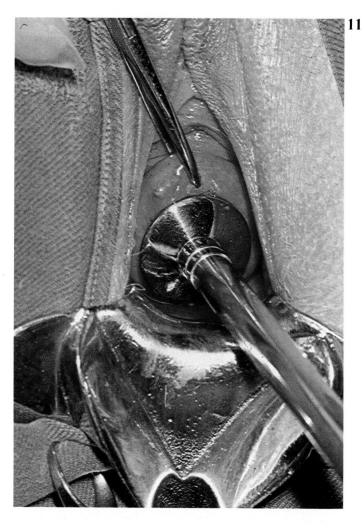

12
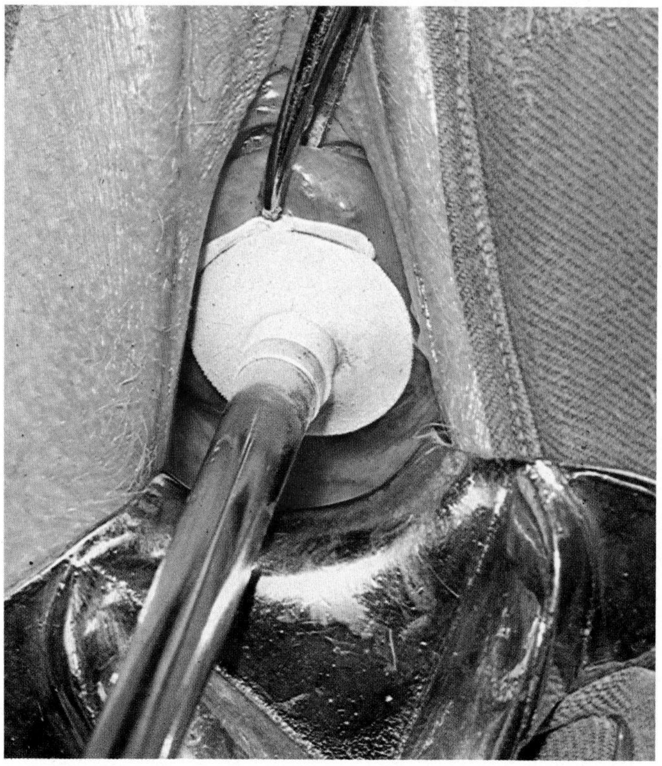

Cryosurgery under general anaesthesia to illustrate application of probe

10 Appearance pre-operatively with probe ready to be applied

11 Probe in place and freezing about to commence

12 Freezing in progress. Ice ball gradually extending outwards

13

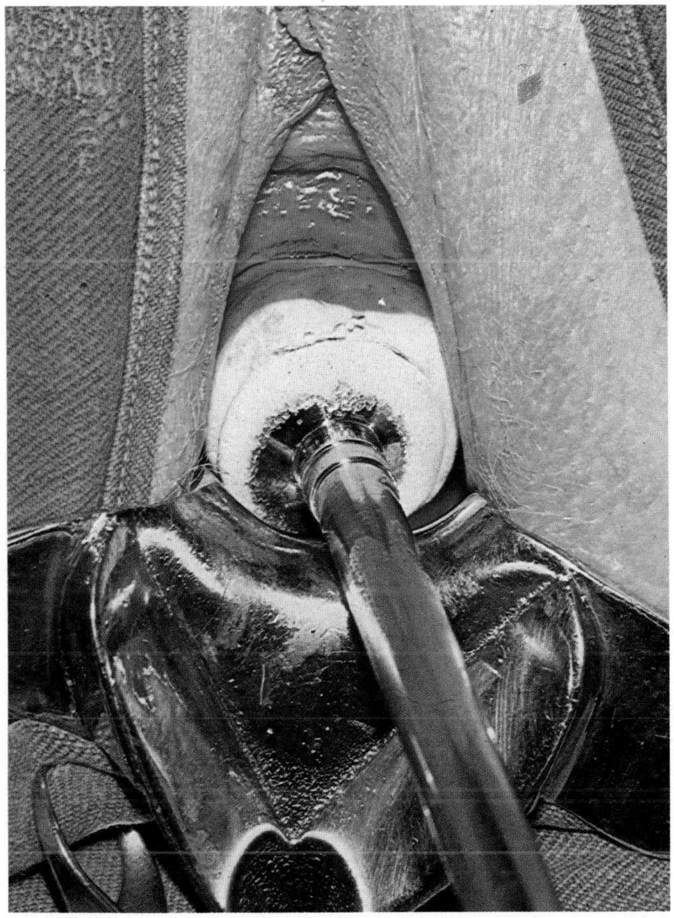

14

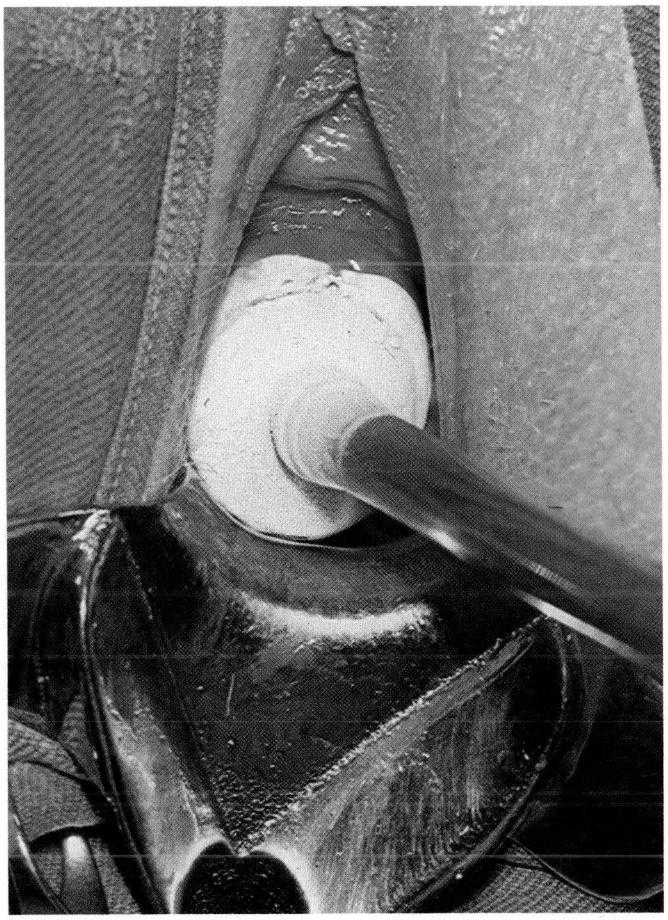

15

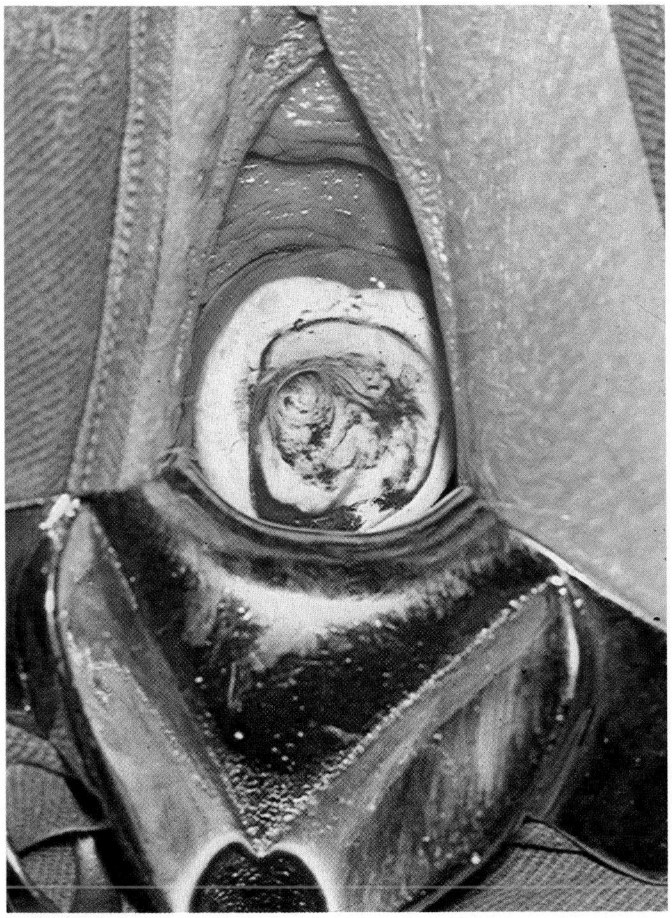

13 Appearance after three minutes of treatment

14 Defrosting commencing. The probe is becoming silver-coloured proximally

15 State of cervix with probe detached

An explanation of the procedure shown in Figures 10 to 15 would be appropriate. The patient shown was having tubal ligation under general anaesthesia and also required cryocautery of the cervix. The shaved vulva, with an Auvard's speculum *in situ*, exposed the cervix and provided ideal conditions for demonstrating the method. Serial photographs were taken and are reproduced.

It is not suggested that general anaesthesia is required or preferred nor even that the vulva need be shaved. That such steps can be omitted is part of the attraction of the method.

4: Removal of sub-mucus fibroid polyp: vaginal excision

A sub-mucus fibroid may be extruded through the cervix by uterine contractions and present vaginally as a polyp of considerable size. In such circumstances the polyp remains attached to the endometrial surface of the uterus by a pedicle of varying thickness. The cervix dilates to transmit the fibroid and remains partially dilated around it or its pedicle. There is usually some interference with blood supply to the fibroid, and surface necrosis and even deeper necrosis is common. There has probably been a history of menorrhagia and this becomes more severe with the protrusion.

If small, the polyp may be twisted off or the pedicle divided with scissors and nothing more is required. But if the pedicle is thick and attached well within the cavity of the uterus then care is required. In such circumstances the pedicle should be ligated and then divided distal to the ligature so that there is no risk of subsequent bleeding and so that the uterine wall is not torn or weakened by the pedicle being avulsed from it.

The case described here is typical and was one of two which arrived at the ward in the same week. The other polyp was much larger and was more haemorrhagic and therefore less suitable for demonstration purposes, but the management was exactly the same. It is surprising how often such fibroids are single and as far as one could tell that was the case in both of these. It is always easy to explore the cavity of the uterus with the finger after such myomectomy because the cervix is well dilated and this is a necessary step in the operation.

A large sub-mucous fibroid presenting at, but not extruded through, a partially dilated cervix is something of a problem. The lower pole is invariably necrotic and abdominal hysterectomy would be both difficult and also dangerous because of the likelihood of sepsis. The management of such cases is to tackle the problem by vaginal hysterotomy in the first place and try to reach the pedicle of the polyp. If that is not possible the polyp should be removed piecemeal and it will then be possible either to proceed to vaginal hysterectomy or resuture the uterine incision once haemostasis is seen to be satisfactory.

1

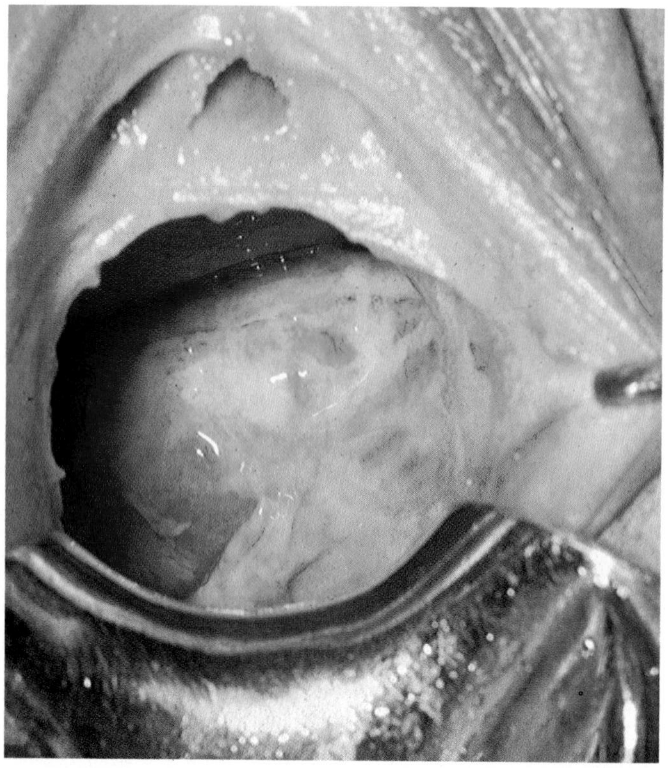

2

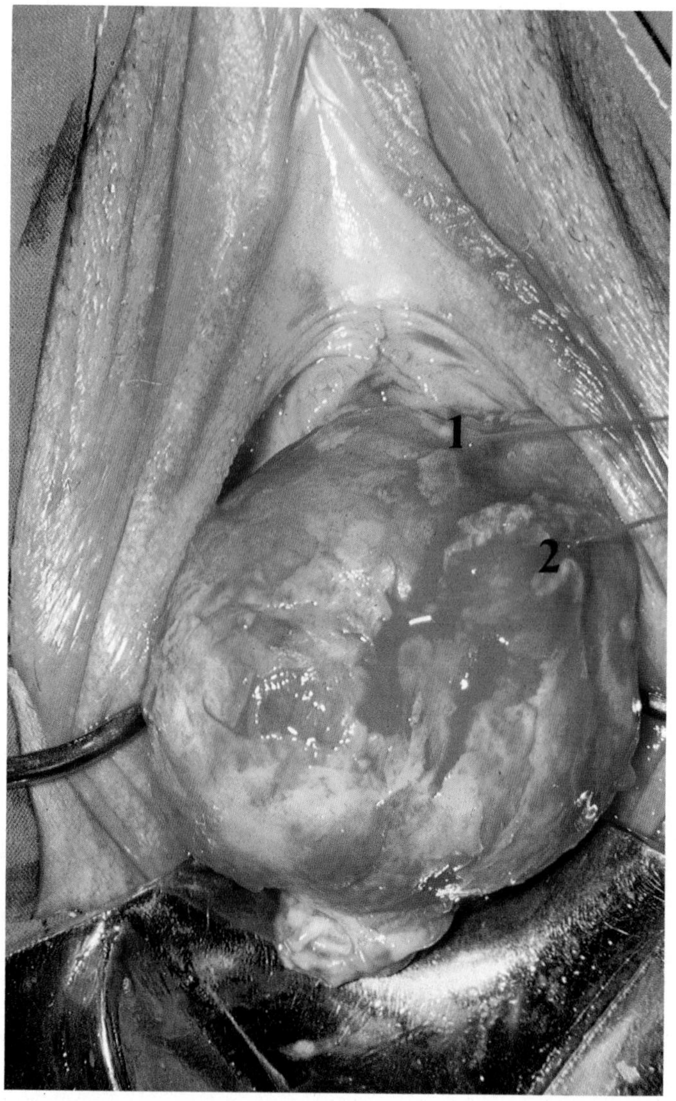

3

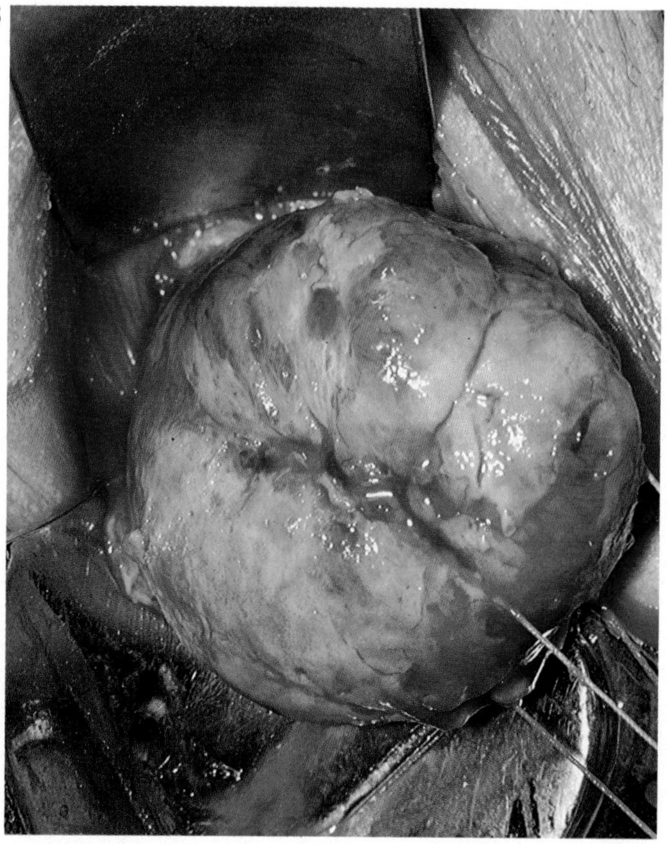

1 General view pre-operatively

The fibroid polyp is seen in the upper vagina when the Auvard speculum is inserted and the labia retracted. There is a covering of lymph over the reddened and vascular myoma and surface necrosis is commencing at several points.

2 Delivery of polyp from vagina (i)

Two holding traction sutures have been deeply placed on the lower pole of the polyp where they were least likely to cut out (**1** and **2**). By traction on these the polyp is being delivered through the introitus. This must obviously be done with care as the tissues are friable and the sutures could easily cut out.

3 Delivery of polyp from vagina (ii)

A further stage in the delivery of the polyp is seen and the areas of necrosis are now more obvious. The retractor on the anterior vaginal wall reveals the edge of the partially dilated cervix through which the polyp has protruded.

4

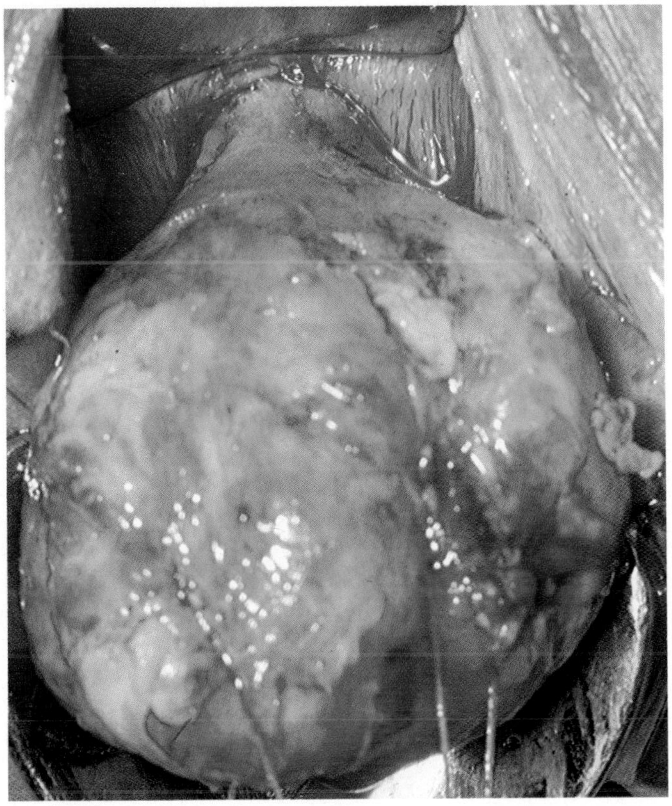

5

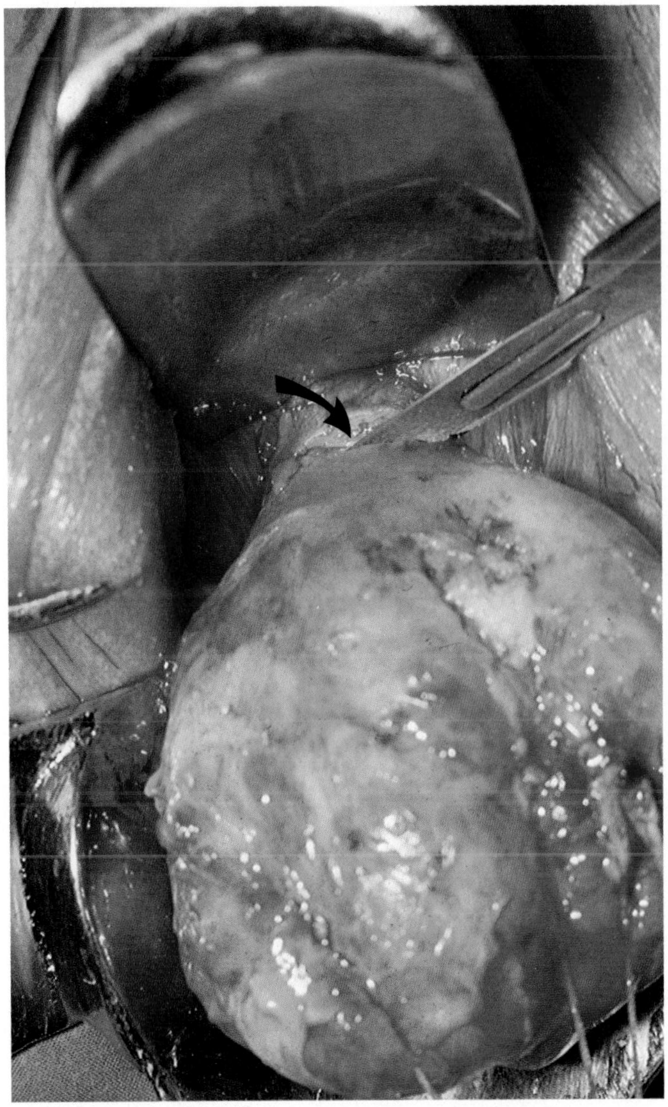

6

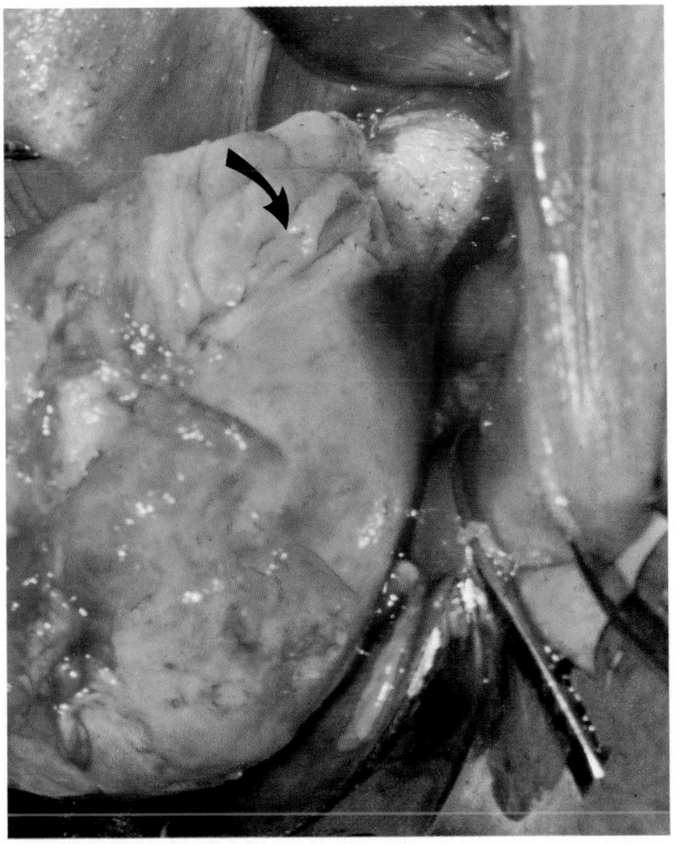

4 Exposure of pedicle of polyp

As the polyp is pulled downward and as the cervix is retracted upwards the pedicle of the polyp comes into view and is seen to be about 1.5 cm diameter as it emerges from the cervical canal.

5 and 6 Division of pedicle

It is important to divide and ligate the pedicle at exactly the correct level. This should be no higher than absolutely necessary so that the uterine wall is not encroached on. On the other hand it is essential to be above the level of the fibroid itself so that myomectomy is complete. A shallow incision is made across the pedicle just clear of the polyp, and there is no sign of encapsulated myoma there. Although unnecessary here the correct level can be checked by making a short incision distally in the body of the polyp when myoma immediately presents through its capsule. These two steps are shown here. The incisions described are arrowed.

7

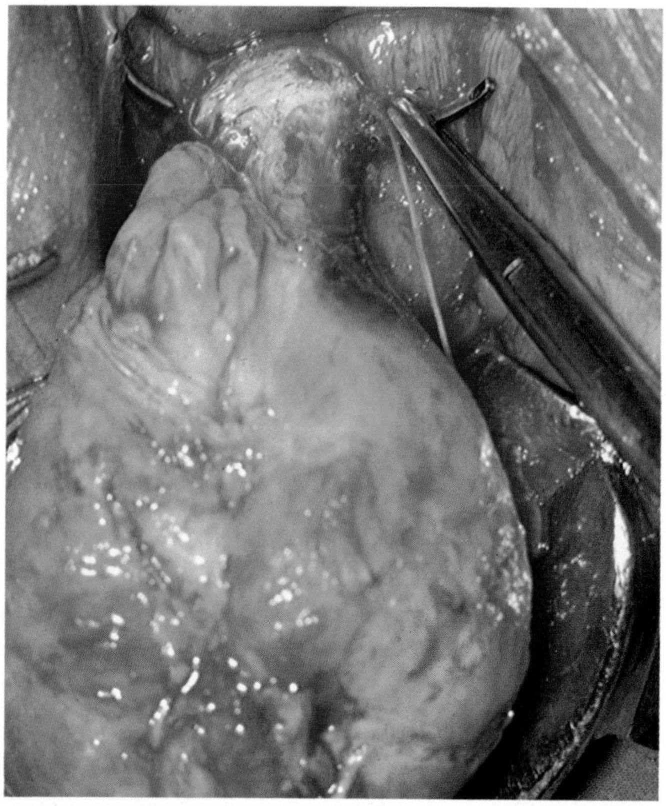

9

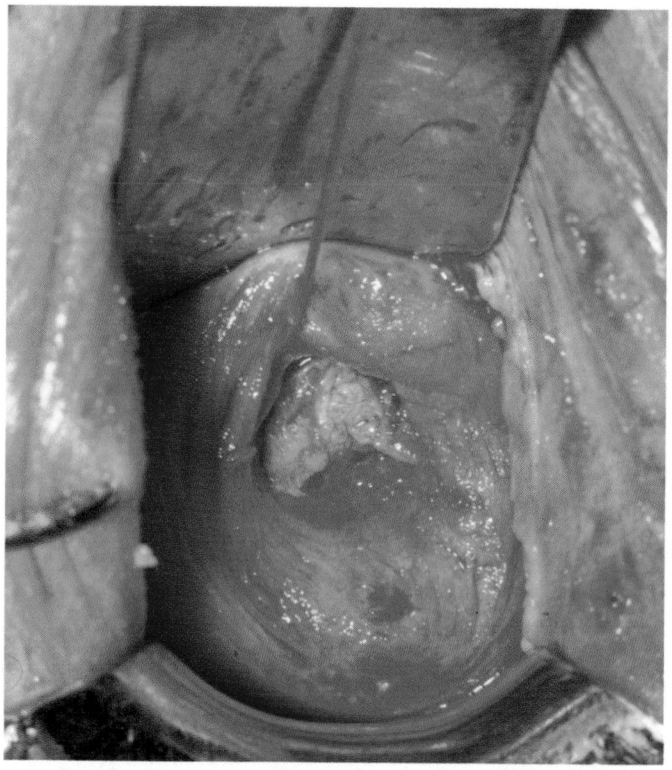

7 Transfixion and ligature of pedicle

A moderately stout round-bodied needle carrying a number 0 PGA suture transfixes the pedicle and is tied off to secure haemostasis. Note how the cervix is retracted while this is in progress and so that ligation can be done under direct vision.

10

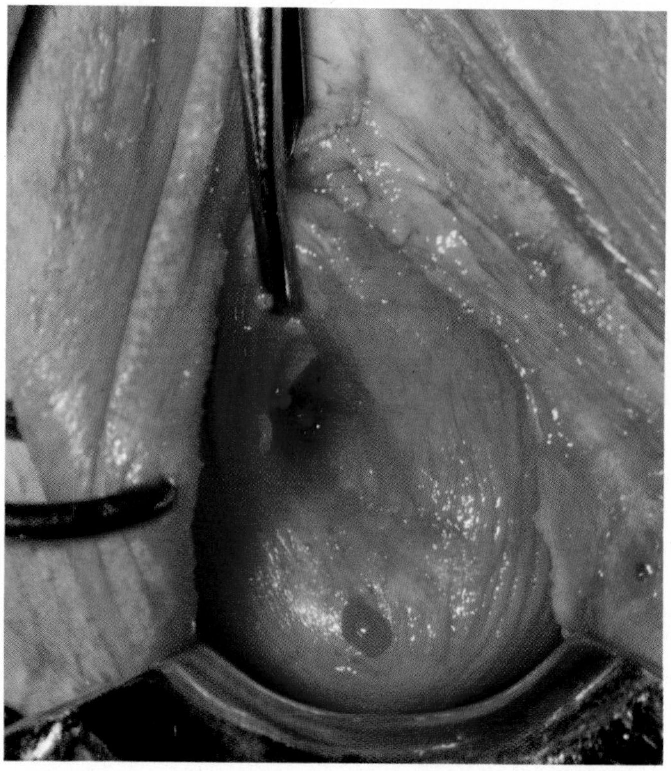

8

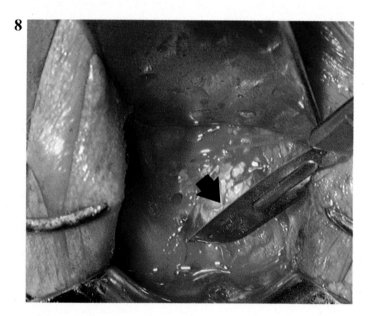

8 Removal of polyp

The remainder of the thickness of the pedicle below the ligature has been cut through by the scalpel and the polyp has fallen clear. The ligated pedicle with the attached uncut suture can be seen as indicated by the arrow.

9 and 10 Pedicle retracting into uterine cavity

The ligated pedicle is seen retracting into the cavity of the uterus through the still dilated cervix. In **9** the stitch is still uncut, the pedicle seems secure and there is no bleeding. In **10** the ligated pedicle has retracted completely out of view into the cavity of the uterus.

11

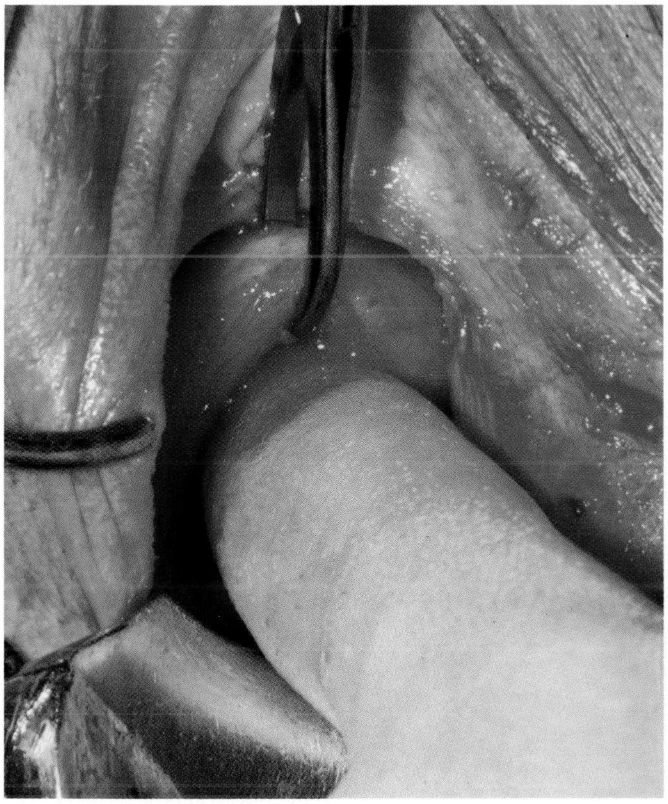

13

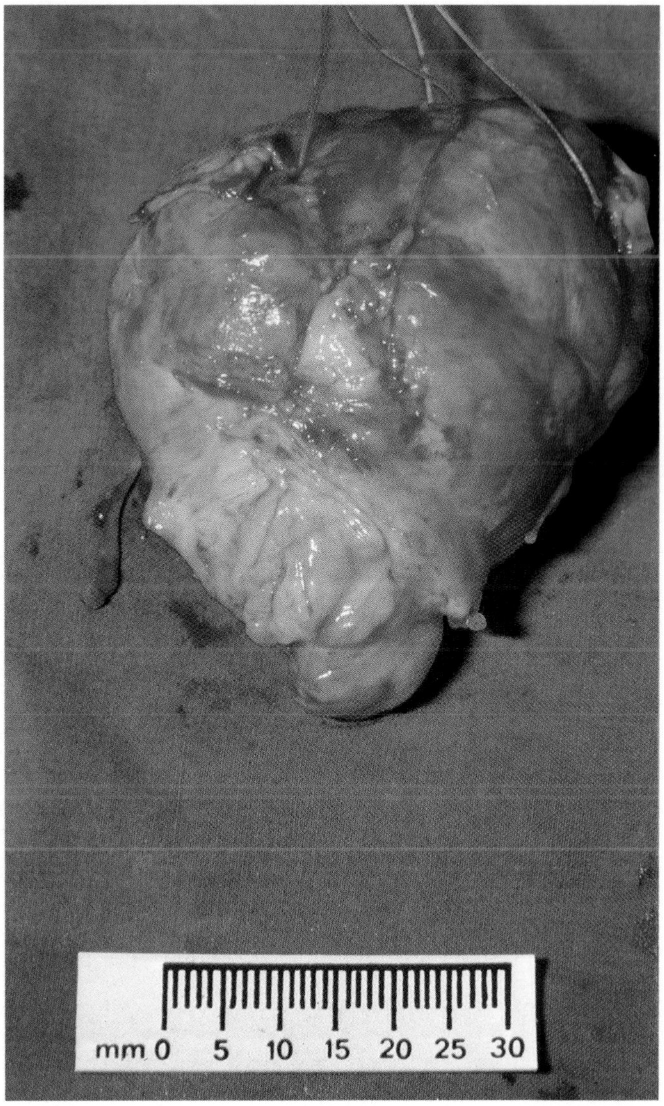

12

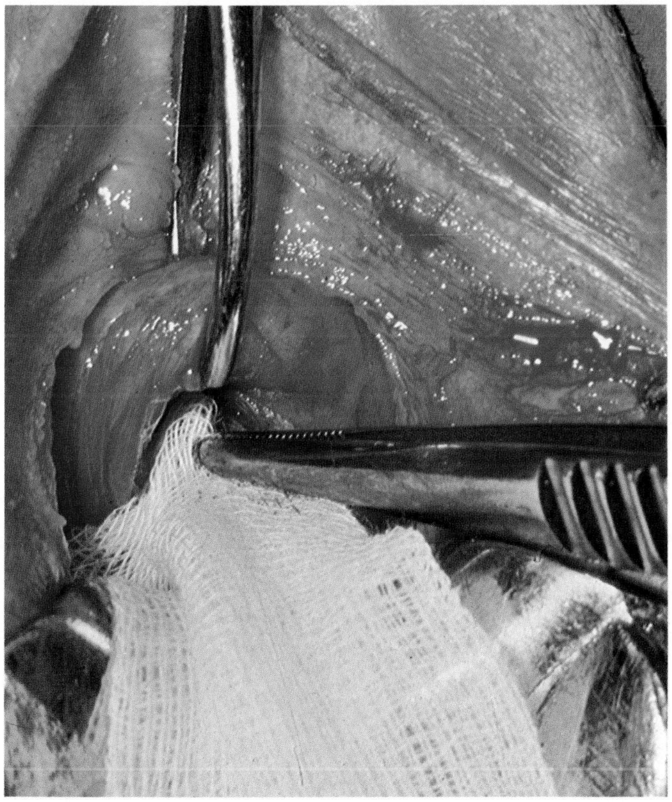

11 Exploration of uterine cavity

It is easy to explore the cavity with the forefinger because the cervix has been well dilated by the prolapsed fibroid. The cavity is quite smooth and there is no evidence of fibromyomata of any size in the body of the uterus.

12 Insertion of vaginal pack

The authors are not enthusiastic about packing the vagina in the normal course of events but consider this may be a reasonable exception. The end of a 7.5 cm wide role of gauze is tucked into the cervical canal to keep it open and the gauze is moderately firmly packed up into the lateral fornices of the vagina. The aim is to keep the cervix open and give the uterus a stimulus to contract over a few hours to encourage haemostasis. It may well be an unnecessary exercise; in any case the pack is taken out after six hours.

13 Appearance of polyp

The fibroid polyp is seen to be approximately 6 cm in diameter with a pedicle of 1.5 cm thickness. Necrosis is minimal and the incision displays the capsule of the fibroid.

Basic instruments required for major vaginal operations

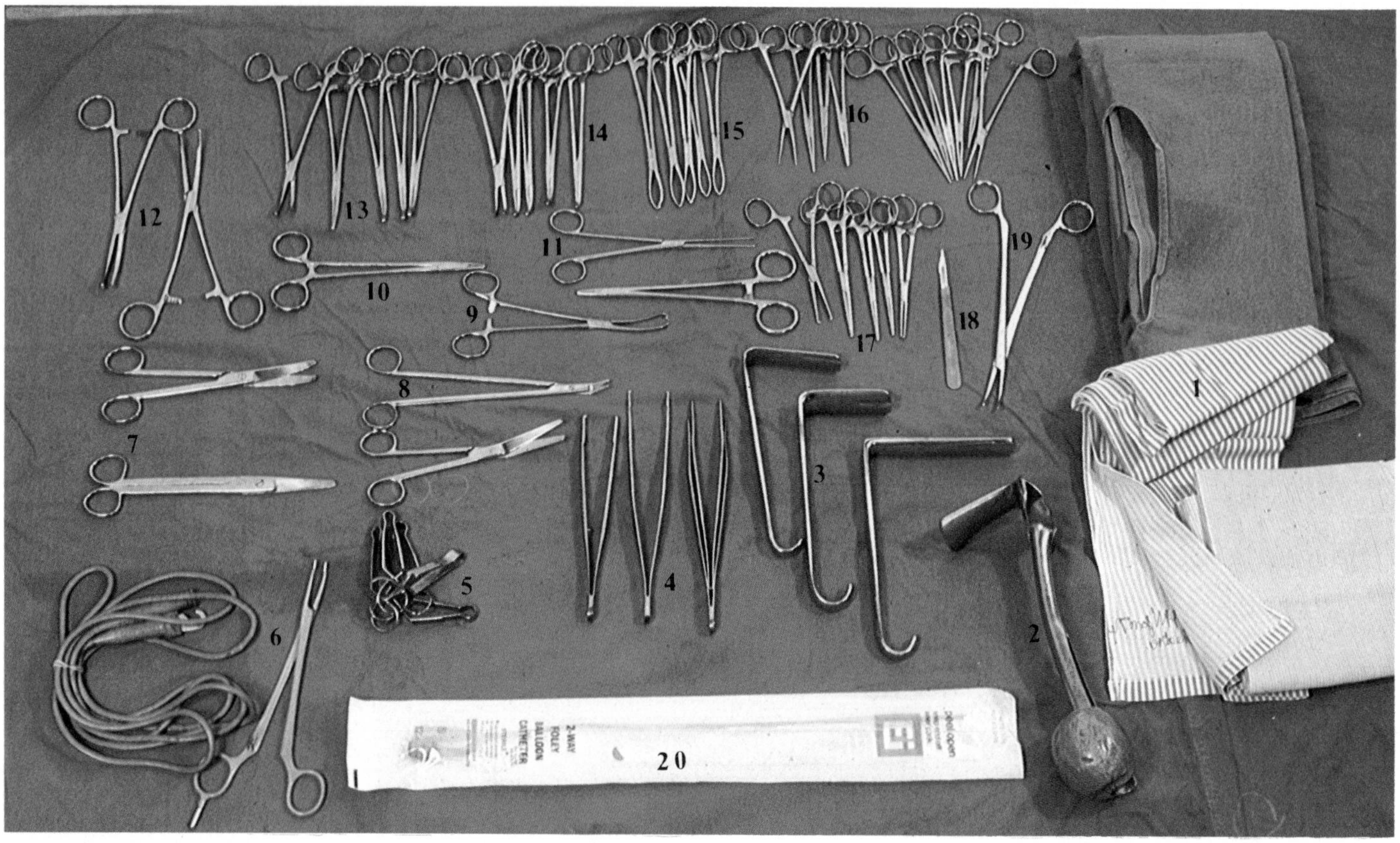

1 Drapes, leggings and exclusion sheet
2 Auvard's speculum
3 Vaginal retractors
4 Dissecting forceps (toothed and non-toothed)
5 Towel clips
6 Diathermy forceps and lead
7 Scissors – curved, straight, angled-on-flat
8 Cleft palate scissors
9 Volsellum
10 Needle holder (Mayo)
11 Sinus forceps
12 Maingot's forceps
13 Curved Oschner forceps (Jessop Hospital pattern)
14 Miles Phillips' forceps
15 Littlewood's forceps
16 Rankin Kelly forceps
17 Spencer Wells forceps
18 Scalpel (Bard Parker)
19 Roberts' forceps
20 Foley catheter

MAJOR OPERATIONS

5: Manchester repair (Fothergill operation): anterior and posterior wall repair

In treating the more severe forms of utero-vaginal prolapse the choice lies between a Manchester repair operation and a vaginal hysterectomy and repair as described in Chapter 8. It is not proposed to debate the merits and demerits of each at present; the operation will obviously be chosen to suit the particular case. Generally speaking, and unless there is need to remove the uterus, it is the authors' opinion that a Manchester repair will cure a prolapse of any degree as efficiently and well as vaginal hysterectomy and repair. Post-operative morbidity and especially bladder dysfunction (i.e. urinary retention) will be less. Technically the vagina will not be shortened as sometimes happens in vaginal hysterectomy. The Manchester repair is particularly suitable for the elderly and medically unfit woman, and can be done quite satisfactorily under local analgesia if necessary.

Once the technique of the operation has been learned it can be done without anxiety about the post-operative course and with minimal disturbance to the patient. It is the standard treatment for prolapse in the hospitals serving the large population of Northern England and it is impossible not to be impressed by the record of the operation and the results achieved. In trained hands the recurrence rate is very small and it should be remembered that the cases treated include patients with chronic bronchitis and obesity who are not fit for vaginal hysterectomy. When catgut is used there is the usual mixed vaginal discharge which is noticed by fastidious patients but has no ill effects. With PGA suture material there is practically no tissue reaction or discharge and the patient can usually go home at the end of a week.

The operation described here includes an anterior and posterior vaginal wall repair. One or other of these latter procedures is required in most vaginal operations and the opportunity is taken here of showing the technique employed.

1

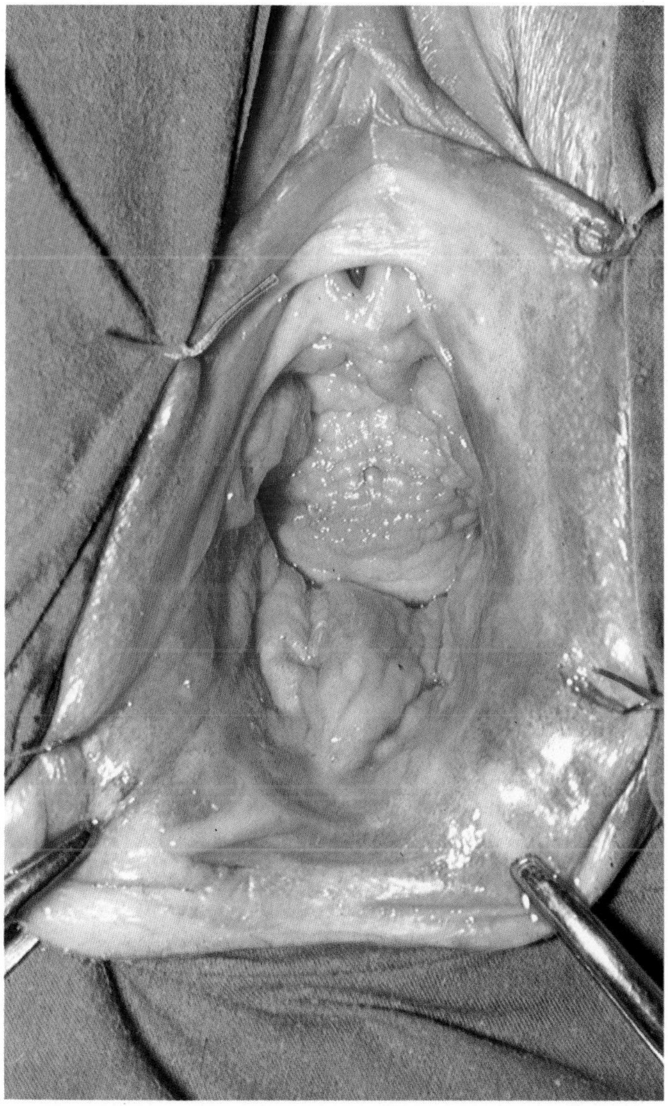

2

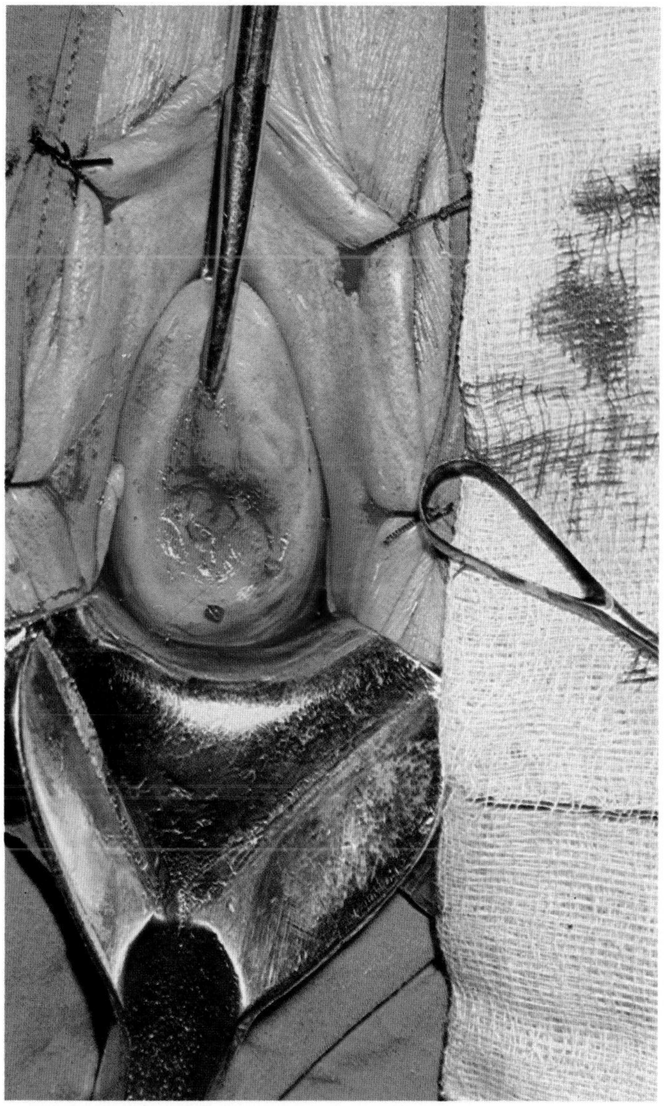

1 A general view

The degree of cystocele, rectocele and deficiency of the perineum in this patient is obvious. Increased exposure and access to the operative area is afforded by suturing the labia minora to the skin laterally and performing a mid-line episiotomy.

2 Preliminary curettage

The cervix descends to the perineum on gentle traction which means that this is a second degree utero-vaginal prolapse. Preliminary curettage is obligatory with no curettings being obtained in this case. The rationale for this procedure has been discussed previously (page 9).

Stage 1: Definition of urethra, bladder base and peritoneal pouches

3

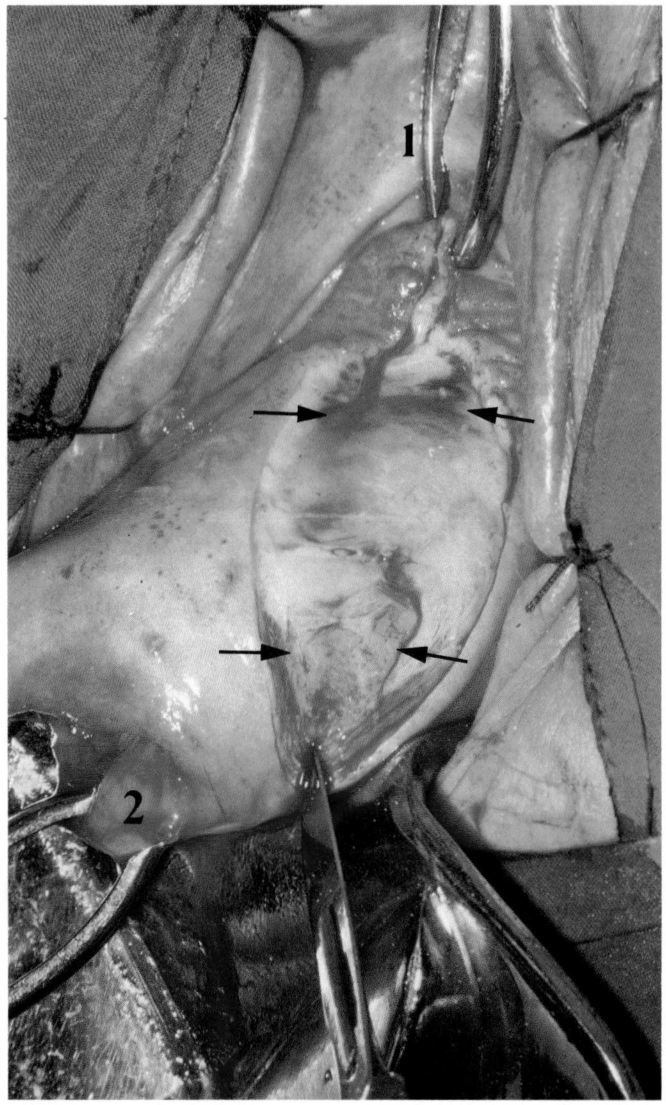

4

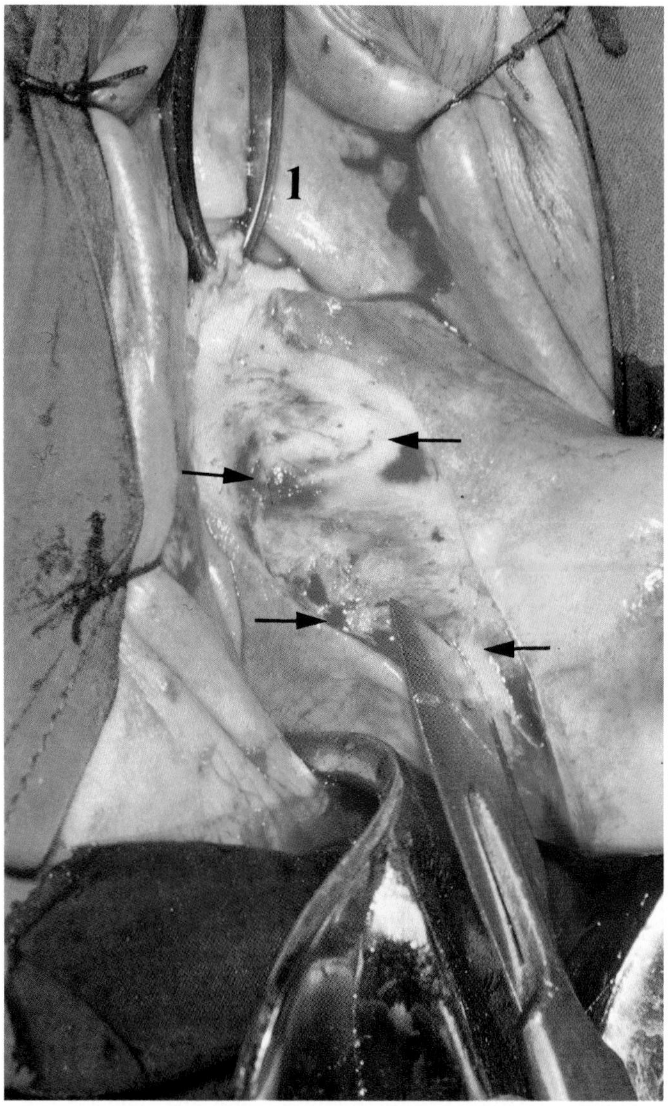

3 Anterior vaginal wall incision (1)

The anterior wall incision takes the form of a triangle with its apex just below the external urethral orifice – forceps (1) – and with its base over the width of the cervix. The incision is being made on the patient's left side and is carried down alongside and half-way round the cervix posteriorly. The depth of the incision is sufficient to divide the skin and the underlying pubocervical fascia. When making the incision the skin is held taut between forceps (1) and forceps (2) on the cervix and the line of the incision is straight. Vasoconstrictive agents have blanched and made prominent the fascial planes of the anterior vaginal wall, the main constituent of which is the pubocervical fascia.

4 Anterior vaginal wall incision (ii)

The corresponding incision has been made on the right side and again demonstrates the two layers of tissue, i.e. vaginal skin and pubocervical fascia. The arrows again indicate the latter.

5
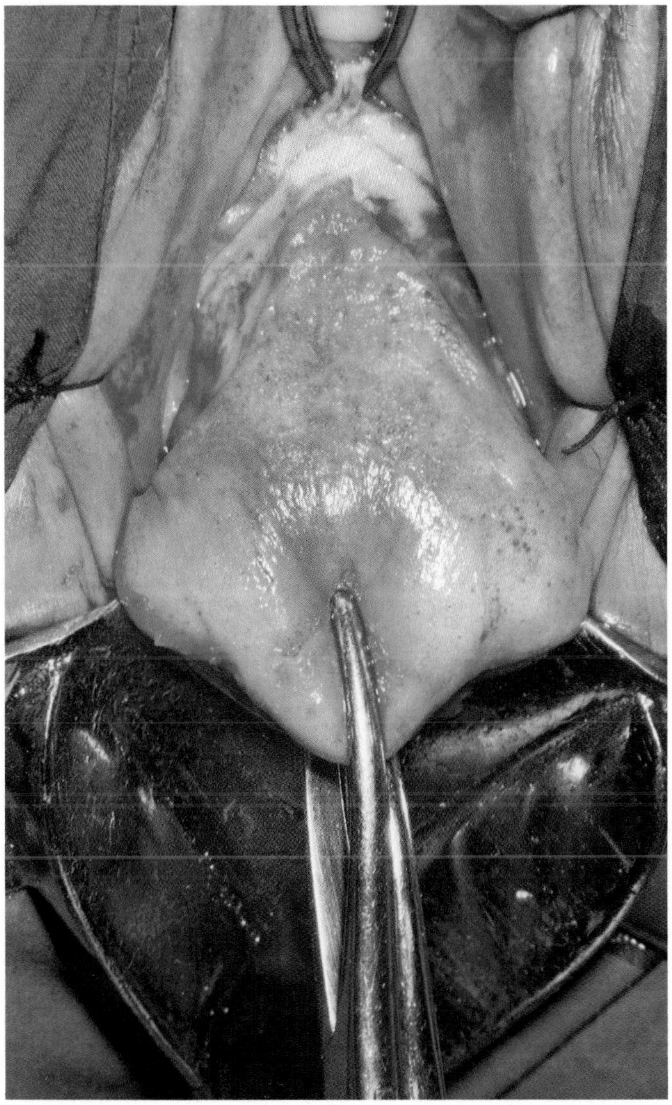

6
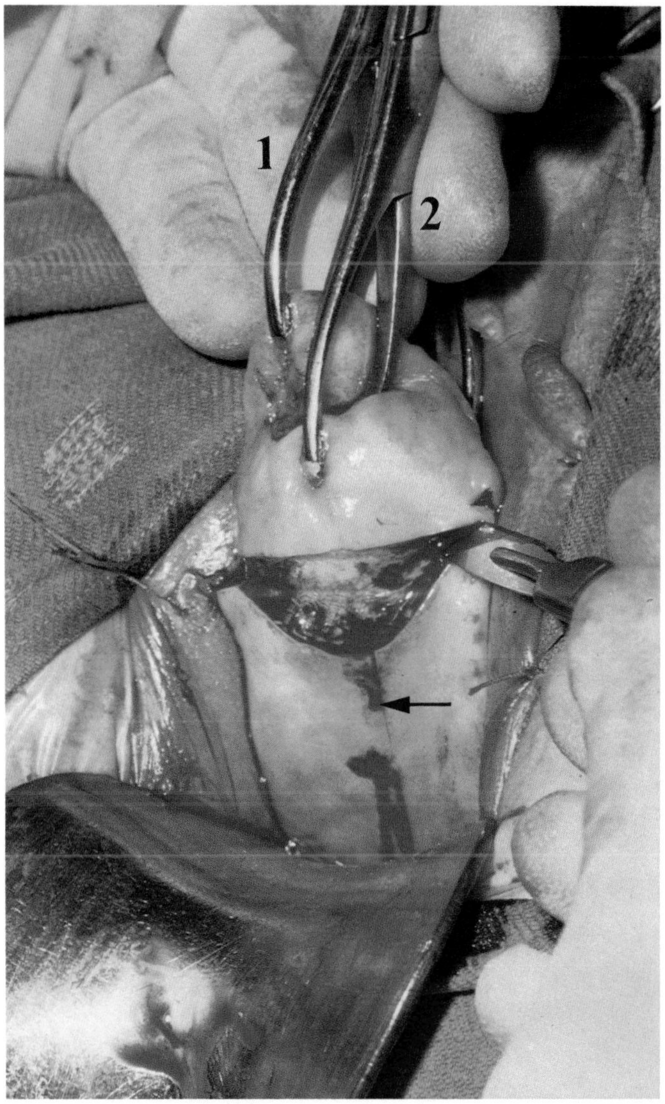

5 Anterior vaginal wall incision (iii)

The comparatively wide apical angle of the triangle is shown. This ensures that the vaginal vault when reconstructed after the completion of the anterior repair will be sufficiently elevated.

6 Joining skin incisions posterior to cervix

The cervix is elevated by forceps (1) and (2) on the anterior and posterior lips respectively, and the lower ends of the two anterior wall incisions are joined across the back of the cervix just at the level where the skin becomes mobile on the cervix. Note the knife scratch on the lower flap (arrowed) which was made before incision to indicate the central point posteriorly. This provides a helpful guide for the subsequent accurate apposition of the resutured vaginal skin.

7

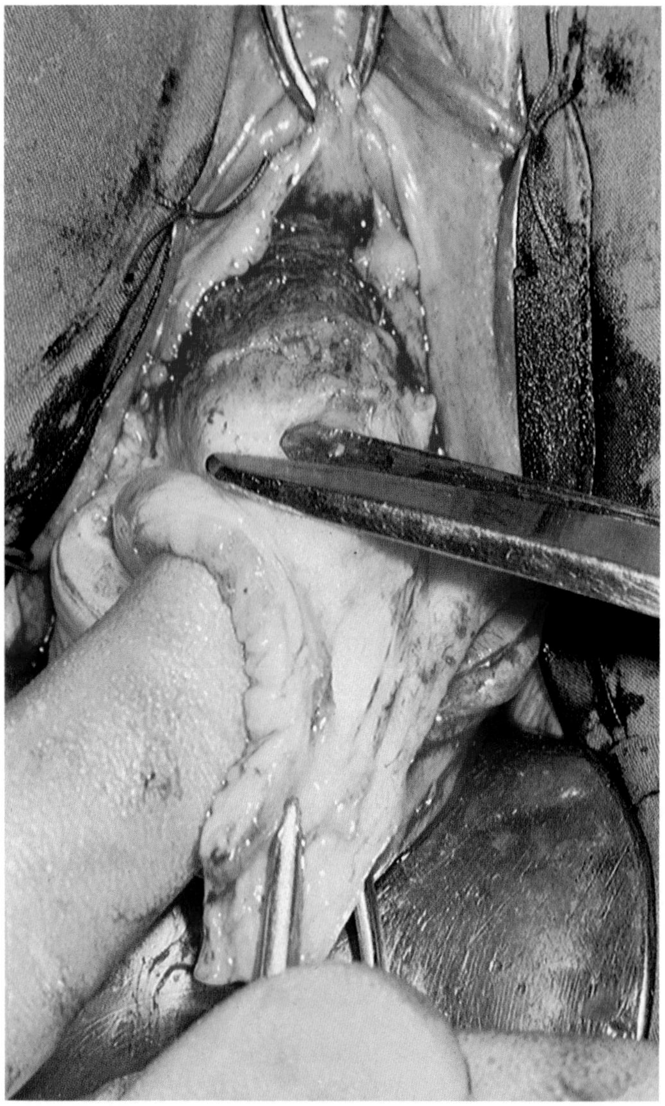

8

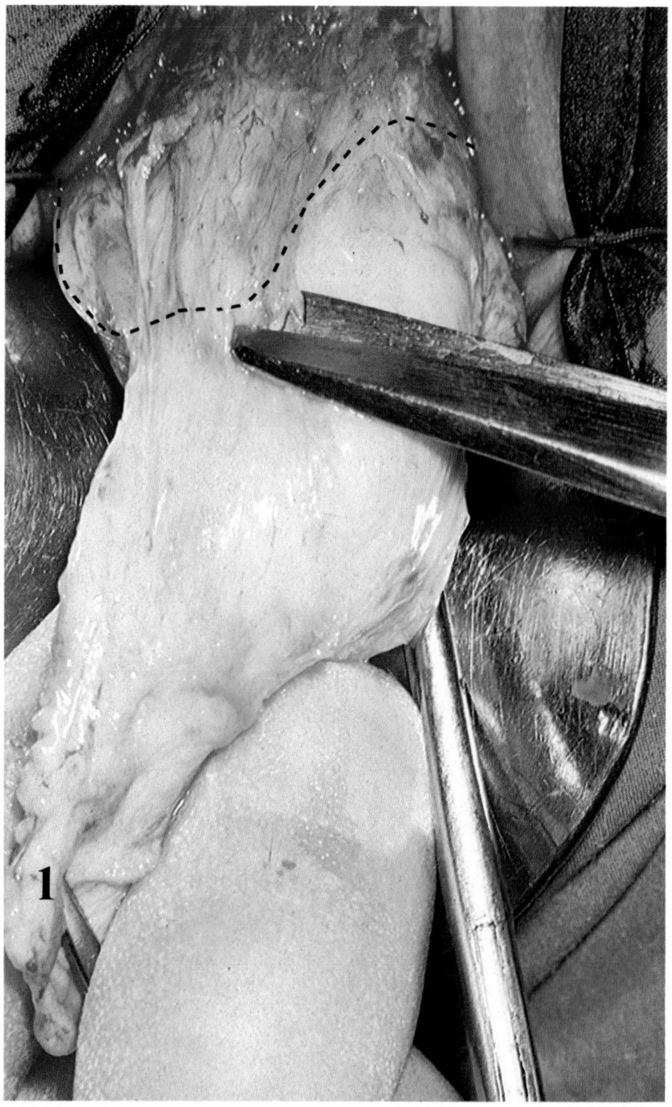

7 Raising the anterior vaginal skin flap

The anterior triangular flap of vaginal skin with its layer of underlying and attached pubocervical fascia is now dissected downwards off the bladder. In the presence of cystocele the fascial layer is invariably incomplete and thinned out medially. Sharp dissection is necessary initially because the skin and fascia are adherent to the upper urethra, but very soon pressure with partially opened scissors is all that is required.

A central plane of cleavage opens up and separation is avascular except for a few small lateral vessels which are sealed with the diathermy. Stripping the flap off the bladder with a swab on a holder or even wrapped around the finger is dangerous and can easily cause tearing of the bladder wall.

8 Mobilisation of bladder (i)

The triangular skin flap is held at its apex by forceps (1) and pulled down from the urethral orifice by forceps to display the bladder base (outlined). The scissors are freeing the bladder from the front of the lower uterus preparatory to inserting a flat retractor to displace and protect it.

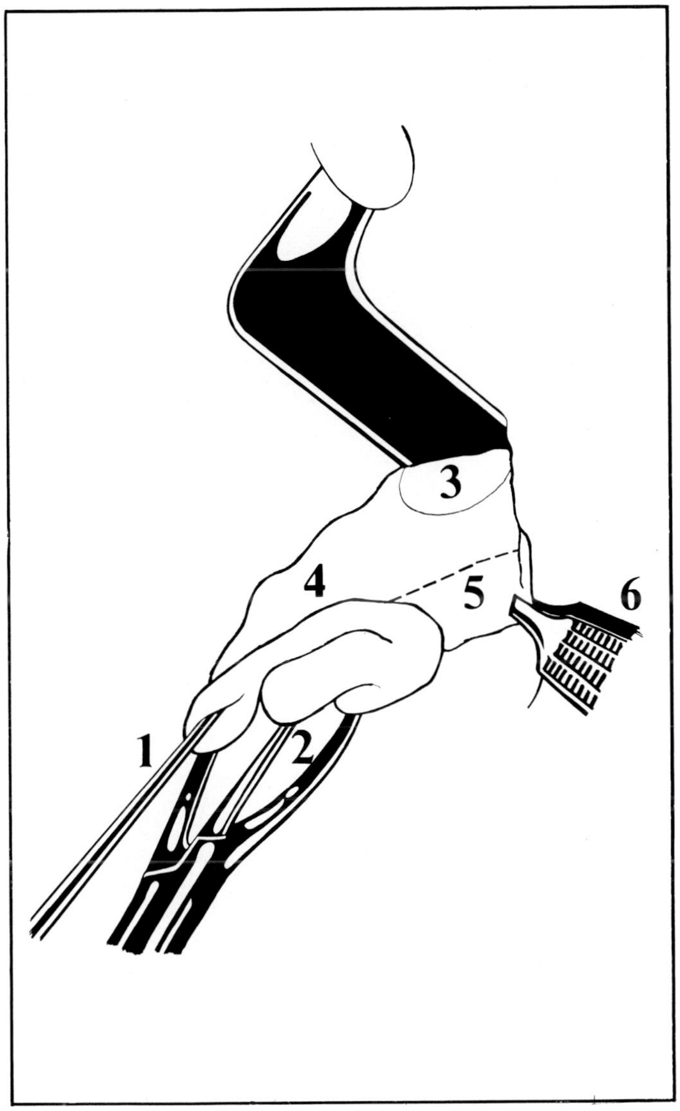

1 Forceps on apex of skin triangle
2 Forceps on posterior lip of cervix
3 Lower edge of utero-vesical pouch
4 Cervix
5 Left cardinal ligament
6 Forceps retracting vaginal skin edge

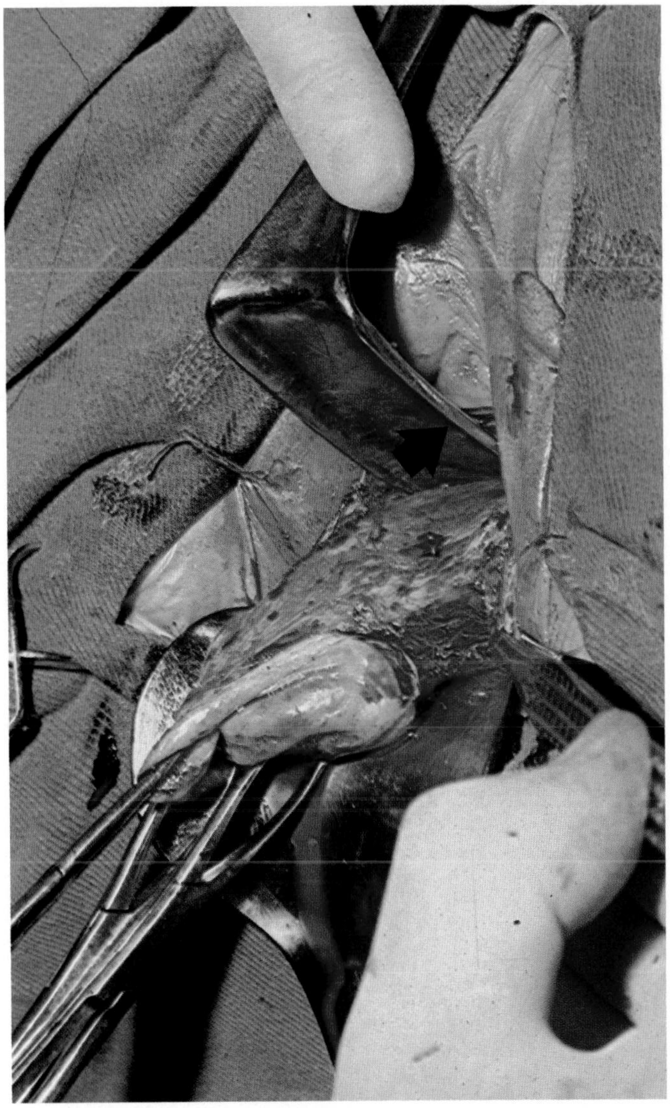

9

9 Mobilisation of bladder (ii)

The triangular skin flap is kept taut by pulling on forceps while a narrow retractor displaces the bladder from the anterior surface of the cervix and lower uterus as indicated by arrow. The lower edge of the utero-vesical pouch can be seen.

10

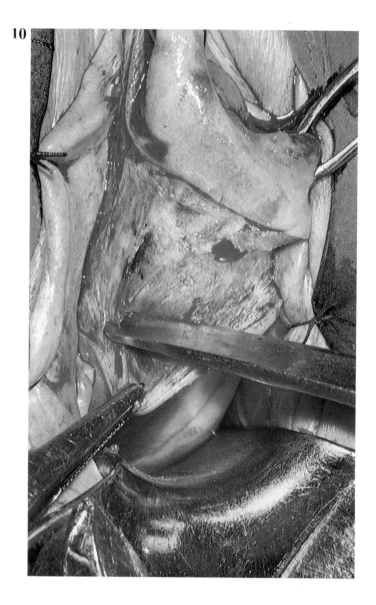

11

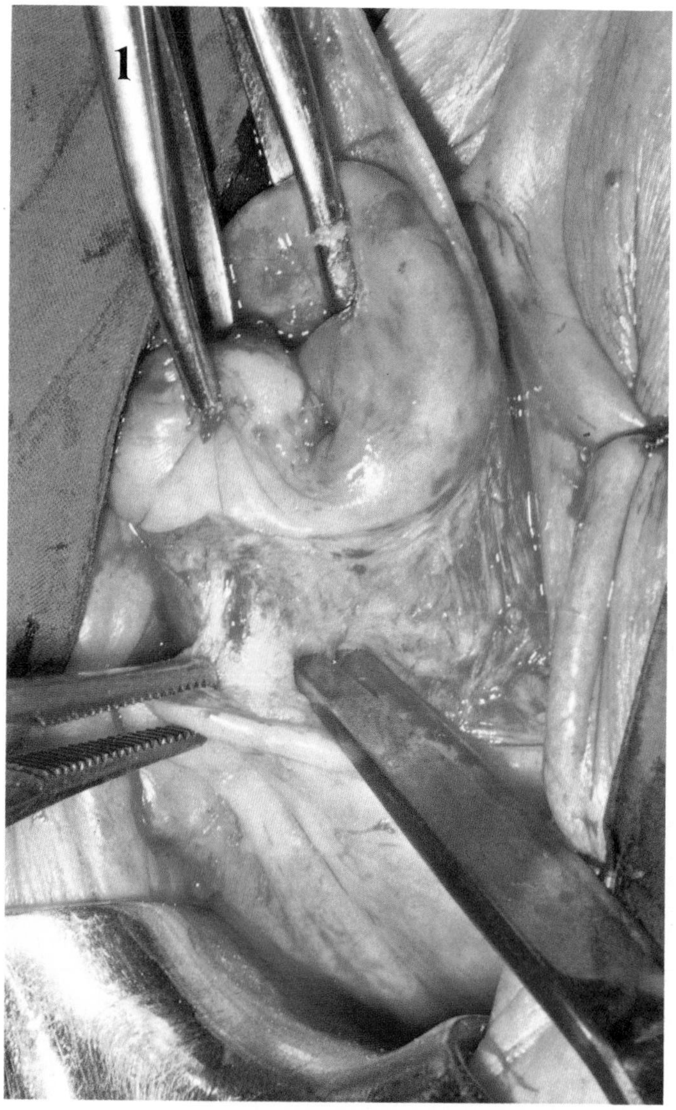

10 Separation of skin from lateral cervix

The upper leaf of vaginal skin is separated off the upper cervix and lower uterus on each side by a combination of scissor cuts and pressure with the partially opened scissor blades. This is an important step because the raised skin flap is destined to cover the cervical stump and it must be sufficiently wide and without tension for that purpose. Separation can be practically avascular once the correct plane is entered.

11 Exposure of utero-sacral ligaments

The process is continued posteriorly in the area overlying the pouch of Douglas and is advanced sufficiently to visualise the pouch itself. Lifting up forceps on the posterior lip of the cervix keeps the utero-sacral ligaments taut and facilitates dissection. The tissue plane is the same as previously demonstrated in **9** and **10** and bleeding is minimal.

12

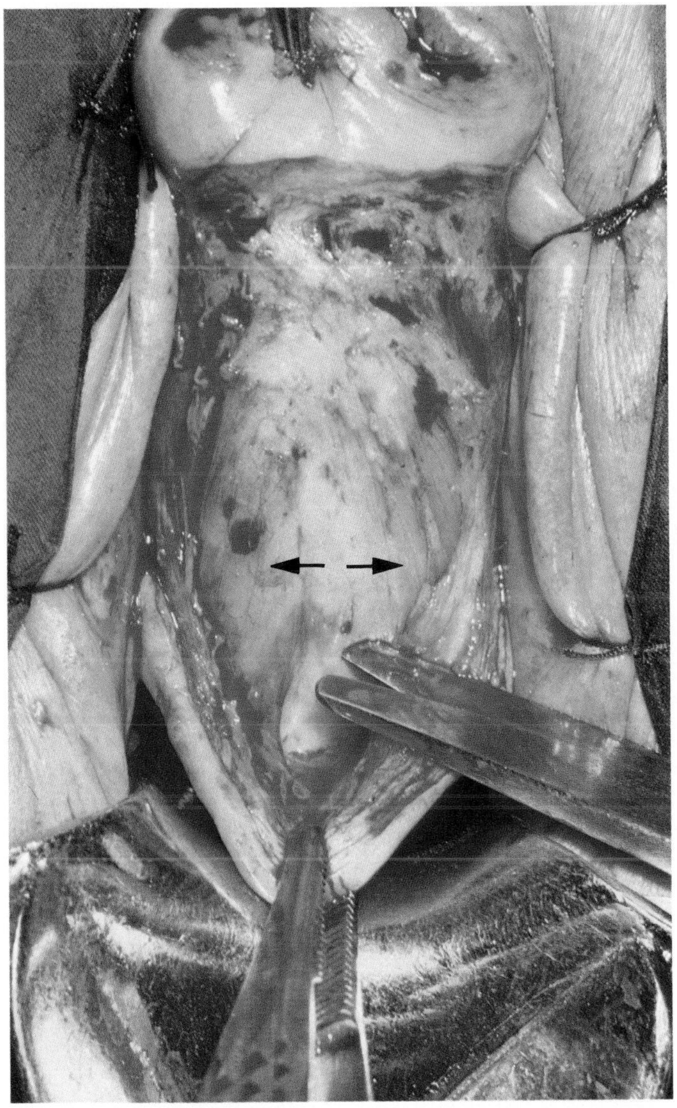

13

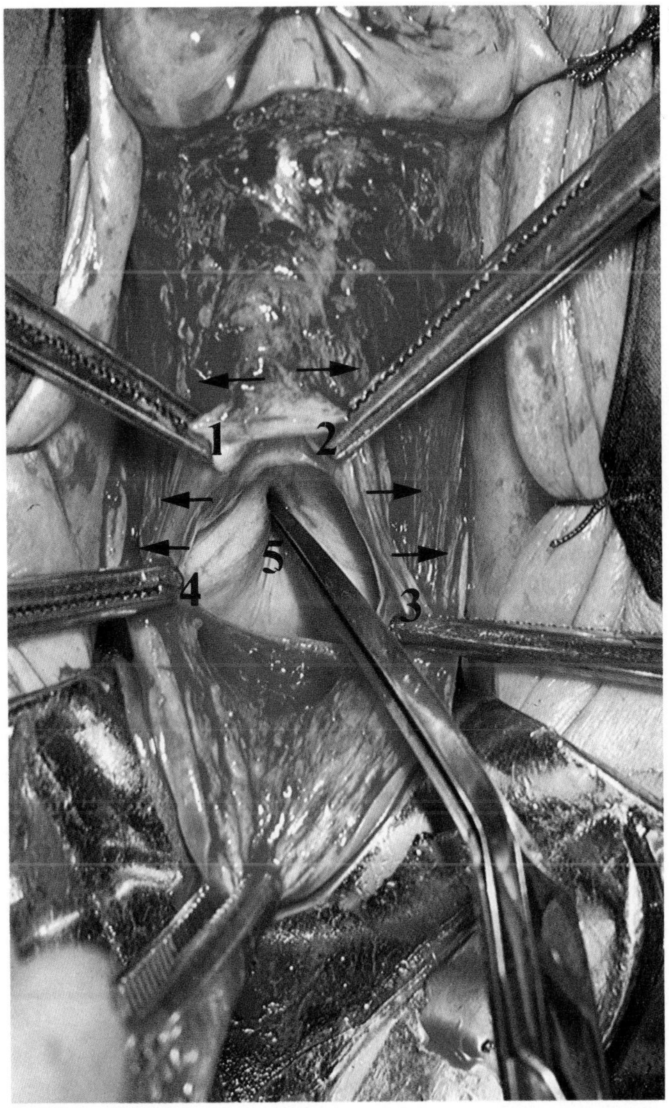

12 Exposure of pouch of Douglas

The pouch of Douglas is indicated by the scissor points and is about to be opened. It appears to be very high but this is because elongation of the cervix invariably accompanies major degrees of prolapse. Even before incision of the pouch the outlines of the utero-sacral ligaments are obvious (marked by arrows).

13 Opening pouch of Douglas

The pouch has now been opened and is held by forceps (1), (2), (3) and (4). It will be dissected up between the utero-sacral ligaments as a hernial sac and the aim will be to secure its closure as high as possible. The utero-sacral ligaments are again marked by arrows. In the photograph the tips of the scissors indent the posterior uterine wall (5).

Stage 2: Obliteration of enterocele sac

14

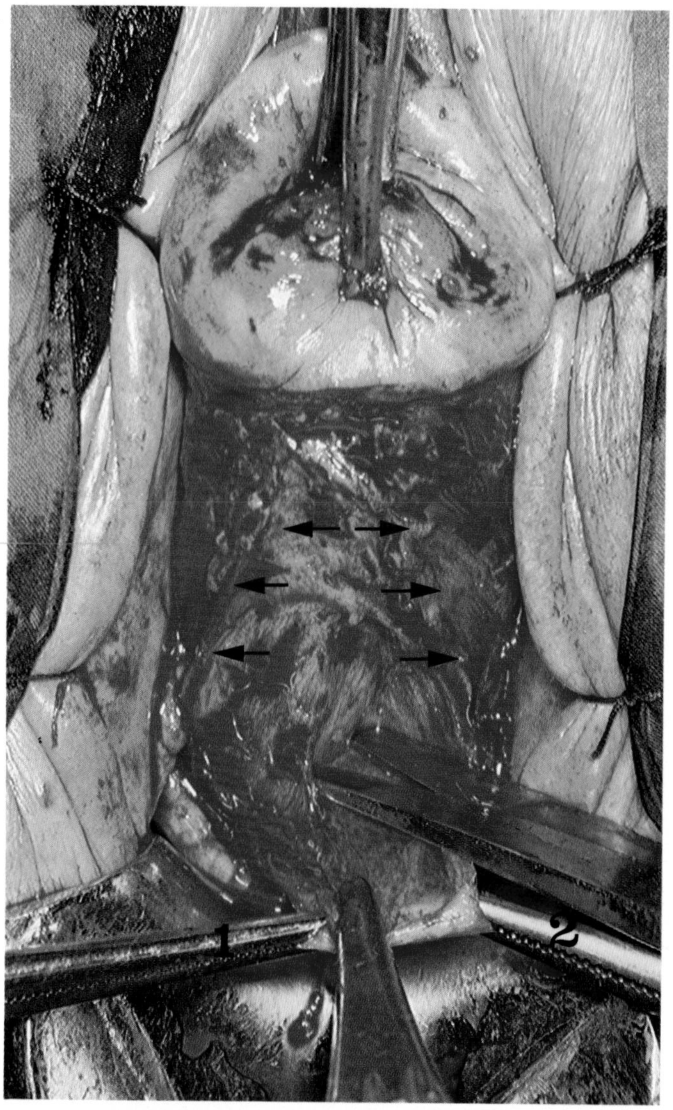

15

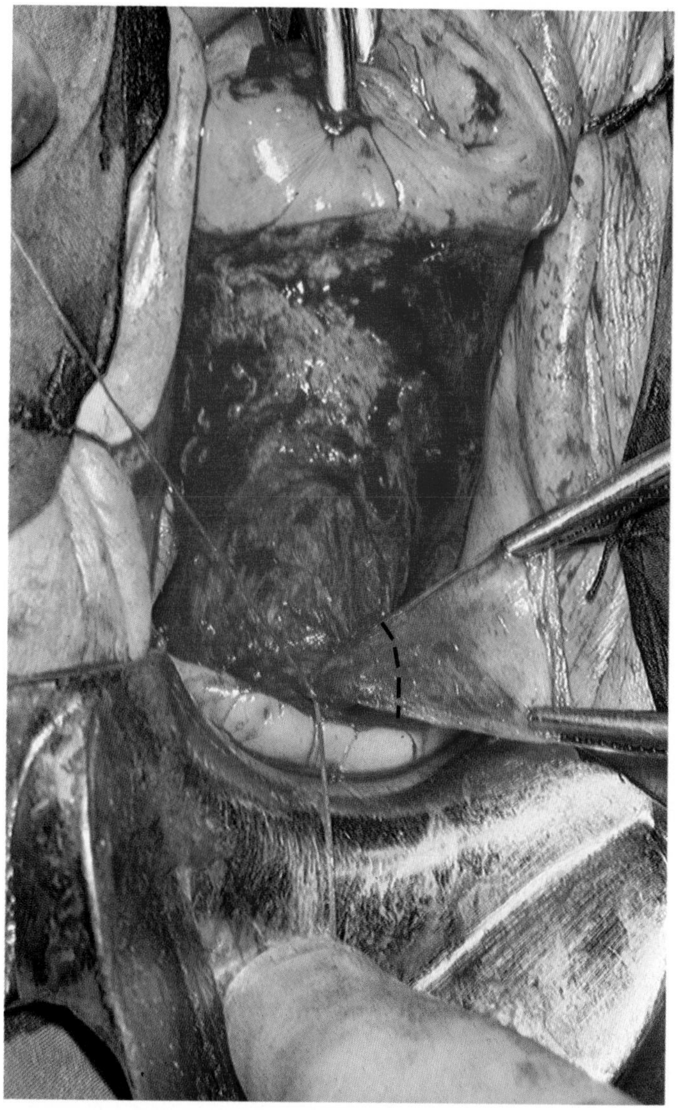

14 Mobilisation of enterocele sac

Dissection of the sac between the utero-sacral ligaments is continued. Forceps (1) and (2) support the upper opening of the sac while the scissors separate it from the ligaments and posterior aspect of the uterus. The open mouth of the sac faces the blade of the Auvard speculum and is not therefore obvious. The outlines of the utero-sacral ligaments are clearly seen and are arrowed.

15 Closure and excision of enterocele sac

The dissected sac has been transfixed and is being ligated in standard fashion as high up as possible. The dotted line indicates where the incision will be made to remove the redundant peritoneum which constituted the sac. The mouth of the sac lies between the two holding forceps.

16

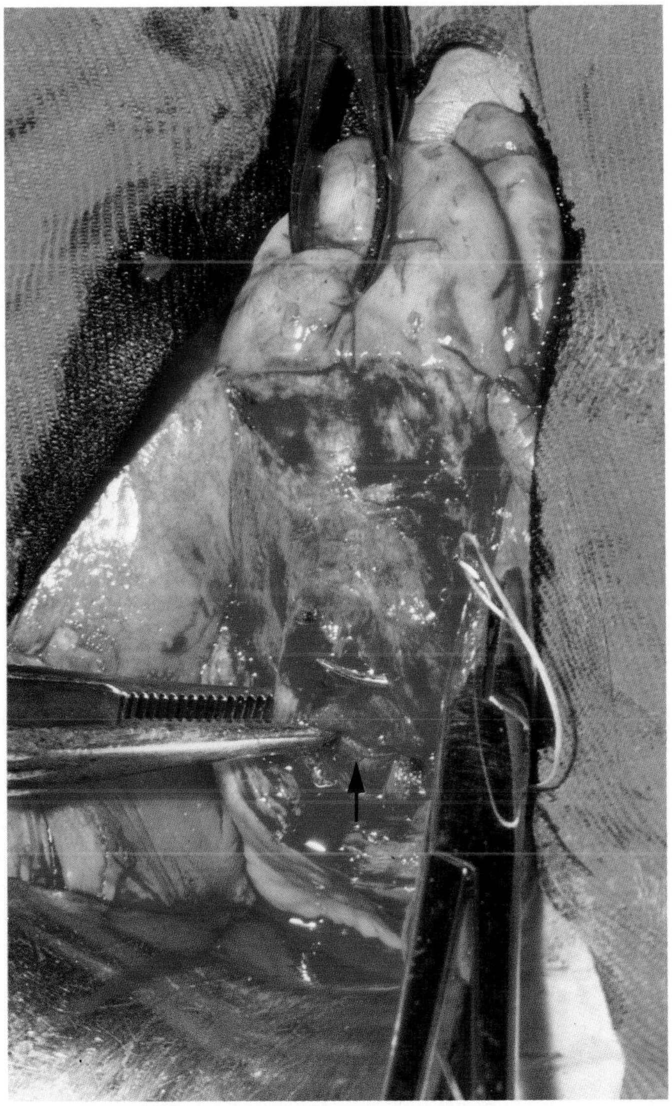

17

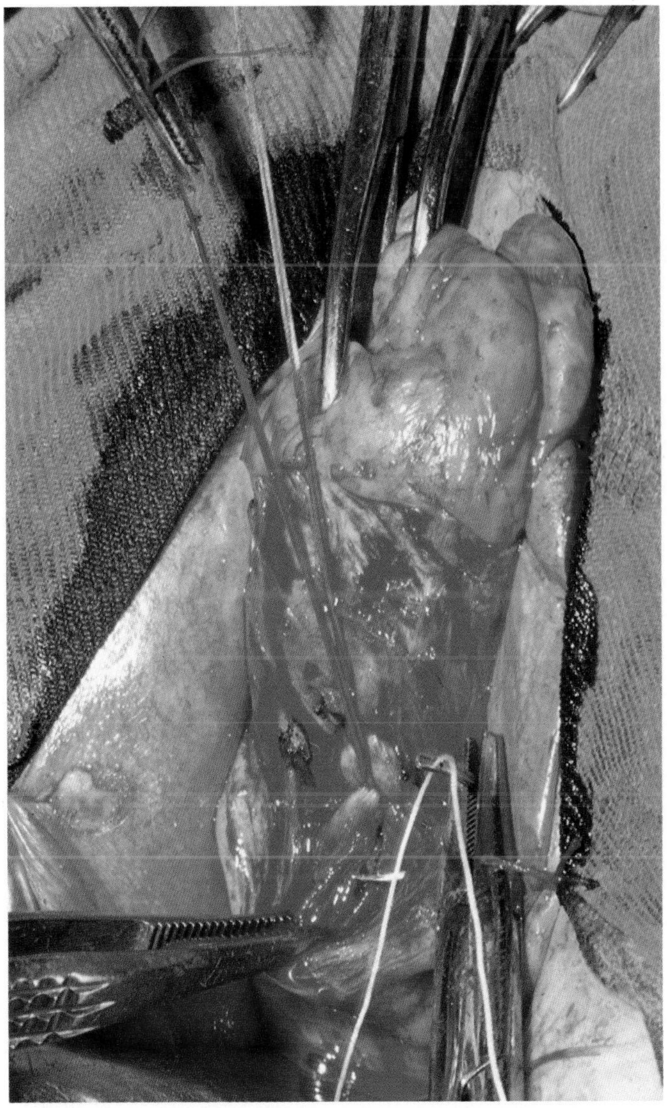

16 Approximation of utero-sacral ligaments (i)

The next and very important step is to approximate the utero-sacral ligaments over the ligated enterocele sac. The left utero-sacral ligament has been picked up on the needle while the right is held in the dissecting forceps. The ligated sac is indicated by an arrow.

17 Approximation of utero-sacral ligaments (ii)

Subsequent approximating sutures are being placed and the ligated enterocele sac is effectively buried under the suture line. Two, or at most three, sutures are required.

Stage 3: Mobilisation of cardinal ligaments

The next stage of the operation involves the definition and detachment of the cardinal ligaments from their insertion into the upper lateral wall of the cervix. Their medial ends are subsequently approximated and fixed to the lower anterior aspect of the uterus and form the main support of the new vaginal vault. It is important that they be defined with accuracy.

18

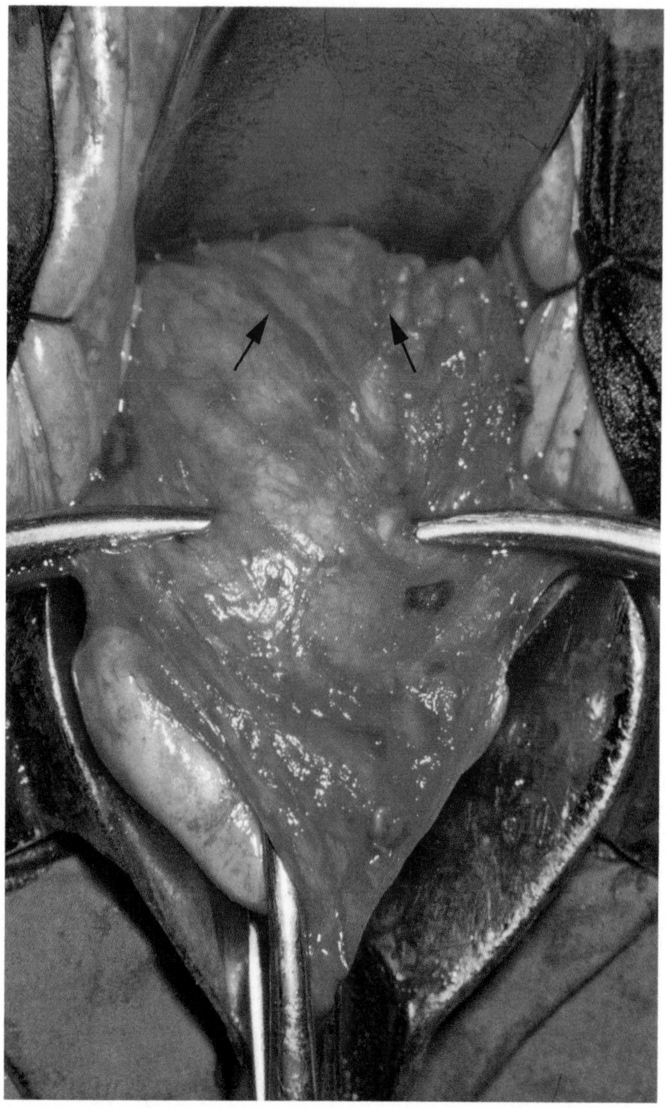

19

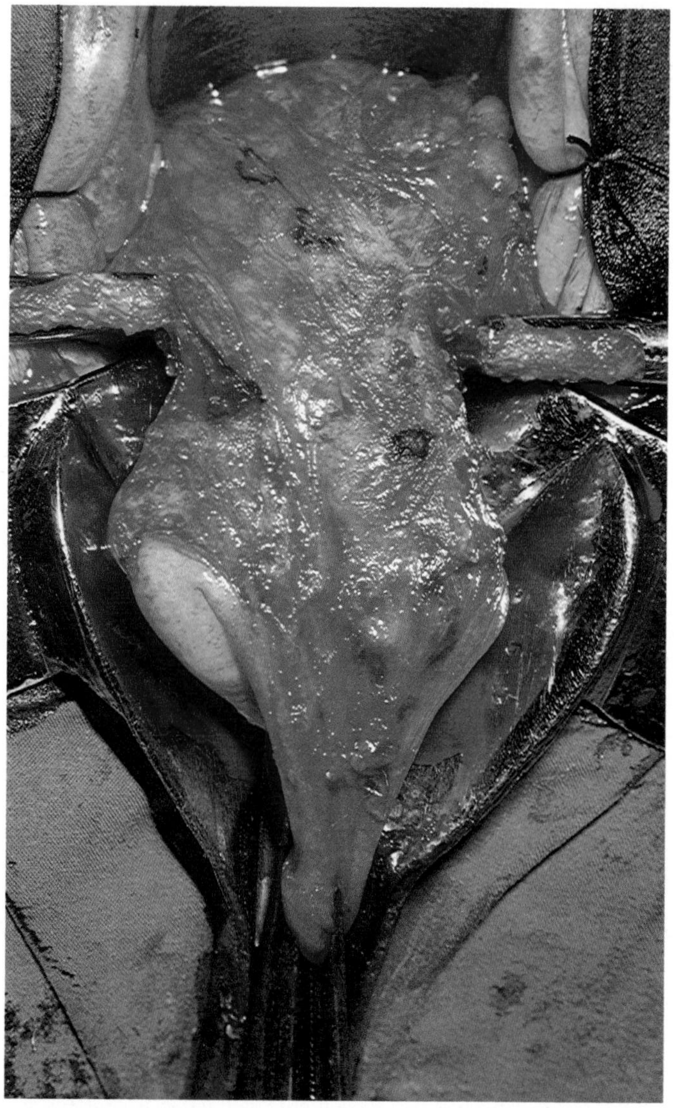

18 Definition and clamping of cardinal ligaments

The cardinal ligaments are shown clamped on both sides by curved Ochsner forceps. The pedicles are easily defined and are largely fibrous although they contain the cervical branches of the uterine vessels. Forceps retract the skin triangle which is still attached and the utero-vesical pouch can be seen in the upper part of the wound under the flat retractor which is displacing the bladder upwards. The lower border of this pouch is arrowed.

19 Separation of cardinal ligaments

The clamped cardinal ligaments have been detached from the cervix with scissors and are seen as free pedicles. Longer and more satisfactory pedicles can be obtained by using the clamping forceps as levers to prise the ligaments back from their uterine attachments. Note how this has been effected on the left side.

20A

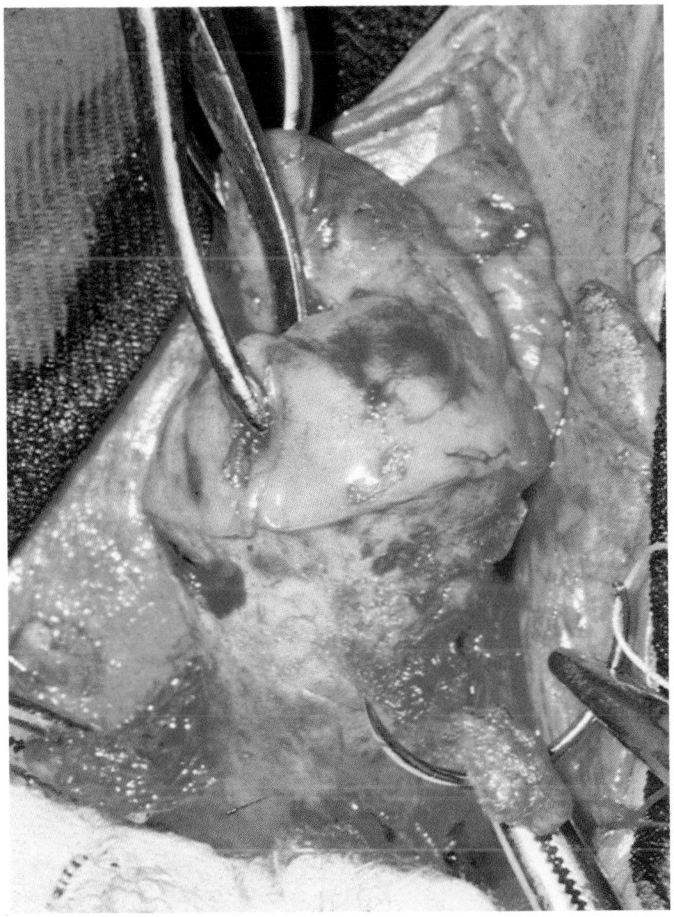

20B

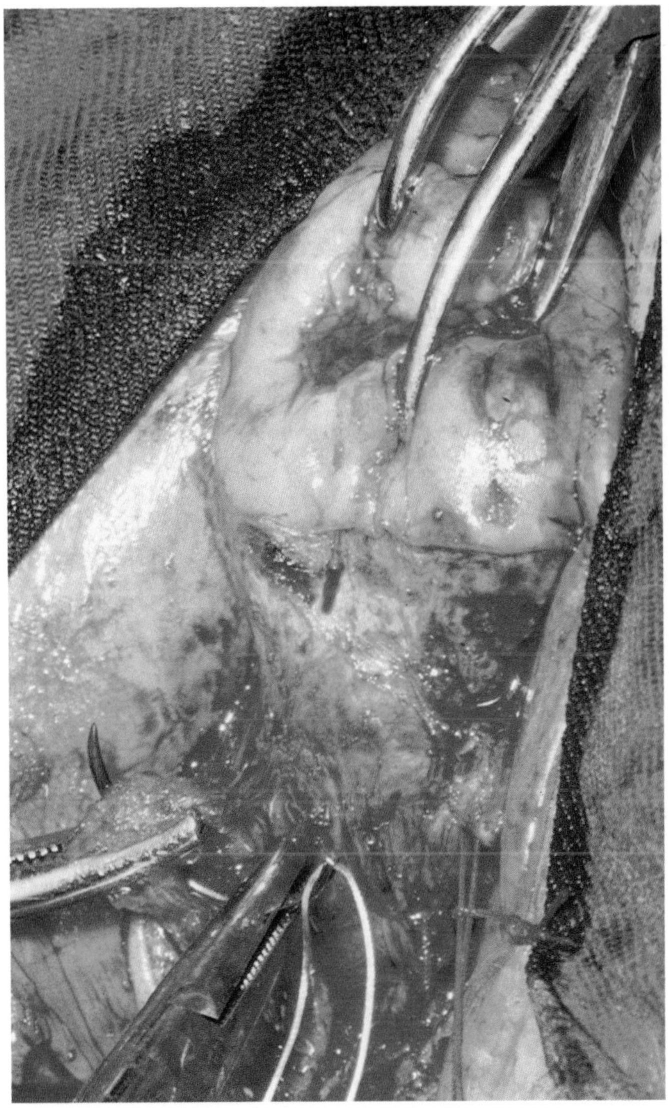

20C

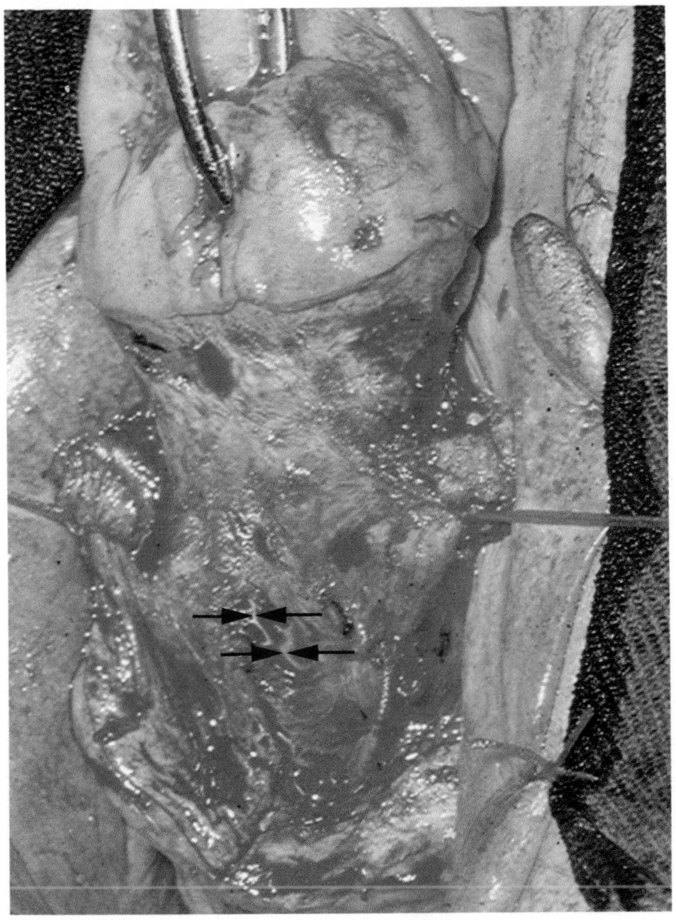

20A–20C Transfixion and ligation of cardinal ligaments

The cervix has been elevated to give access to the pedicles. Here they are being transfixed and will be ligated in standard fashion. In **20C**, each cardinal ligament is held by a long suture which is fixed to the drapes. The area between the approximation line of the utero-sacral ligaments now covers the closed enterocele sac (as arrowed). The stage is now set for amputation of the cervix and reconstruction of the vault of the vagina.

Stage 4: Amputation of the cervix

The main reason for amputation of the cervix is to obtain access to the medial ends of the cardinal ligaments. These ligaments will form the main support of the new vaginal vault when subsequently sutured to the lower anterior uterine wall. There are generally additional benefits from amputation of the cervix, notably where there is an accompanying 'erosion' or lacerations following childbirth.

21A

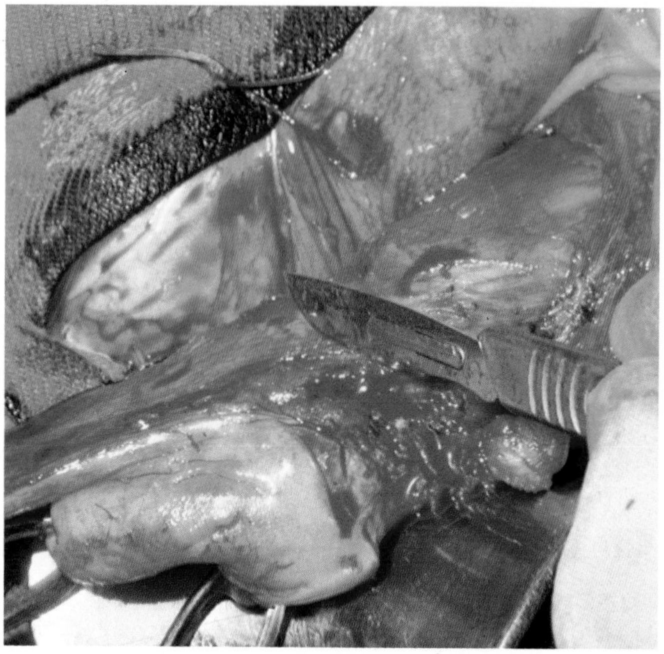

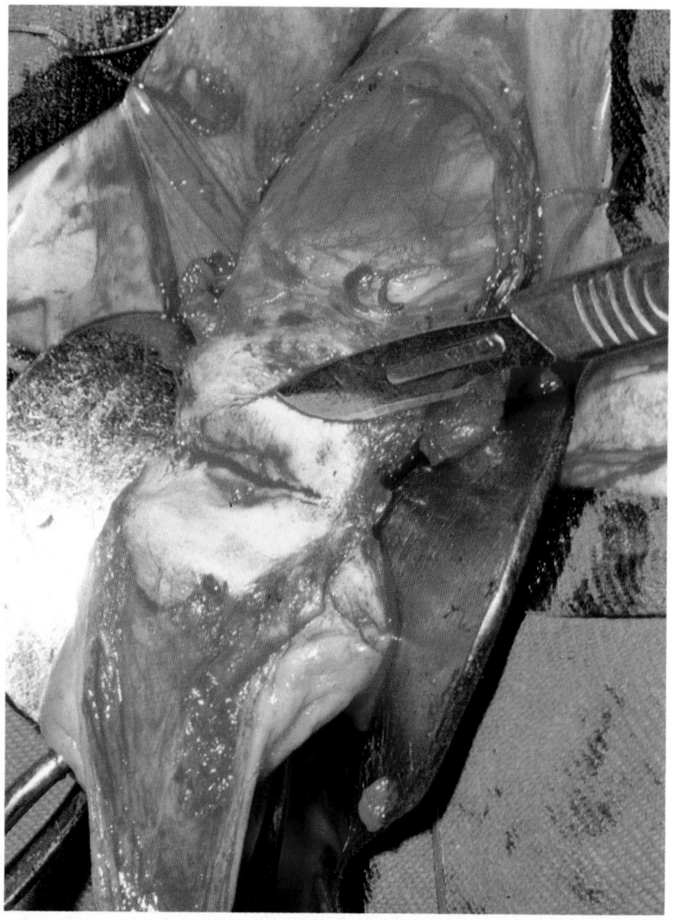

21B

21A–21C Amputation of the cervix

Figure **21A** shows the level of the incision. The cervix is completely removed except in patients hoping to have a further pregnancy. The incision is first carried through the anterior wall of the cervix into the canal as shown in **21B**. The assistant grasps the anterior wall of the cervical stump with a Littlewood's forceps and the surgeon completes the amputation through the posterior wall as shown in **21C**. In women desirous of future pregnancy no more than one-half of the cervix is amputated.

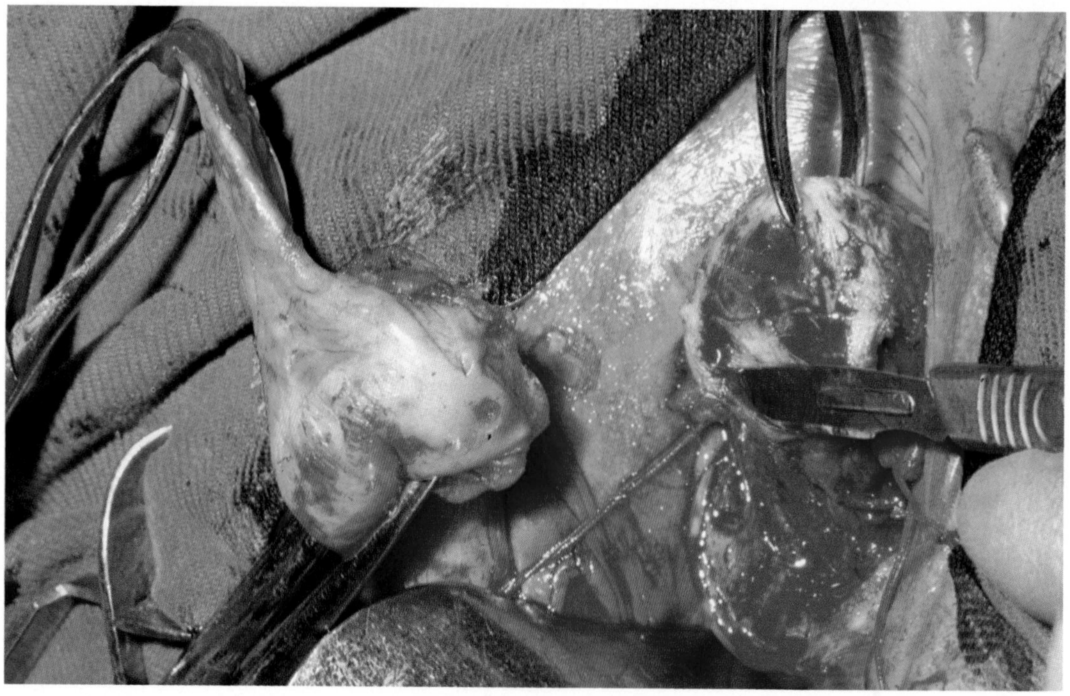

21C

Stage 5: Reconstruction of the cervix

The next stage of the operation is to cover the cervical stump by utilising the free skin flap. A definitive procedure must be followed if this is to be completed accurately.

This technique involves:

1 Insertion of a *Sturmdorf* suture posteriorly
2 Insertion of two lateral *investing* sutures
3 Covering of the anterior cervix by what is termed a *crown* suture.

The purpose of the Sturmdorf suture is to cover the posterior aspect of the bare cervical stump with the loose skin flap. Specialist gynaecologists are familiar with the stitch, which has various applications in cervical surgery but those in general surgical practice or in training may not be familiar with it.

22A

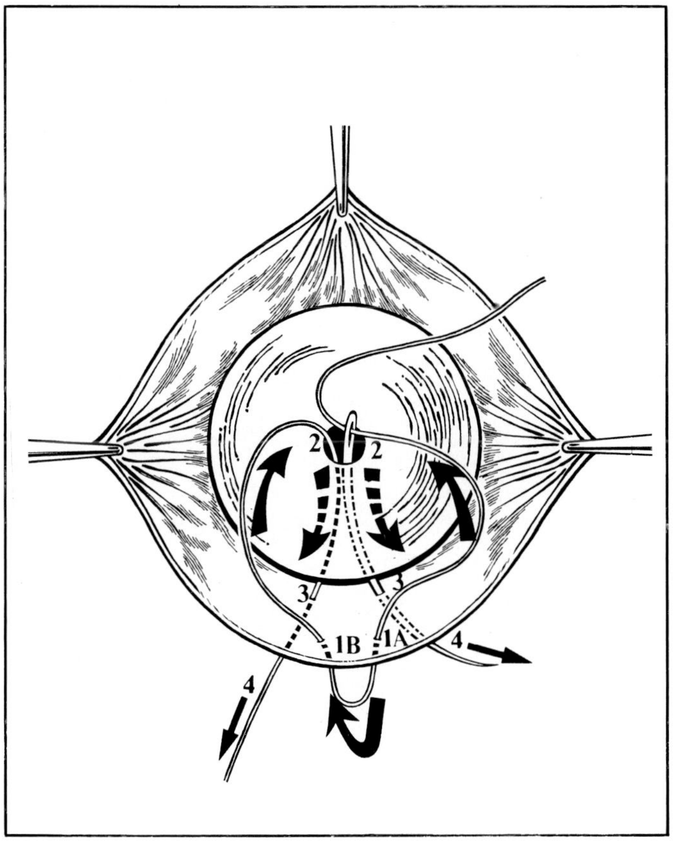

22B

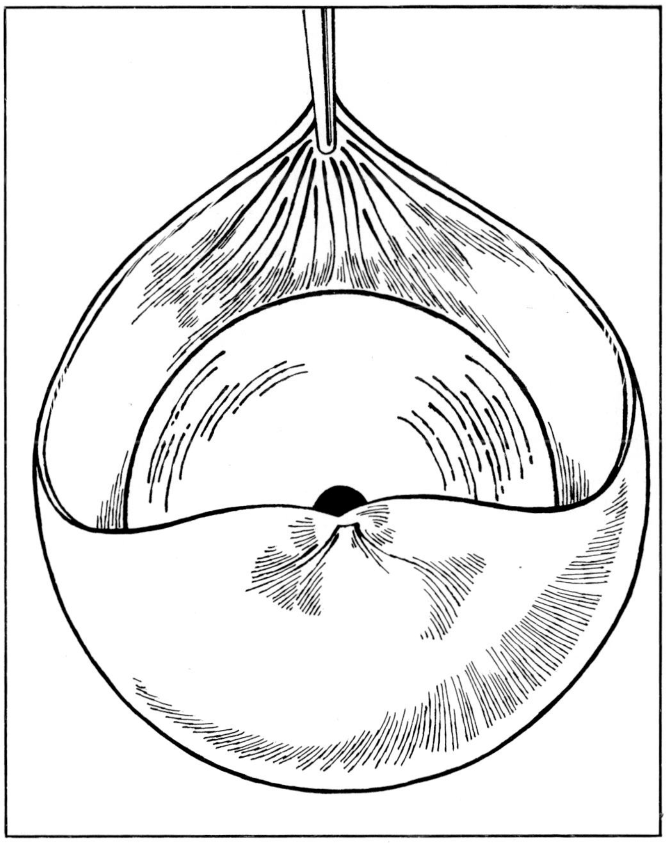

22A shows the route taken by each end of the suture after it has picked up the mid-point of the edge of the posterior skin flap. The stitch commences by traversing the skin edge at 1A and some surgeons prefer to throw a double hitch or tie a knot at this point. In any case this is the mid-point of the suture length and each half will be inserted separately on each side. One end is taken and inserted in the progression marked on the diagram 1–4: the other free end is then likewise inserted.

22B shows the effect when the stitch has been pulled up tight and tied off. Since the stitch embraces the major part of the cervical stump between its two halves or ends it has value as a haemostatic agent and there is no need to worry about vessels bleeding from the end of the stump while it is being inserted. The diagrams will also serve as reference charts where there is any doubt about the photographic illustrations.

23

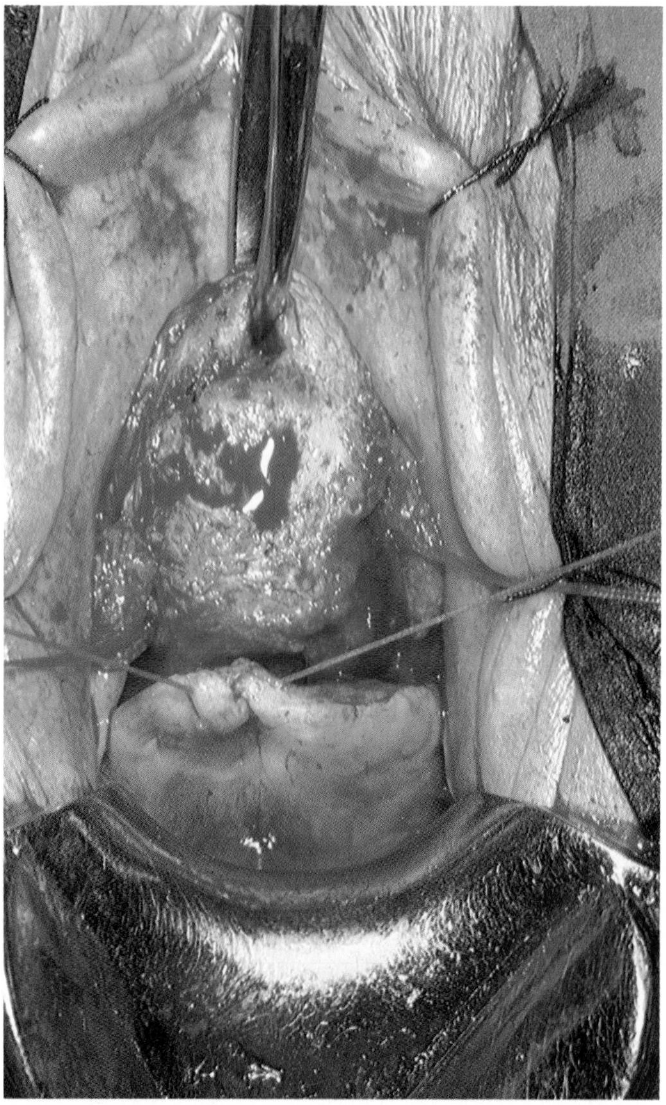

24

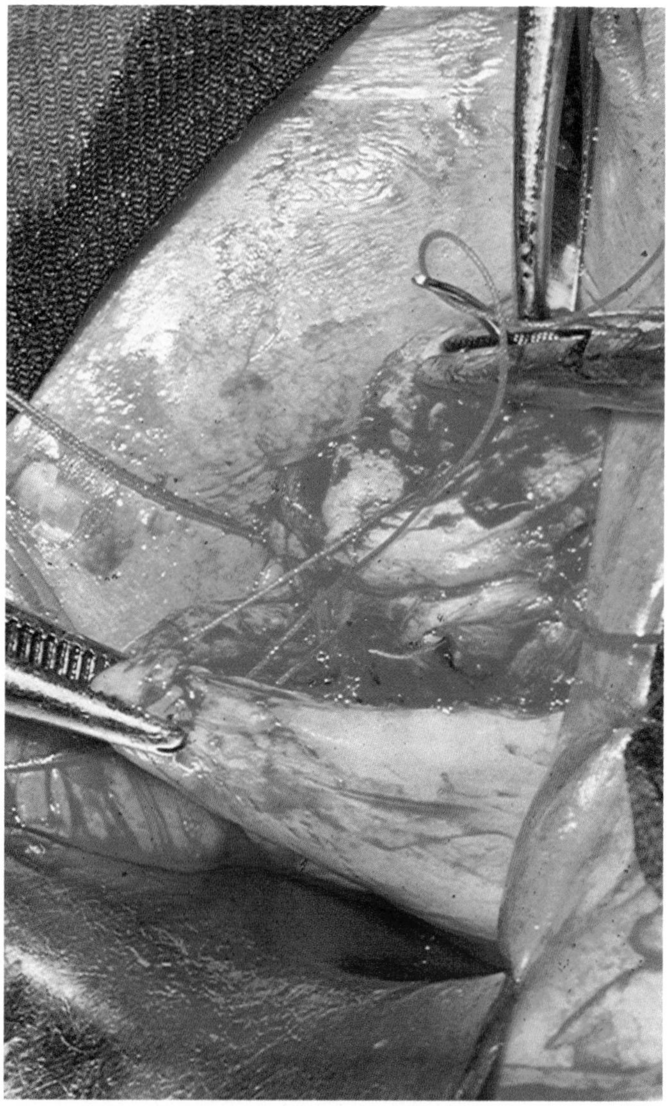

23 Sturmdorf suture (i)

The posterior skin flap is picked up at its mid-point as indicated by the skin scratch and a double loop hitch is inserted, leaving the ends of equal length. PGA No. 0 suture is used. There may be some bleeding from the cervical stump at this stage but it will soon be controlled by the stitches. This manoeuvre corresponds to 1A–1B in diagram **22A**.

24 Sturmdorf suture (ii)

The needle carrying the stitch on the patient's right side is introduced just inside the cervical canal and transfixes the posterior wall of the stump from within outwards. It enters the wall just at the lower edge of the canal but emerges higher up at a distance of 1.5 cm above the lower edge of the posterior surface. It is now ready to pierce the skin flap as that is lifted up to cover the raw area. Since this is the right side the stitch deviates to the right and comes through the cervical wall in the 7 o'clock position. The cervical stump is shown drawn to the left to facilitate this step. This corresponds to 2 and 3 in diagram **22A**.

25

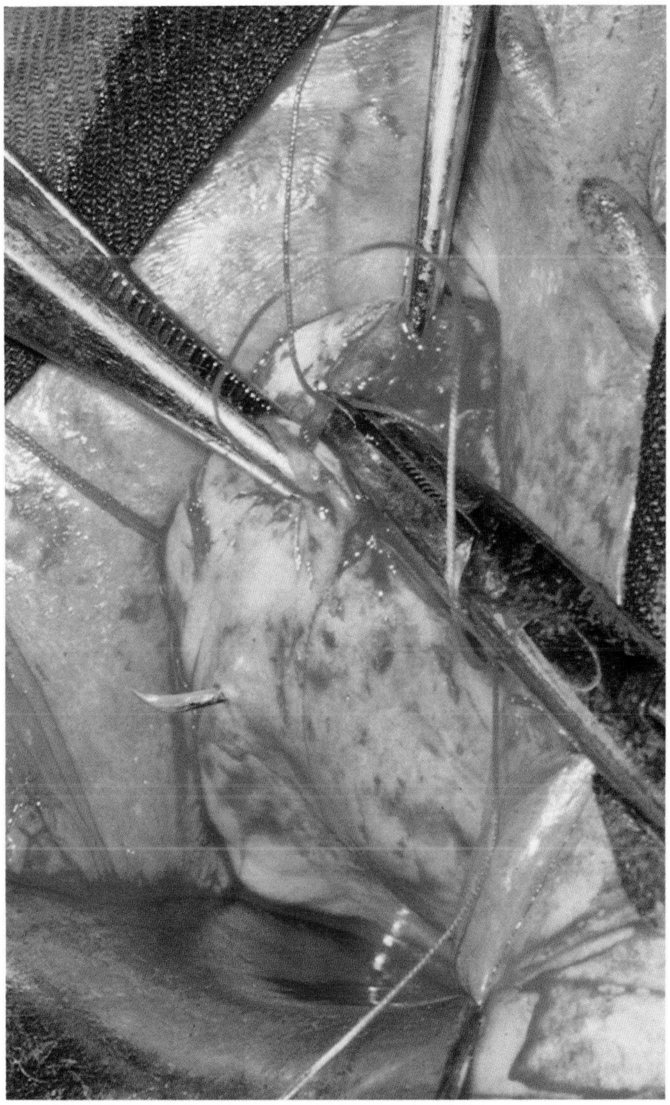

26A

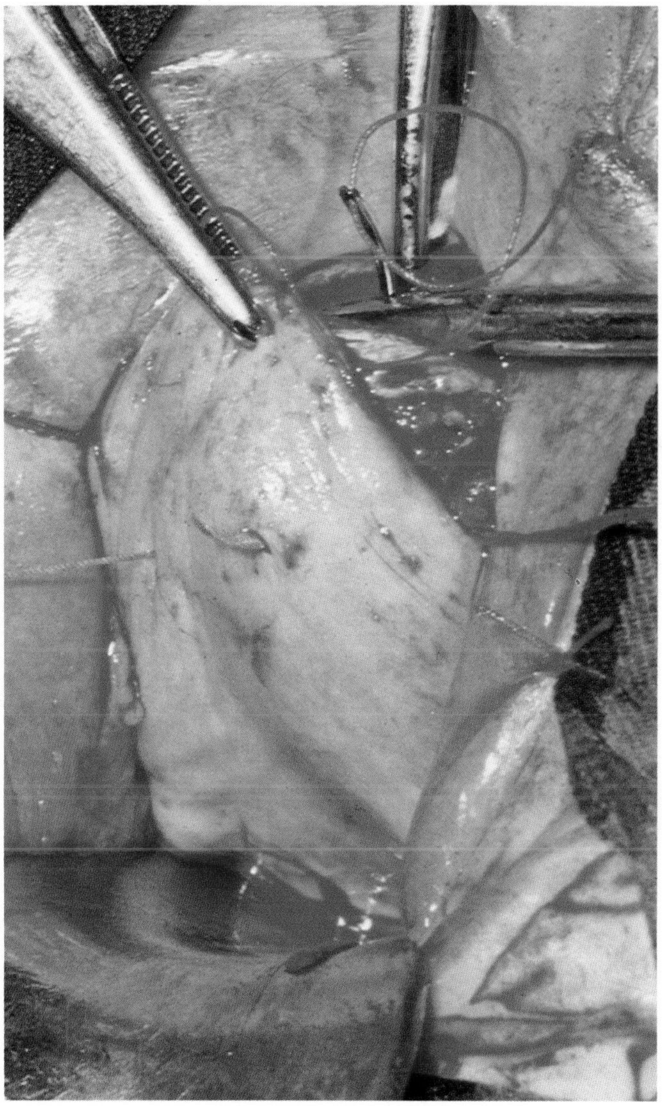

25 Sturmdorf suture (iii)

The needle emerges through the posterior skin flap on the right side at a distance of 2 cm from its edge and slightly to the right of the mid-line as indicated by the skin scratch. The skin flap is held up in position and the effect of the Sturmdorf stitch is becoming obvious. This corresponds to step 4 in diagram **22A**.

26A Sturmdorf suture (iv)

The needle emerges through the skin flap on the patient's left side in the 5 o'clock position, 2 cm from the skin edge. This corresponds to 3 and 4 in diagram **22A**.

26B

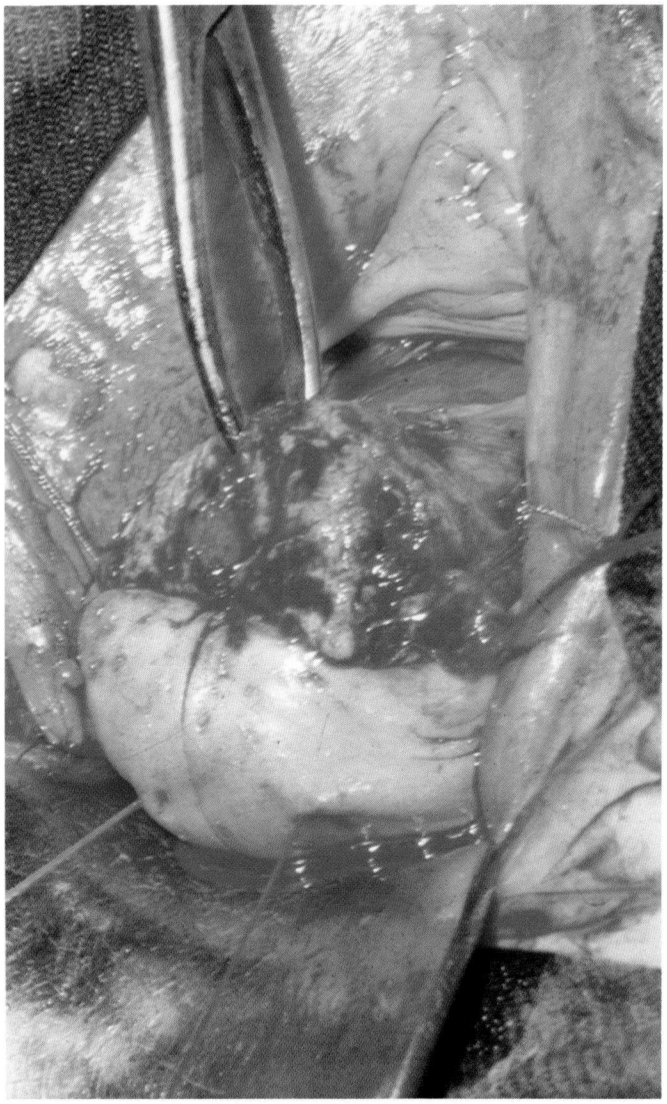

27

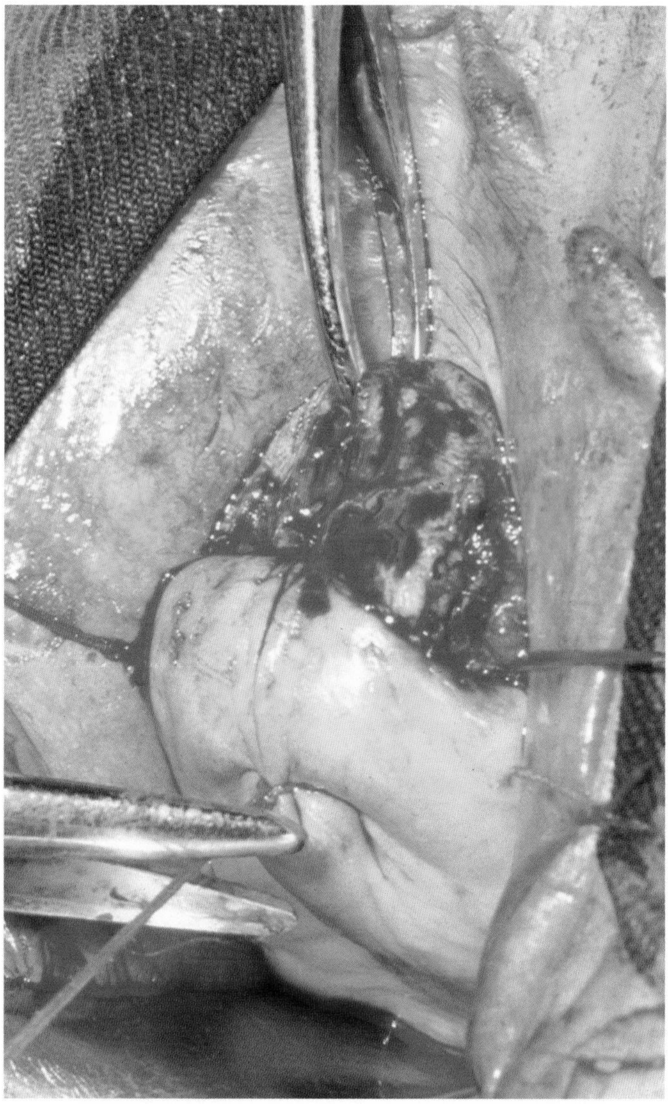

26B Sturmdorf suture (v)

Both ends of the Sturmdorf suture are in place and ready to be tied.

27 Sturmdorf suture (vi)

The stitch has now been tied and is being cut short. The whole posterior lip of the cervical stump has been re-invested with vaginal skin which is closely applied to the raw surface. This corresponds to diagram **22B**.

Stage 6: Lateral investing sutures

The lateral sutures are designed to cover the raw stump of the cervix on each side from the loose skin flap which has already been used postero-medially for the Sturmdorf stitch. The suture and the needle carrying it is so placed that it has the effect of rolling the edge of the skin flap inwards towards the cervical canal. These stitches also have haemostatic effect.

28

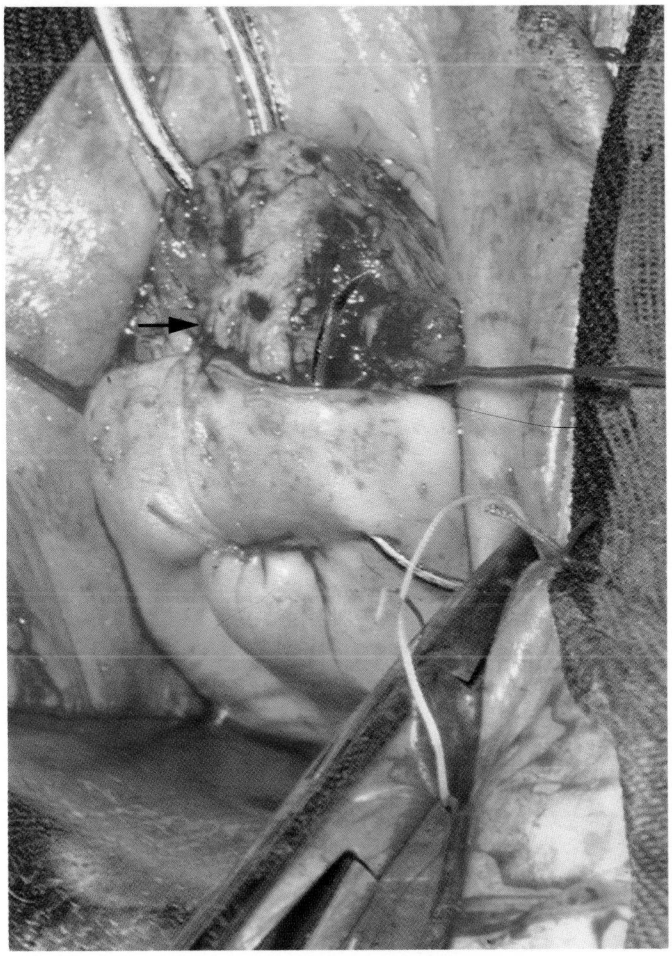

29

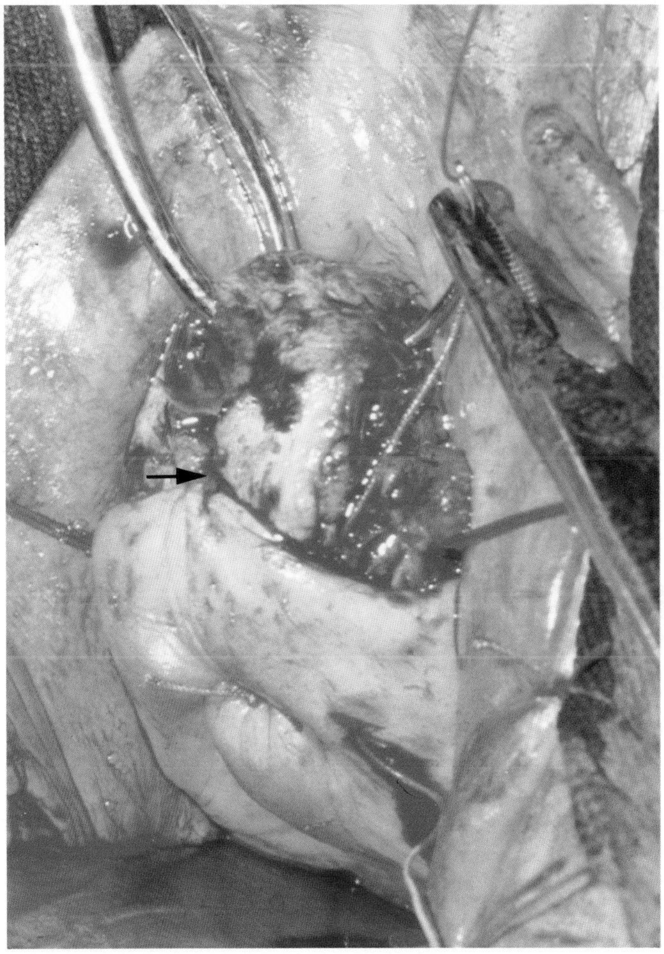

30

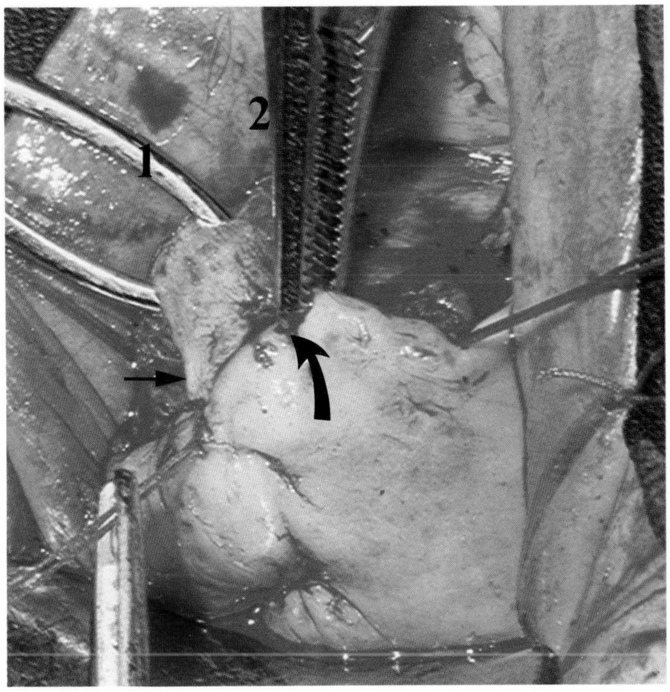

28 Lateral investing suture (left i)

The needle is shown traversing the skin flap at a distance of 1.5 cm from its edge in the direction of the canal and in the 4 o'clock position relative to the cervix. The cervical canal is indicated by an arrow here and in **29** and **30**.

29 Lateral investing suture (left ii)

The needle holder is reapplied and the cervical stump is transfixed from without inwards and aiming for the centre of the canal in the 2 o'clock position relative to the cervix.

30 Lateral investing suture (left iii)

The stitch is tied while the assistant holding the cervix by forceps (1) rolls and encourages the skin flap medially with forceps (2) to cover the raw area. As the stitch is tied it fixes the skin in that position and the completed suture lies horizontally in the 3 o'clock position. The curved arrow indicates the direction in which the skin edge is encouraged medially.

31A

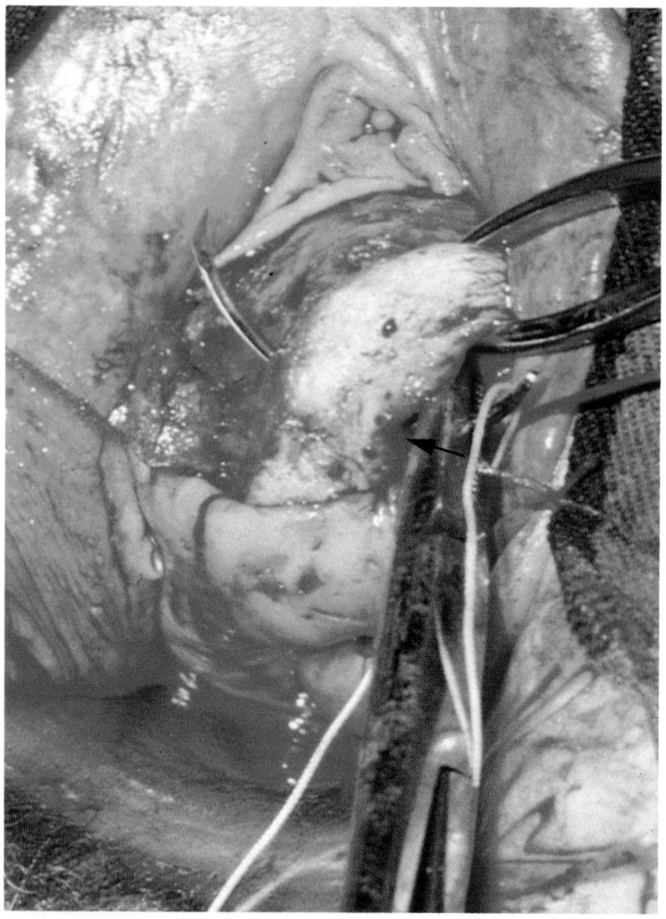

31B

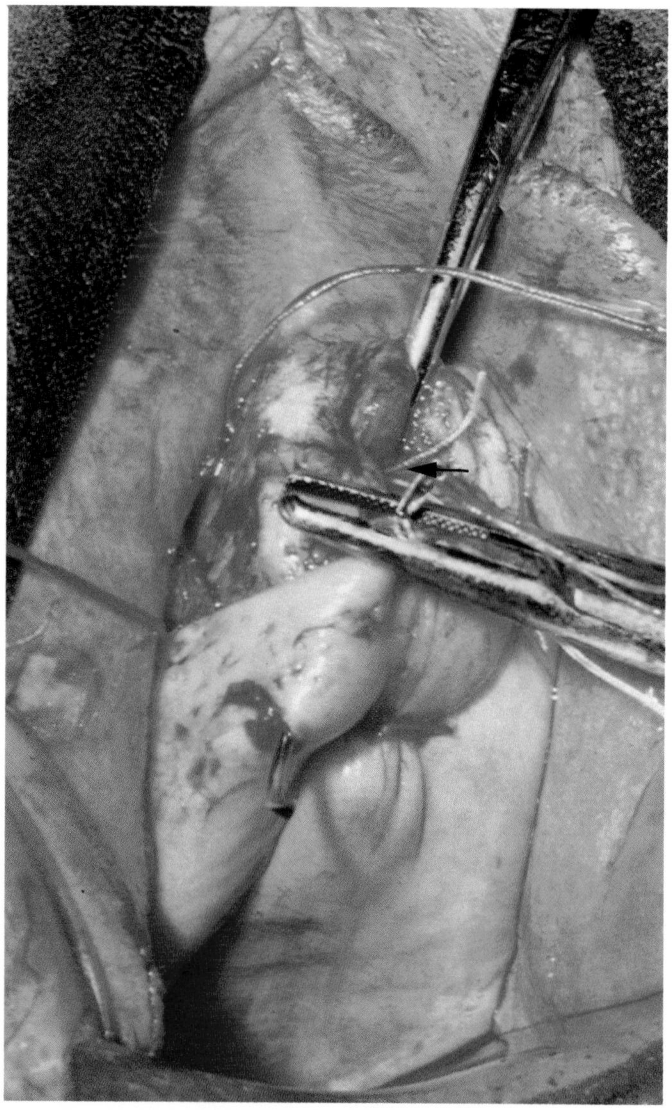

31C

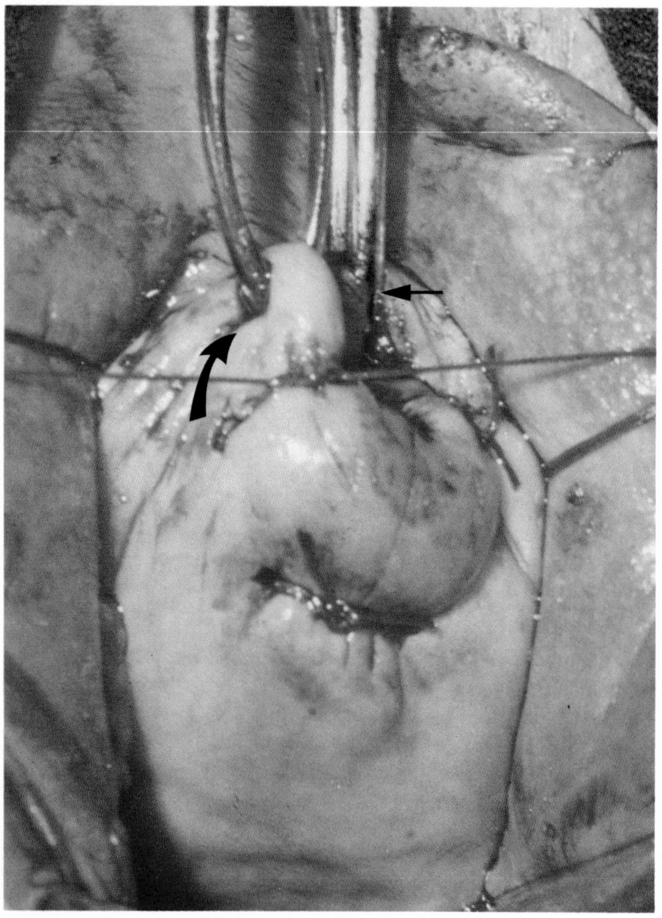

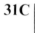

31A–31C Lateral investing suture (right)

The three illustrations repeat the manoeuvre shown on the left side, but in this case and to suit the surgeon's hand, it is carried out in reverse order. In **31A** the needle goes through the cervix from within outwards at 10 o'clock; in **31B** it pierces the skin edge at 8 o'clock; and the resultant completed suture shown in **31C** falls in the 9 o'clock position. The arrows indicate the cervical canal and the curved arrow in **31C** shows the direction in which to advance the skin edge.

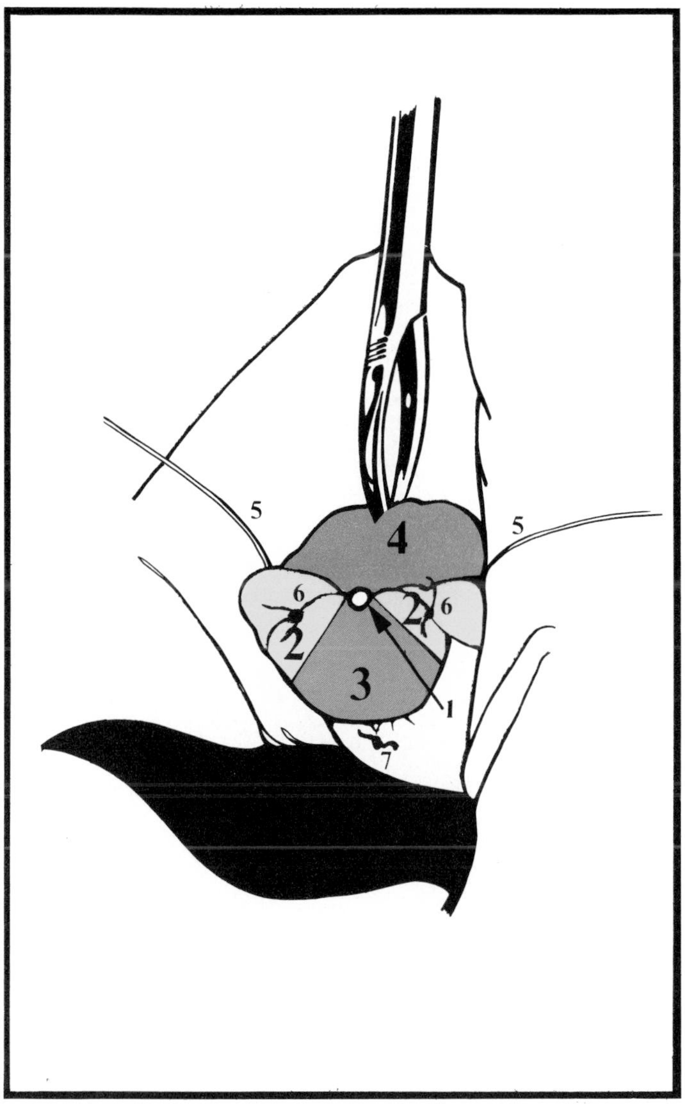

1 Cervical canal
2 Area covered by lateral sutures
3 Area covered by Sturmdorf suture
4 Area to be covered by Crown suture
5 Sutures on cardinal ligaments
6 Lateral sutures (tied)
7 Sturmdorf suture (tied)

32

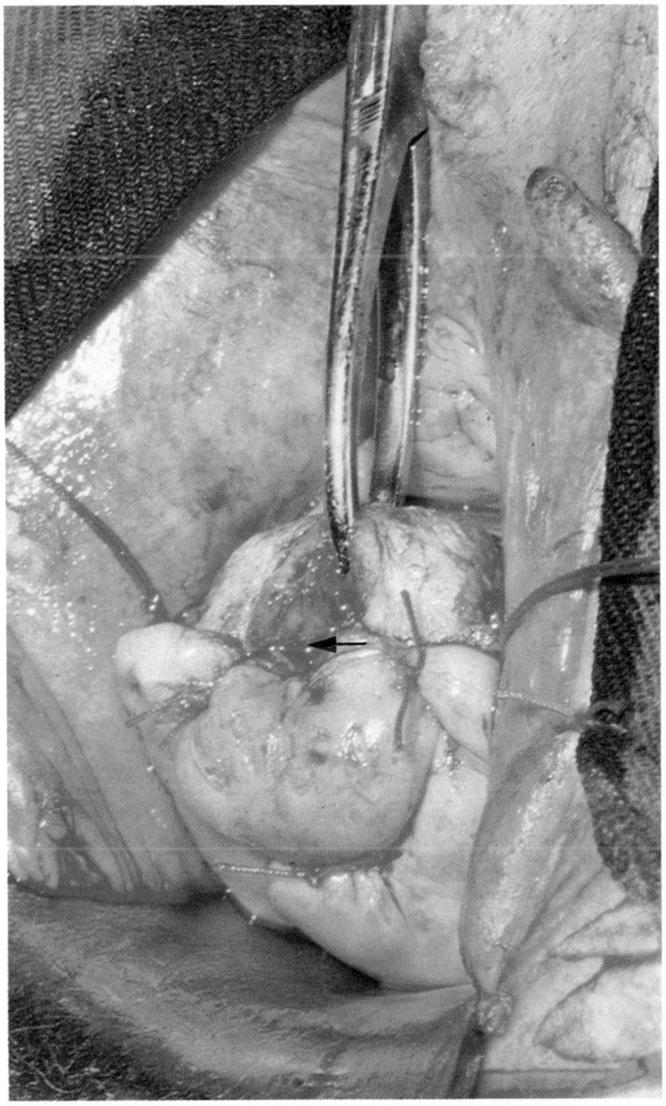

32 Posterior and lateral investment completed

The Sturmdorf and lateral sutures are shown in place and cut short. The anterior lip is ready to be covered by the crown suture.

Stage 7: Crown suture

33A

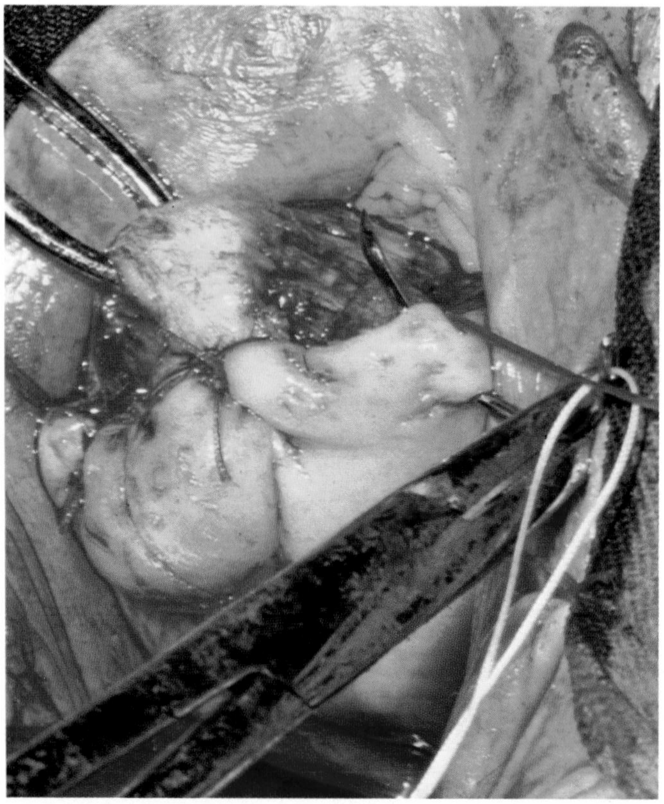

33B

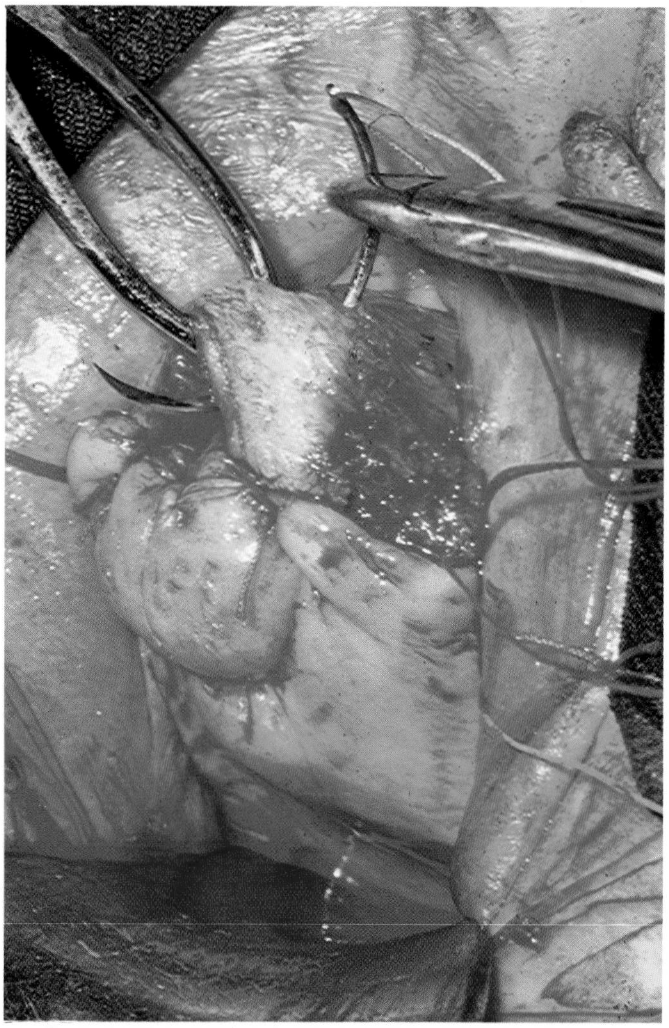

33C

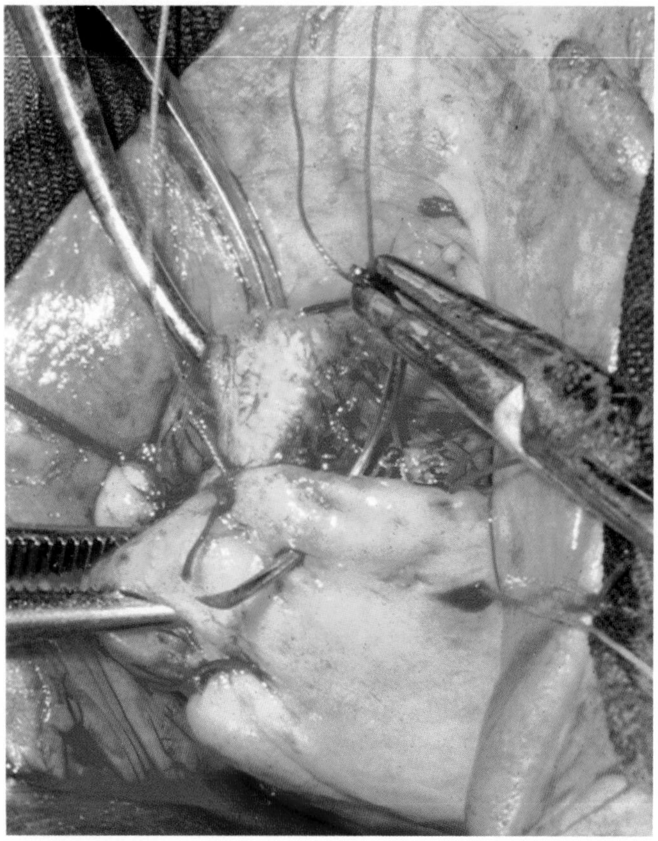

The purpose of the stitch is to approximate the free skin edges in the mid-line over the cervical stump in such a way as to invest the remainder of the raw surface with skin. There are various ways of doing this, generally by a figure of eight or X stitch across the mid-line which traverses the anterior wall of the cervix in each direction. These are all satisfactory enough but the method described is preferred because it gives a neater appearance and avoids scarring by investing the cervix completely and closely with vaginal skin.

33A–33C Crown suture (i)

In **33A** the needle traverses the skin flap from without inwards, 2 cm from the lateral cervical stitch and 1 cm from the skin edge.

In **33B** the needle has been reapplied and transfixes the full thickness of the anterior wall of the cervical canal in the mid-line from above downwards. Its course is 1 cm from the lower edge and the needle emerges in the cervical canal.

In **33C** the needle picks up the left skin flap from within outwards at a distance of 1 cm from the previous point or halfway between it and the left lateral cervical stitch.

34A

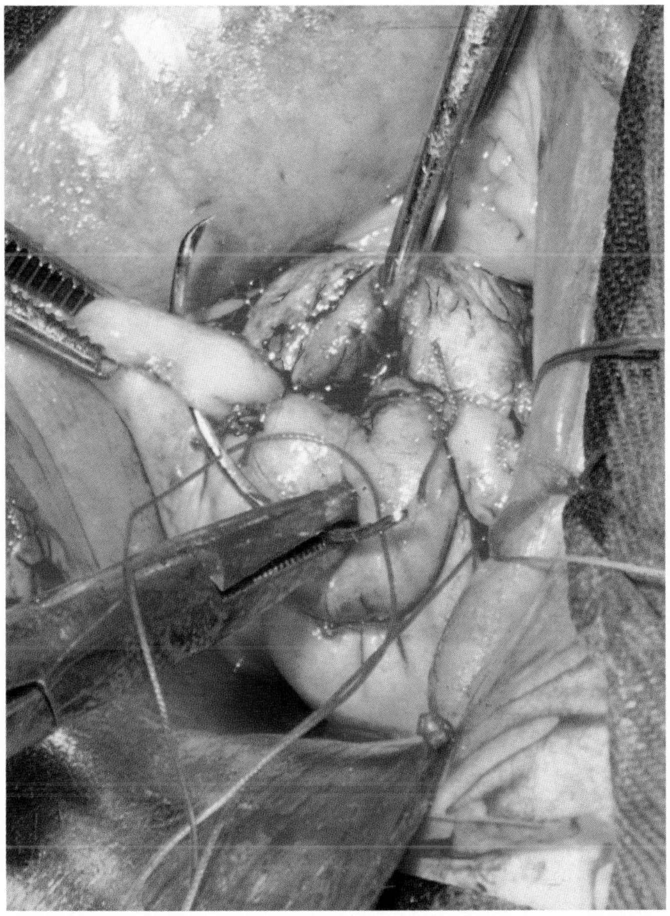

34B

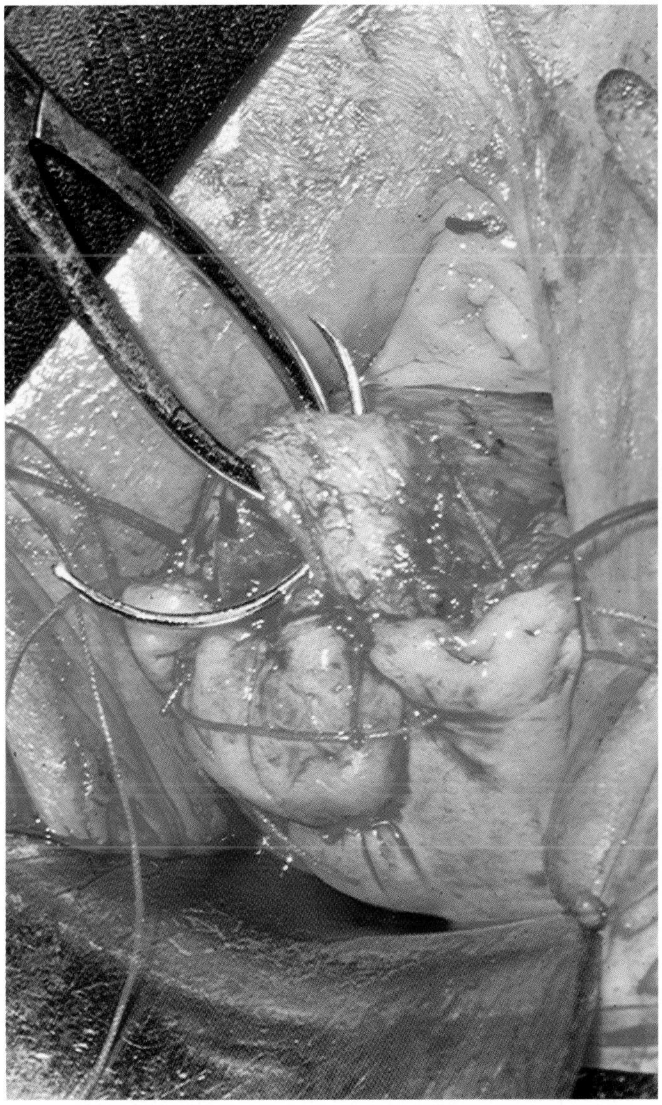

34C

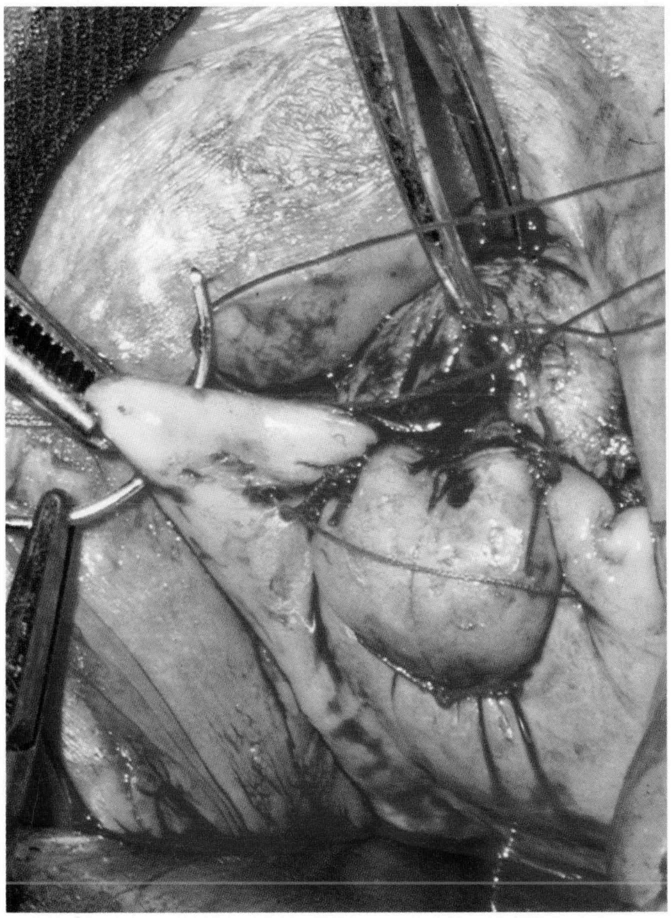

34A–34C Crown suture (ii)

Figure **34A** shows the needle holder reapplied. The suture is taken to the opposite side where it traverses the right skin flap from without inwards at a distance of 1 cm from the right lateral cervical stitch and 1 cm from the free skin edge. Forceps still hold the anterior lip of the cervix at its mid-point.

In **34B** the needle returns to the anterior wall of the cervix which it traverses exactly as before but in the opposite direction i.e. from below upwards. It enters the cervical canal and emerges on the front of the cervix 1 cm from its edge in the mid-line. It therefore lies alongside the suture previously inserted from above downwards.

Figure **34C** shows the needle emerging from within outwards 1 cm from the free edge of the skin flap on the right side and 1 cm above the previous point of entry on that side.

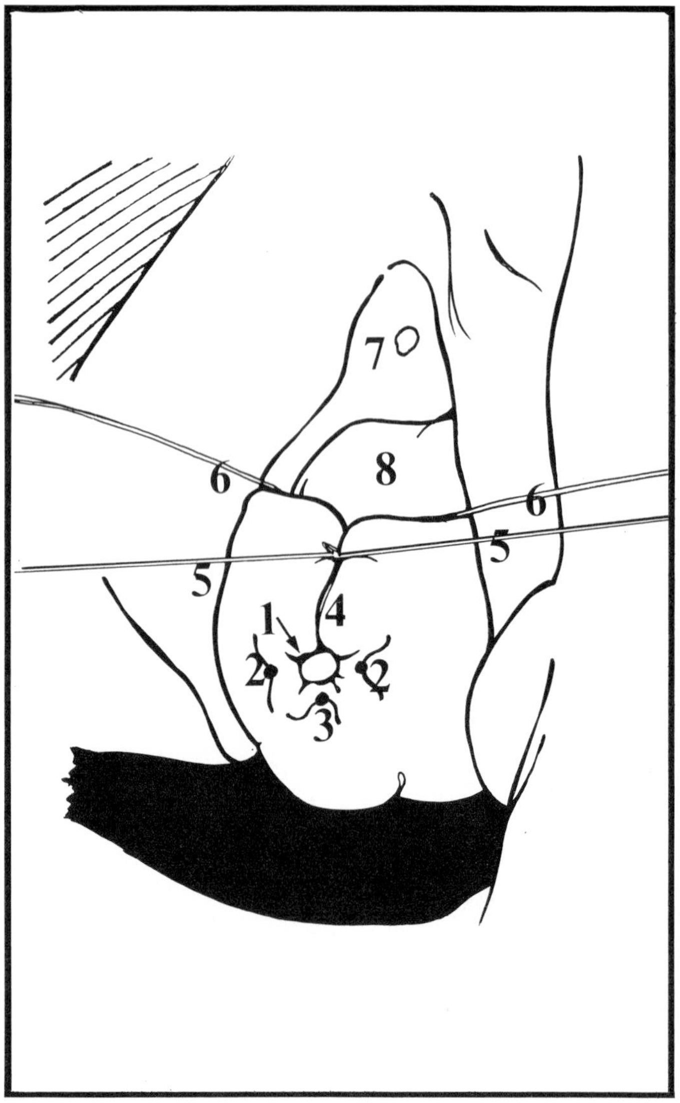

1 Cervical canal
2 Lateral cervical sutures
3 Sturmdorf suture
4 Approximated skin edges
5 Crown sutures drawn tight
6 Cardinal ligament sutures
7 Urethral orifice
8 Anterior surface of uterus

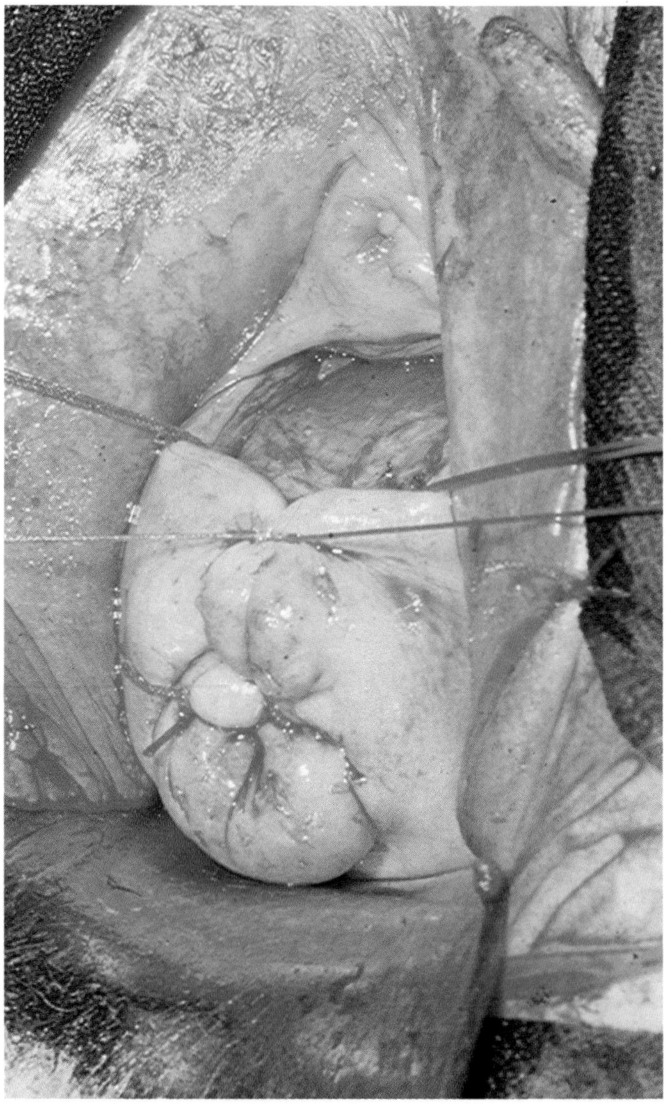

35

35 Crown suture (iii)

The two ends of the stitch are drawn tight and a neat covering of the cervix is shown. The crown suture is not tied at this stage so as not to interfere with the placing of the important Fothergill suture.

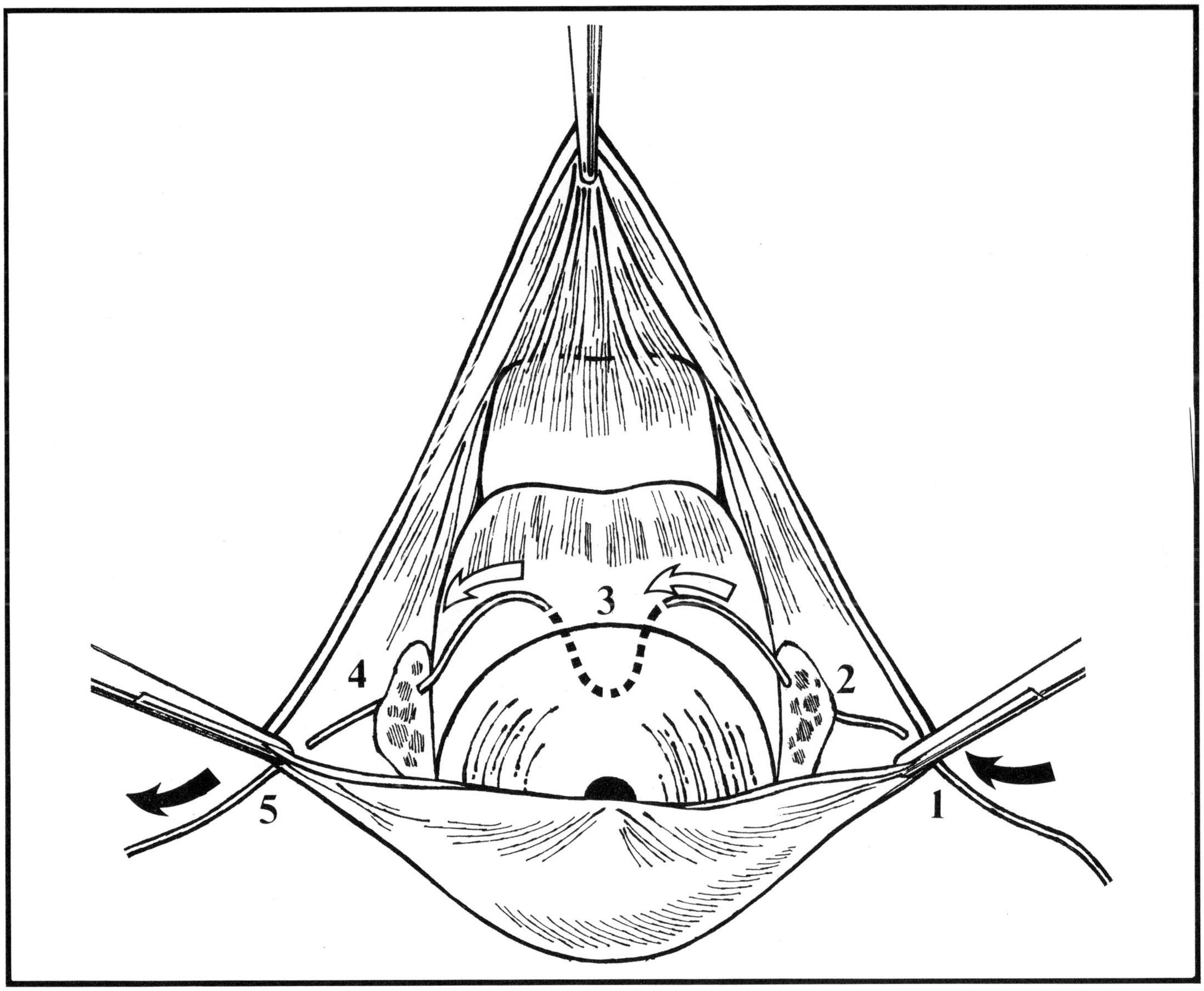

36

Stage 8: The Fothergill suture

Insertion of the Fothergill stitch is the most important step in the operation because success depends on accurate application of the cardinal ligaments to the anterior aspect of the cervical stump or lower uterus. It will create the main support of the new vaginal vault. Diagram **36** indicates the course taken by the suture carrying needle and will serve as a reference when studying the progression of photographic illustrations.

1 Transfixion of left skin flap (illustration **37**)
2 Transfixion of left cardinal ligament (illustration **38**)
3 Transfixion of lower uterine wall (illustration **39**)
4 Transfixion of right cardinal ligament (illustration **40**)
5 Transfixion of right skin flap (illustration **41**)

37

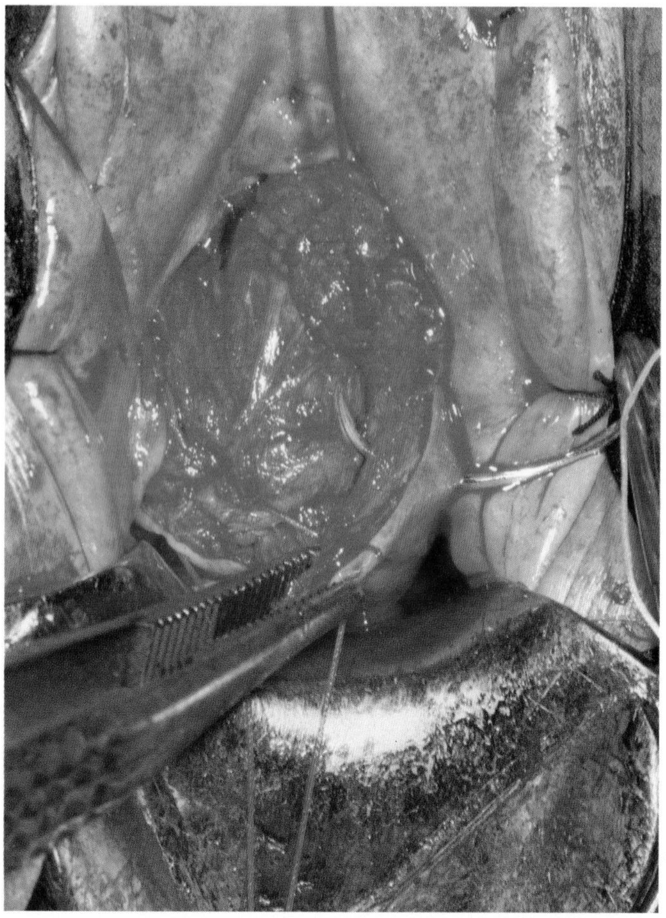

38

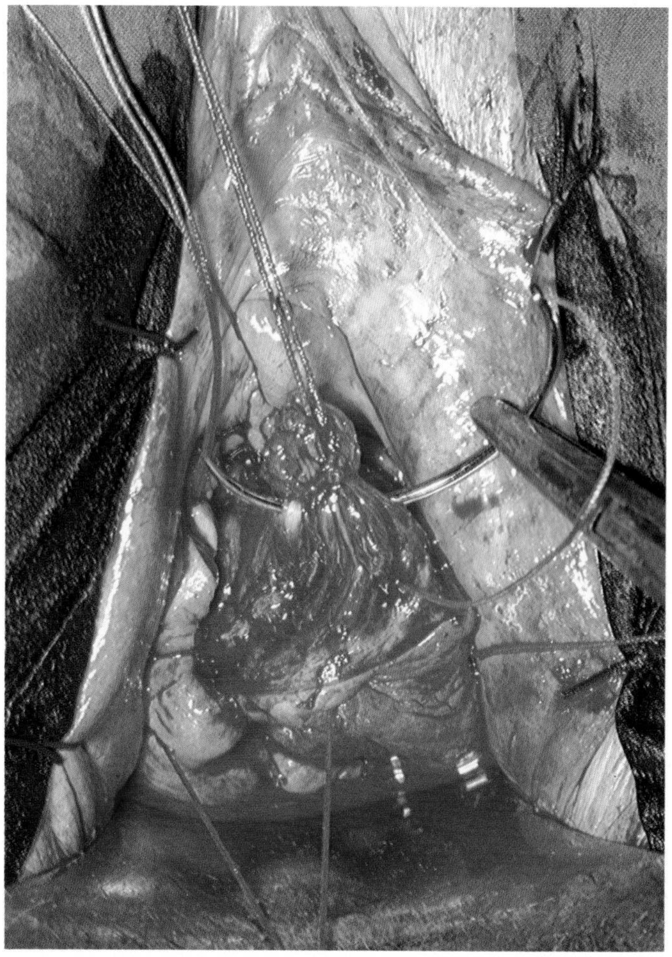

39

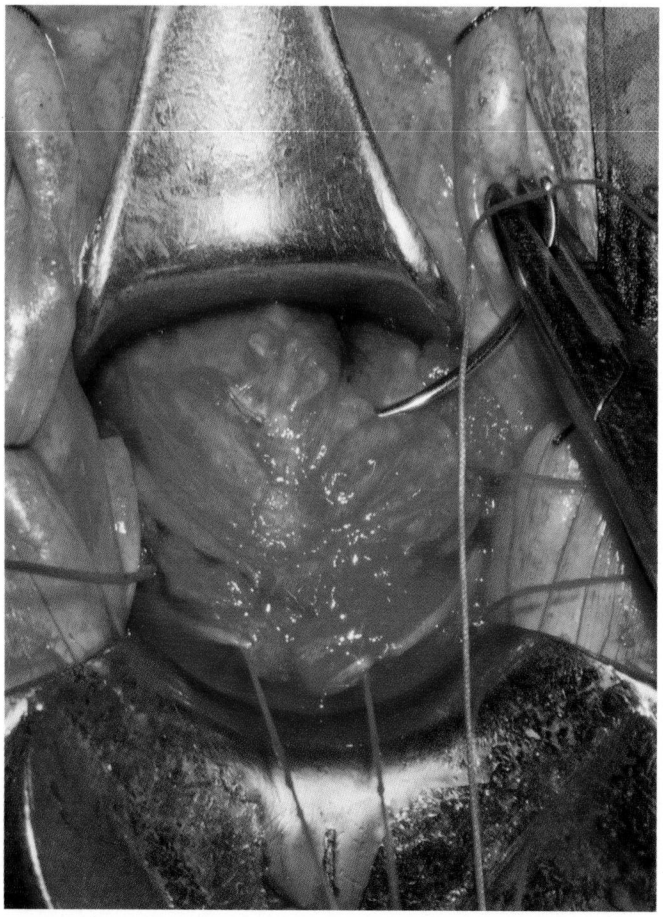

37 Insertion of Fothergill suture (i)

The needle first picks up the skin flap from without inwards on the patient's left side at a distance of 2 cm from the medial edge and 1.5 cm above the crown suture. The point is seen emerging from under the flap. PGA No. 1 suture on a round-bodied needle is used.

38 Insertion of Fothergill suture (ii)

The needle passes through the left cardinal ligament just proximal to its ligature, the long ends of which support it while it is being transfixed.

39 Insertion of Fothergill suture (iii)

The next step is to take a firm bite of the anterior aspect of the lower uterine wall in the mid-line – the illustration shows the depth of the needle track. It is not necessary or desirable to go through the anterior wall of the cervix into the canal and come back again. The bladder is retracted upwards out of the way and the lower border of the utero-vesical pouch is just visible.

40
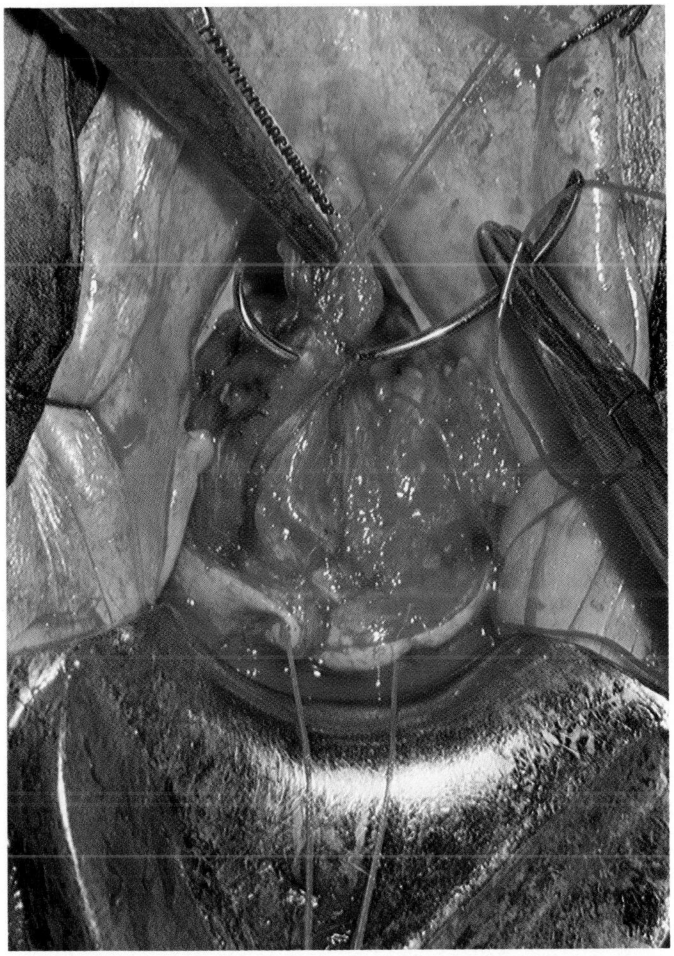

41
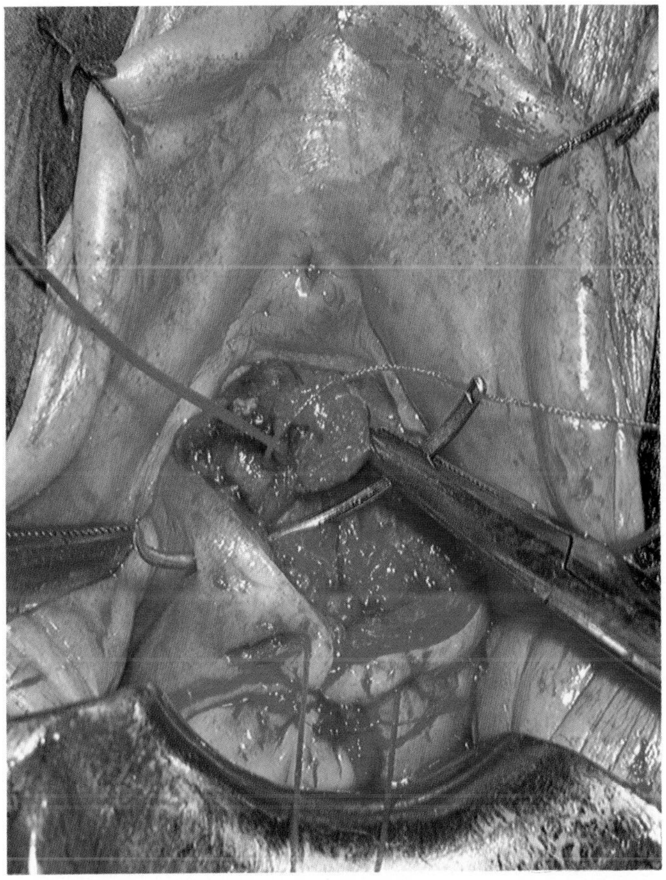

42
 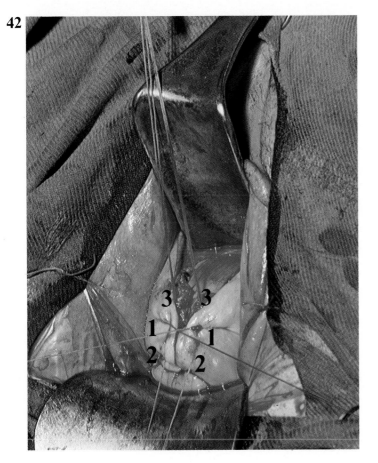

40 Insertion of Fothergill suture (iv)

The right cardinal ligament or pedicle is transfixed exactly as on the other side.

41 Insertion of Fothergill suture (v)

The stitch emerges through the right skin flap 2 cm from the medial edge and 1.5 cm above the crown suture. The Fothergill suture is now in place and ready to be tied.

42 Insertion of Fothergill suture (vi)

With the ends of the suture crossed and held taut the principle of the stitch is demonstrated. The cardinal ligaments are brought into apposition with each other and fixed to the anterior surface of the uterus. They are firmly secured in that position and at the same time covered by the skin edges as the stitch is drawn tight. The anterior vault of the vagina ascends as the cardinal ligaments are tightened in their new position and retroversion of the uterus which usually accompanies prolapse is corrected. The numbers 1 indicate the untied Fothergill suture, 2 indicates the untied crown suture, and numbers 3 indicate the holding sutures on the cardinal ligaments.

43

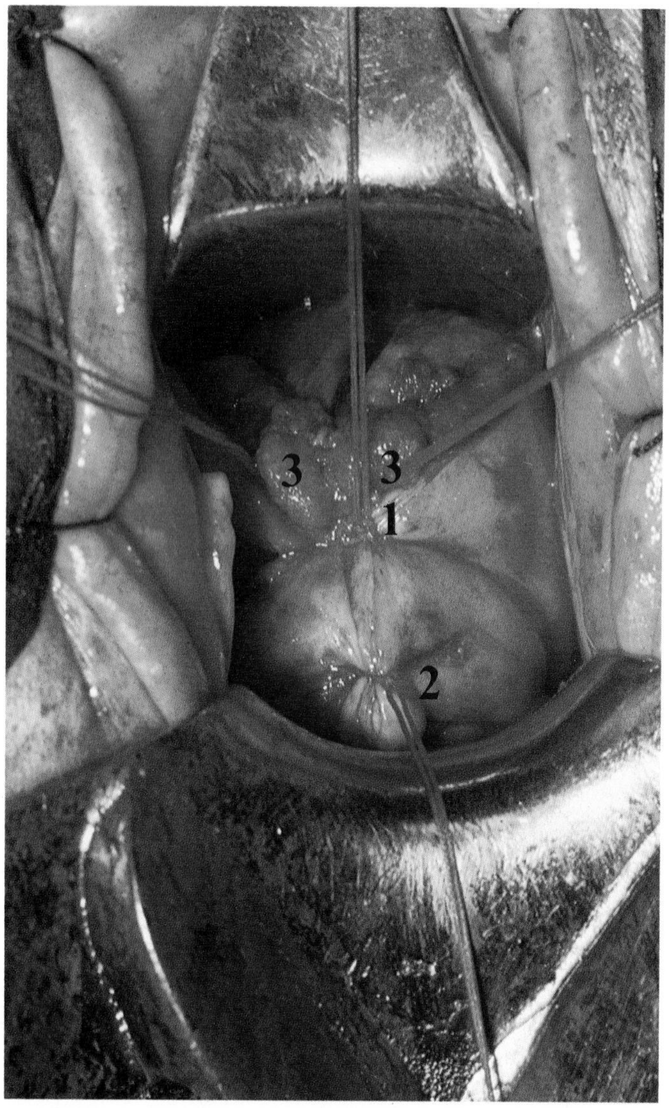

44

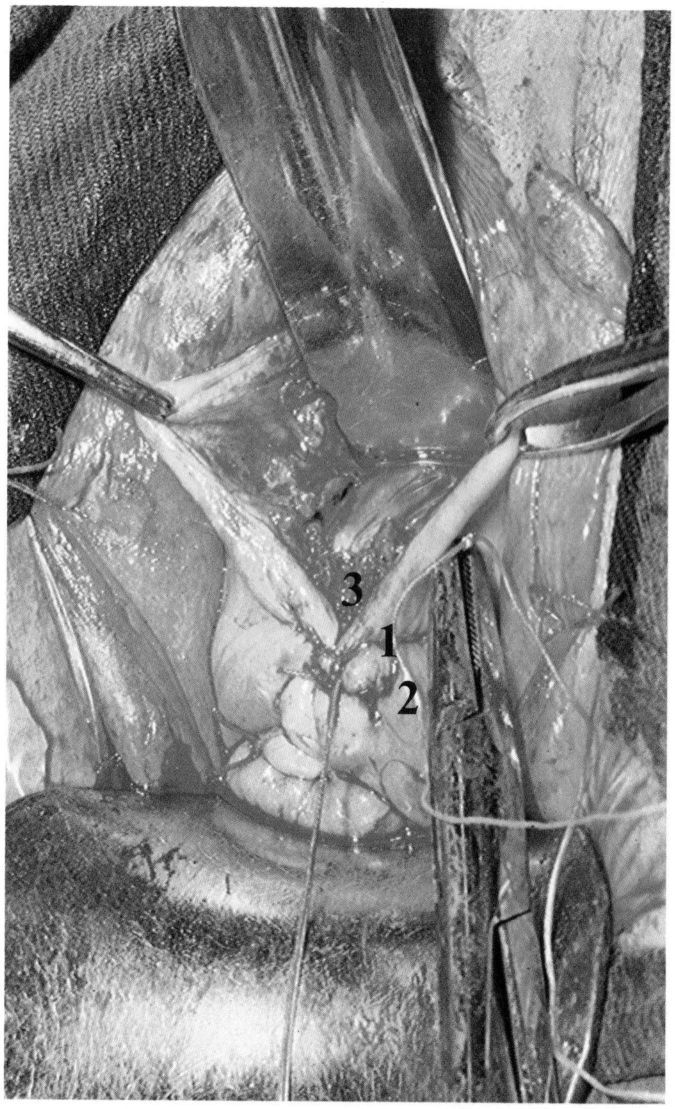

43 Insertion of Fothergill suture (vii)

The Fothergill suture has been tied (1) as has the crown suture (2). The cardinal ligament pedicles still retain their long ligatures (3).

44 Reinforcing Fothergill suture

We recommend the insertion of a second or reinforcing Fothergill stitch. This is placed in exactly the same way as the main stitch and at a distance of 1 cm above it. The same structures are traversed by the needle in the same order but the cardinal ligaments are picked up distal to the ligatures and no great amount of anterior uterine wall is included. The stitch eliminates dead space, fixes the cardinal ligaments snugly on to the front of the uterus and safeguards the main suture while the anterior vaginal wall is repaired. The bladder is protected by the retractor which exposes the anterior aspect of the uterus. The needle tip is seen emerging at the completion of its course. The numbers here relate to the same structures as those numbered in illustration **43**.

Stage 9: Anterior vaginal wall repair

As explained in the introduction to this volume the anterior vaginal wall repair is an essential part of the operation and is directed towards correcting cystocele and urethrocele. The technique illustrated and described is applicable in all other circumstances where such a repair is indicated.

The principles of the operation are first to separate the skin layer from the underlying pubocervical fascia in the whole length of the incision on both sides. Secondly, the edges of the pubocervical fascia thus defined are stitched together in the mid-line to support the bladder base and urethra from the urethral meatus to the anterior aspect of the uterus or the vaginal vault. The skin layer is subsequently approximated by a series of inverted mattress sutures to further support the lower urinary tract and eliminate cysto-urethrocele.

45

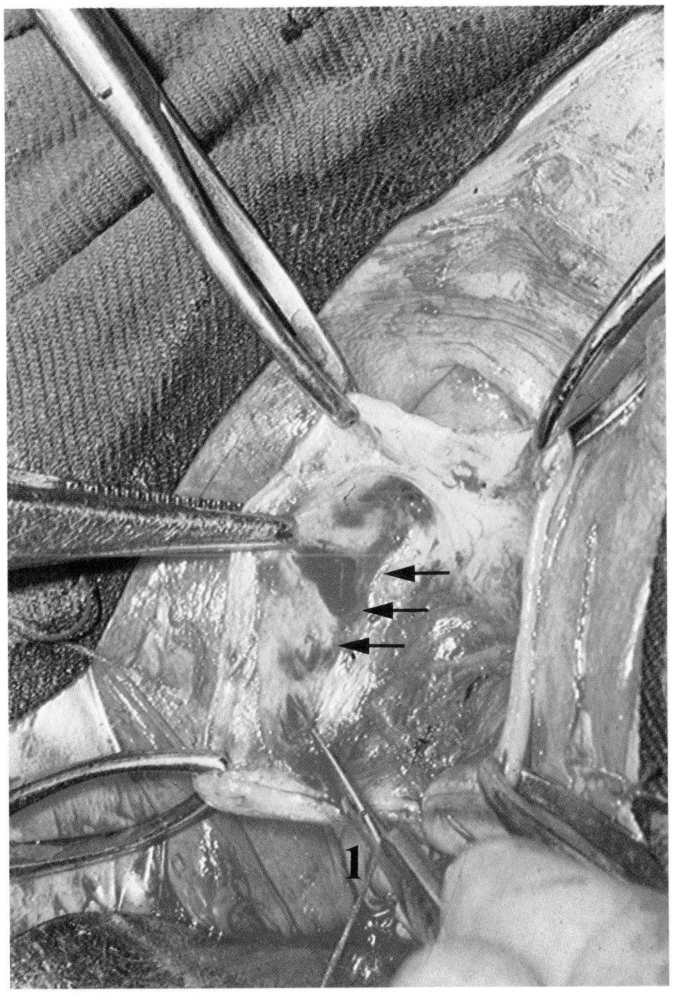

46

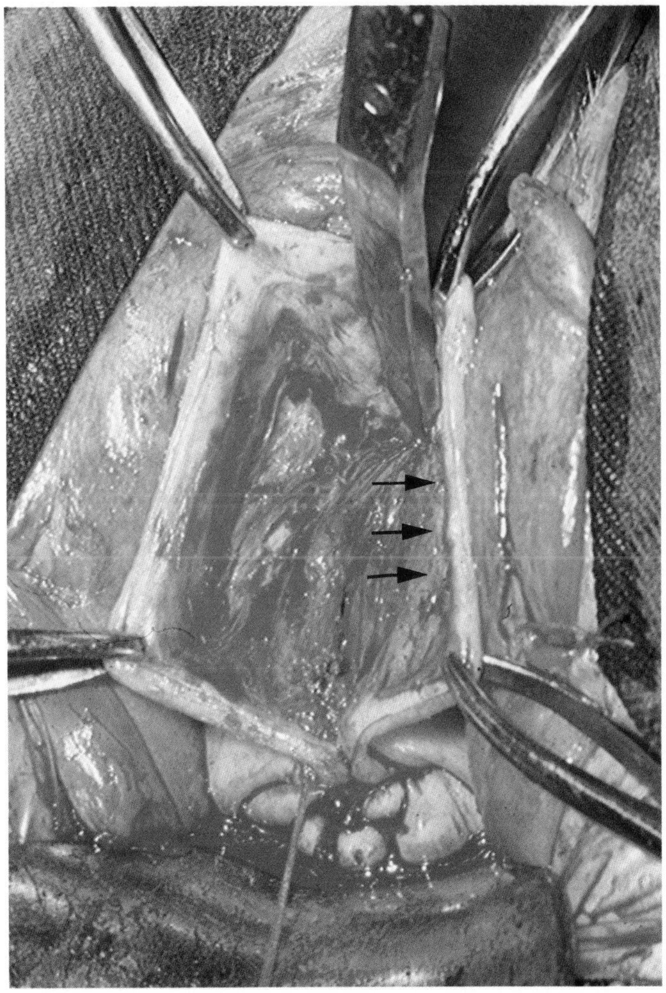

45 Definition of pubocervical fascia (right)

With the skin edges held in Littlewood's forceps (four in number) the surgeon finds, by sharp dissection, the plane between the skin and pubocervical fascia on the right side. This is achieved by starting separation of the two layers with a small-bladed scalpel in the lower vagina near the urethral meatus and working laterally until the plane of cleavage is encountered. This part of the operation should be done gently and slowly taking care not to buttonhole the skin by being too superficial or opening the venous sinuses by being too deep. In the illustration the fascia is seen falling medially as the plane is opened up and any further separation can be made by blunt dissection. It is carried back along the full length of the incision. Note the long suture (1) of the reinforcing Fothergill stitch at the vault. The arrows indicate the edge of the pubocervical fascia.

46 Definition of pubocervical fascia (left)

The same procedure has been carried out on the left side and the closed scissors are being used as blunt dissectors. The edges of the pubocervical fascial layer are clearly indicated by arrows.

47

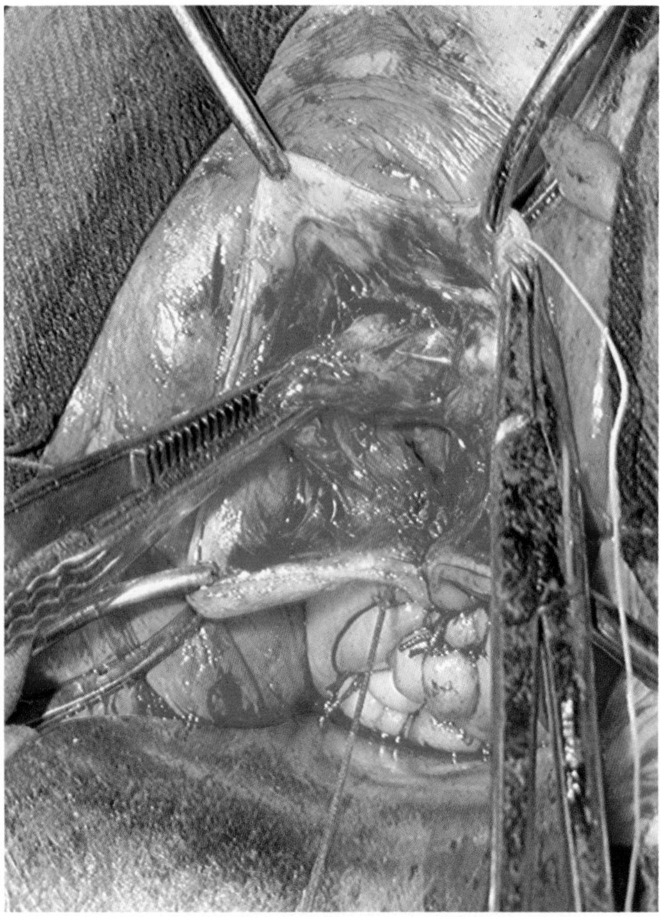

48A

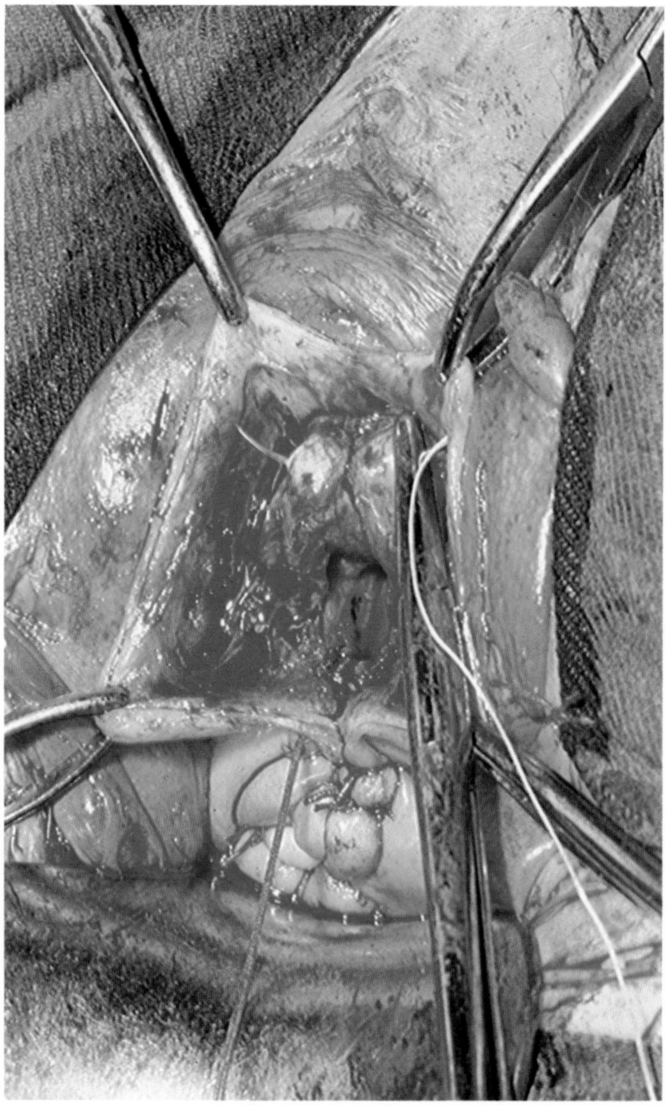

48B

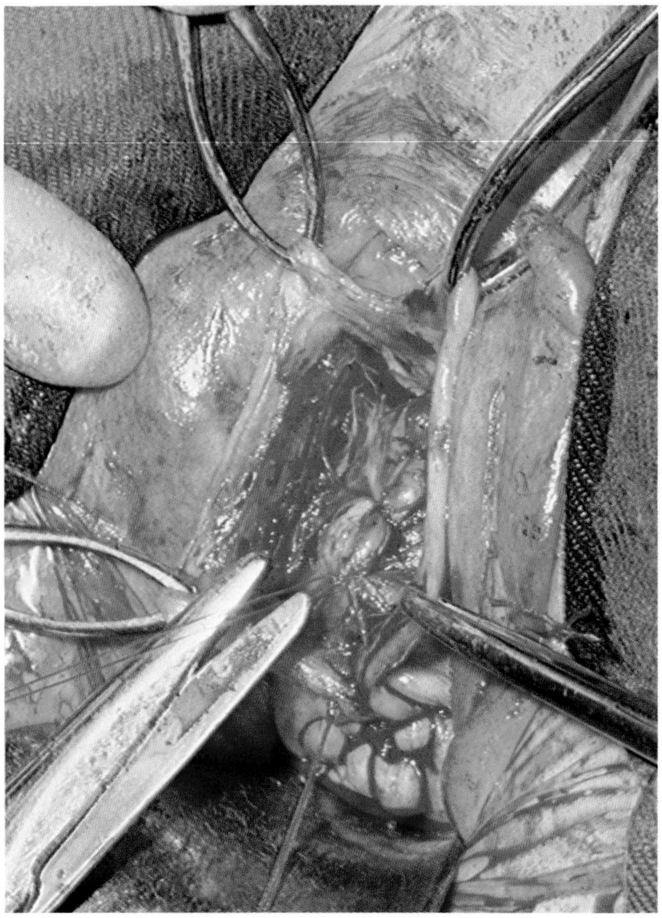

47 Suture of pubocervical fascia (i)

The edges of the pubocervical fascial layers are approximated in the mid-line by PGA No. 00 suture carried on an atraumatic needle. The stitches are at a distance of 1 cm from each other and may be continuous or interrupted. They pick up a good bulk of tissue as shown in the photograph. The left edge has been transfixed by the needle and the right edge is held in the dissecting forceps.

48A and 48B Suture of pubocervical fascia (ii)

Further stages in the repair of the fascial layer are shown. In **48A** the first stitch is in place and ready to be tied. In **48B** the final stitch is being cut short. The suture line is both reparative and haemostatic and creates a firm layer of pubocervical fascia under the urethra and bladder.

49
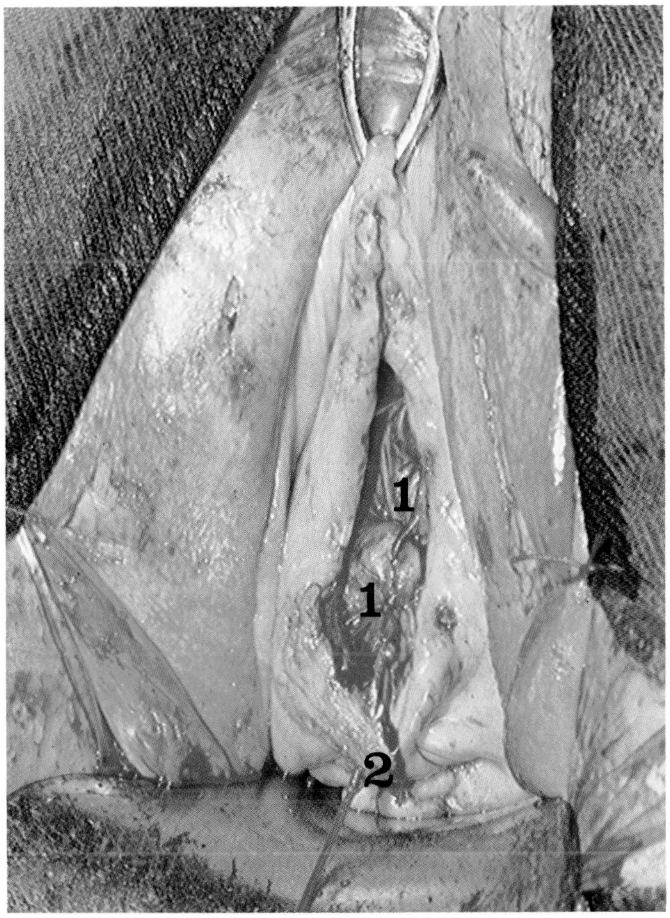

50
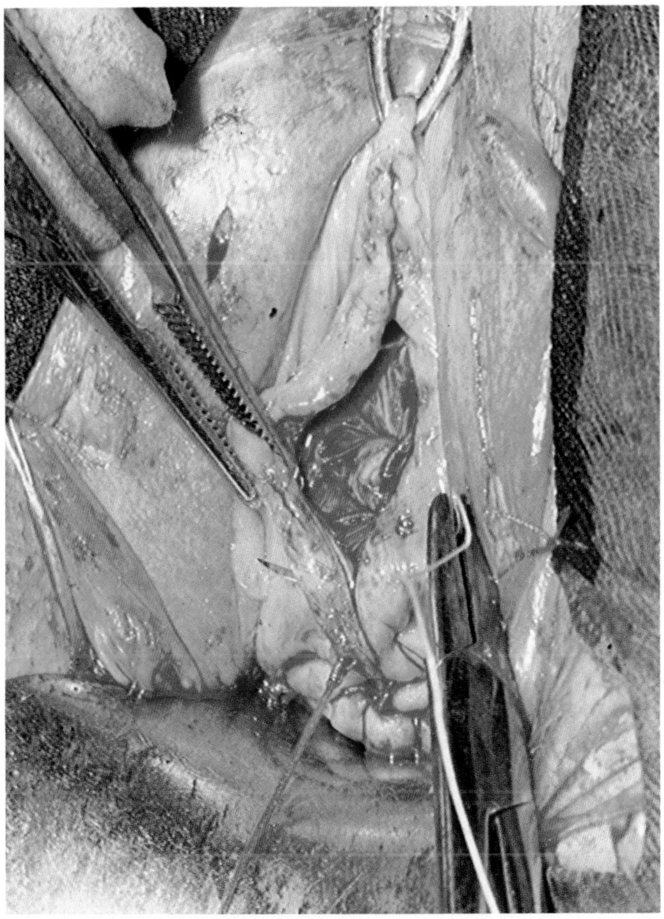

49 Anterior vaginal wall closure (i)

The skin edges are ready for suture and the repaired pubocervical fascia can be seen in the wound. Note that there is no excess or shortage of skin and this can be expected when a triangle is excised as described.

1 The repaired pubocervical fascia
2 The reinforcing Fothergill stitch

50 Anterior vaginal wall closure (ii)

Closure commences above by a series of interrupted PGA No. 0 sutures on an atraumatic needle. The first stitch is being inserted.

51 Anterior vaginal wall closure (iii)

Inverted mattress sutures are used routinely and placed at a distance of 1 cm from each other. The mattress effect brings a raw skin area of 0.5–1 cm wide from each side into apposition and ensures a firm suture line which will not stretch. A neat result is obtained and subcutaneous haematomata are avoided.

51
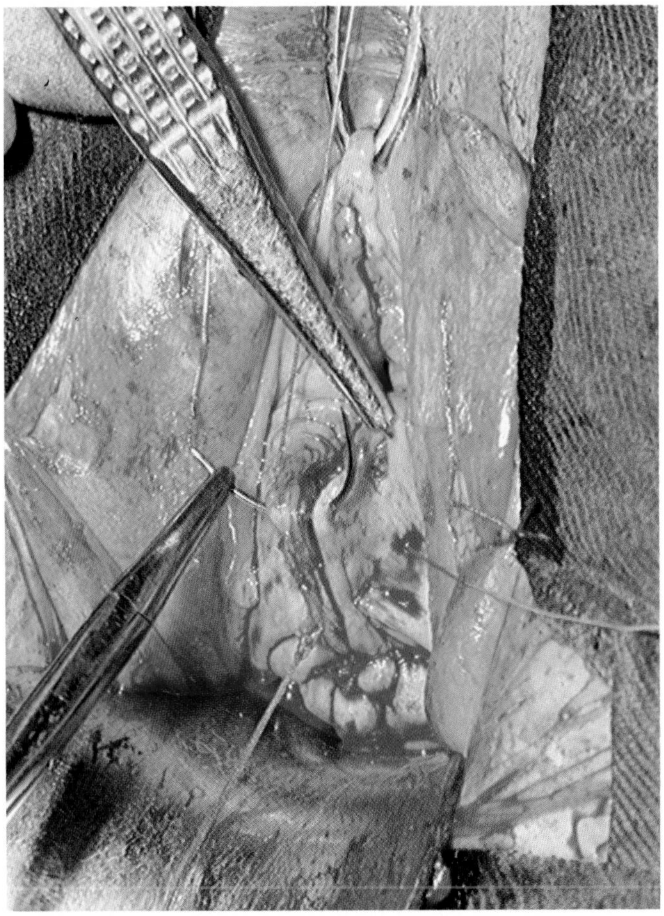

52

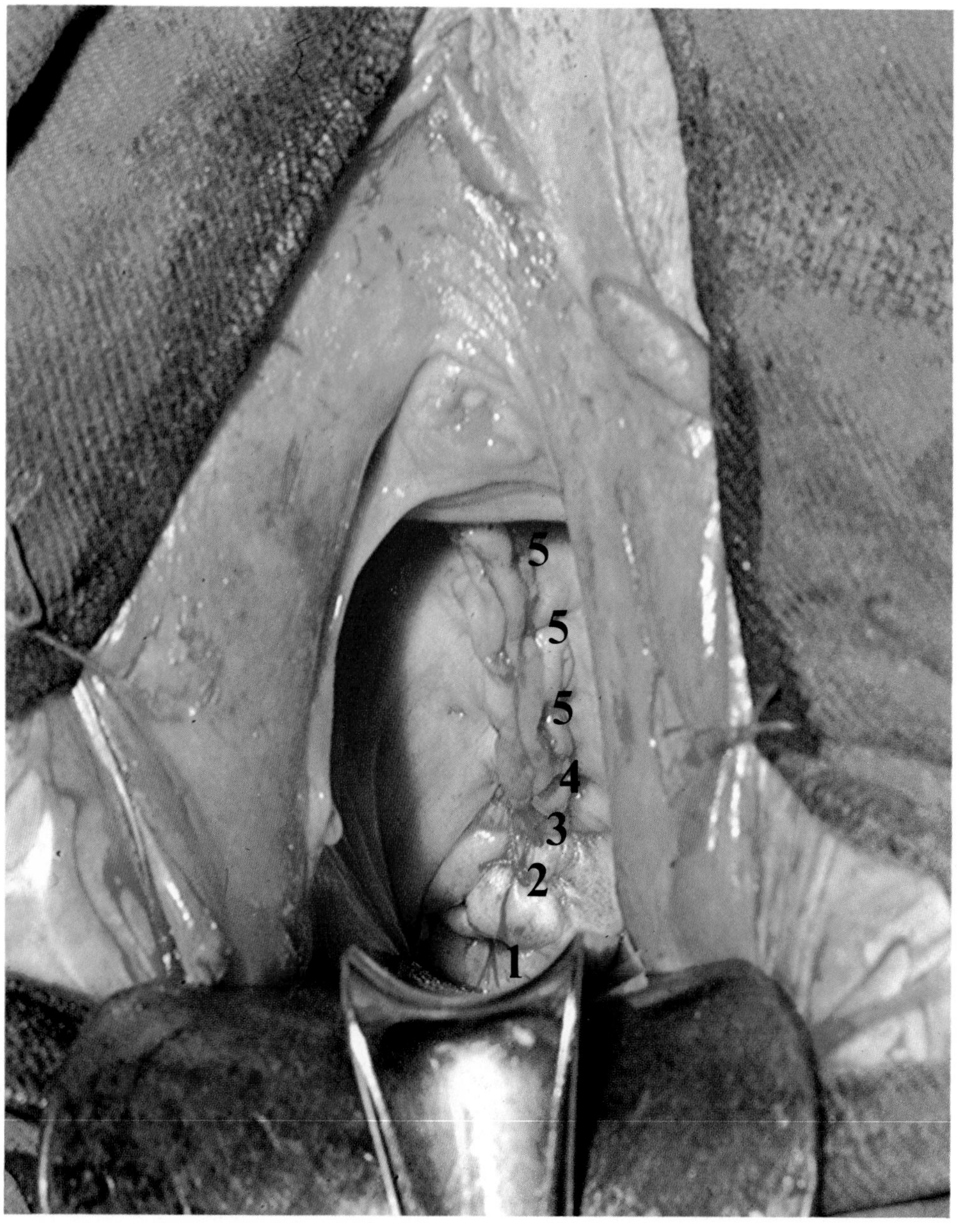

52 Anterior vaginal wall closure (iv)

The anterior vaginal wall is shown closed. The lumen of the vagina is adequate and uniform throughout its length and the anterior fornix is high. The wound is quite dry.

1 Cervical canal
2 Crown suture
3 Fothergill suture
4 Reinforcing Fothergill suture
5 Inverted mattress sutures closing anterior vaginal wall skin

Stage 10: Posterior vaginal wall repair

Where a Manchester (Fothergill) repair is indicated it is nearly always necessary to complete a posterior vaginal wall repair both to correct any degree of rectocele and to restore deficiency of the perineum. There has been a tendency to omit posterior repair on the grounds that dyspareunia is sometimes a problem in post-menopausal women who make up the majority of those having this operation.

As a result, the benefits of the Manchester operation have sometimes been diminished by this omission. We are convinced that the posterior wall should be attended to in most cases and given careful consideration in all. It was pointed out that anterior vaginal wall repair is a necessary component of almost all vaginal operations and the same applies to posterior repair and perineorrhaphy. The technique described here is applicable in all such circumstances.

The principles of the operation are first to excise a somewhat narrow triangle of skin and the underlying attenuated pre-rectal fascia from the posterior vaginal wall to expose the rectum as far as the introitus. An inverted and smaller triangle of skin is then raised from the perineum to expose the levator muscles anteriorly and the external anal sphincter posteriorly. The vaginal skin on each side is dissected free from the pre-rectal fascial layer and the medial edges of the latter fascia are sutured together in the mid-line to support the rectum and eliminate rectocele. The posterior vaginal wall skin is then closed by a continuous suture. The perineum is repaired by defining the edges of the levator muscles and fixing them together by deep interrupted sutures, and the skin of the perineum is closed by a subcutaneous stitch.

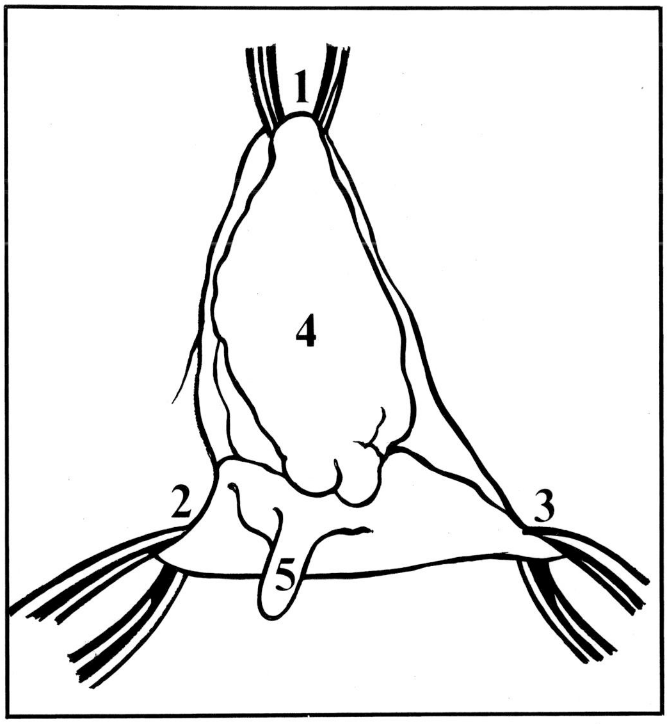

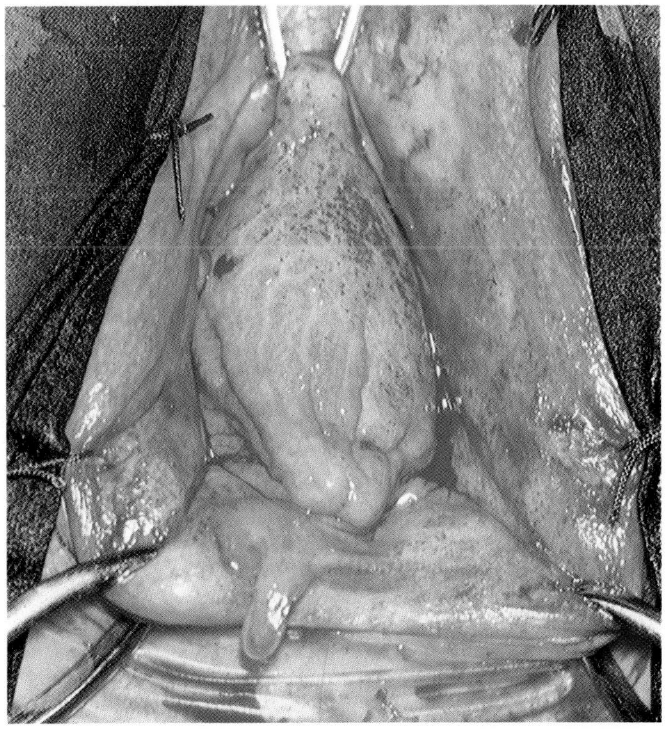

53

1 Forceps on upper edge of rectocele
2 and 3 Forceps at introitus
4 Bulge of rectocele
5 Skin tag from previous perineal laceration

53 General view pre-operatively

The considerable degree of rectocele and perineal deficiency is obvious. A triangle of redundant skin will have to be removed from the posterior vaginal wall but the angle at the apex should not be too wide lest it cause a deficiency of skin resulting in narrowing at the introitus or localised contraction higher up. The angle should be narrow with a correspondingly narrow base at the introitus.

The area requiring attention is outlined by a triad of forceps, (1) on the upper edge of the rectocele, (2) on the right side of the introitus posteriorly and (3) on the left posteriorly. The points of application of (2) and (3) are about 2 cm from the mid-line and the impression made on the skin by the blade of the Auvard's speculum is a useful guide to where they should be placed.

54

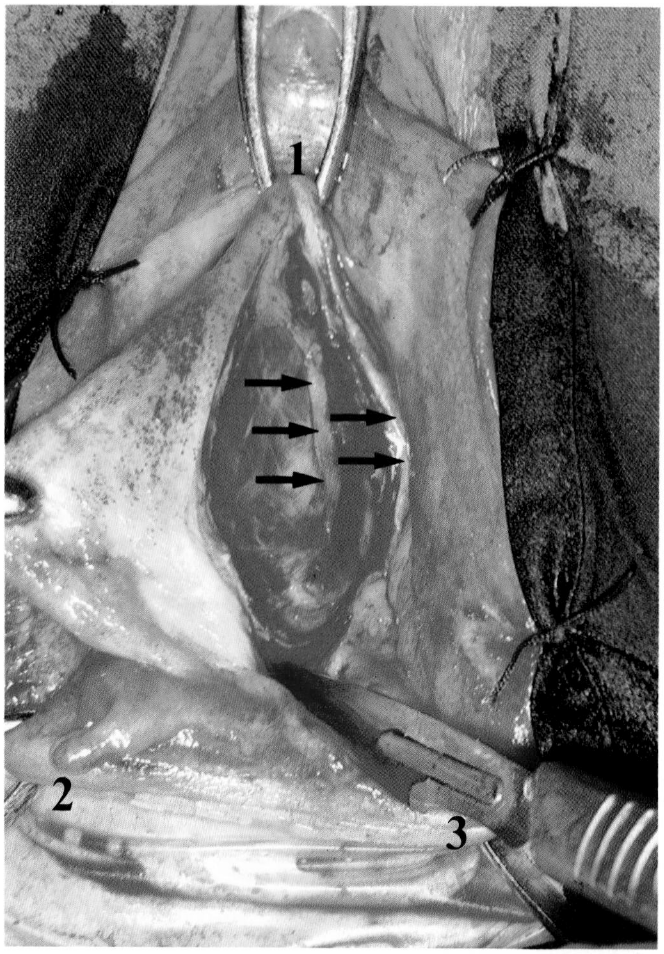

55

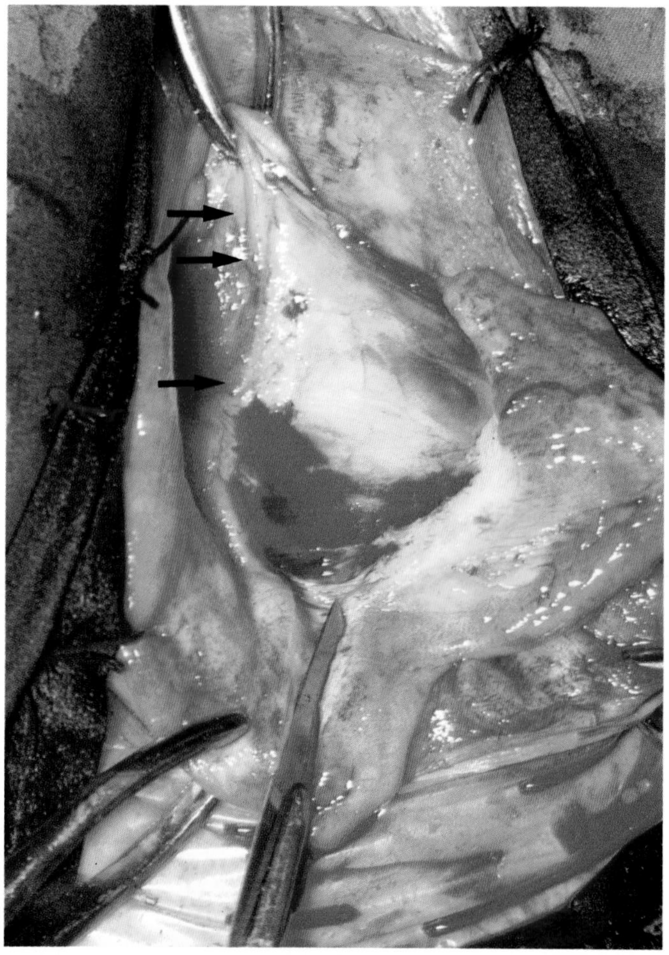

56

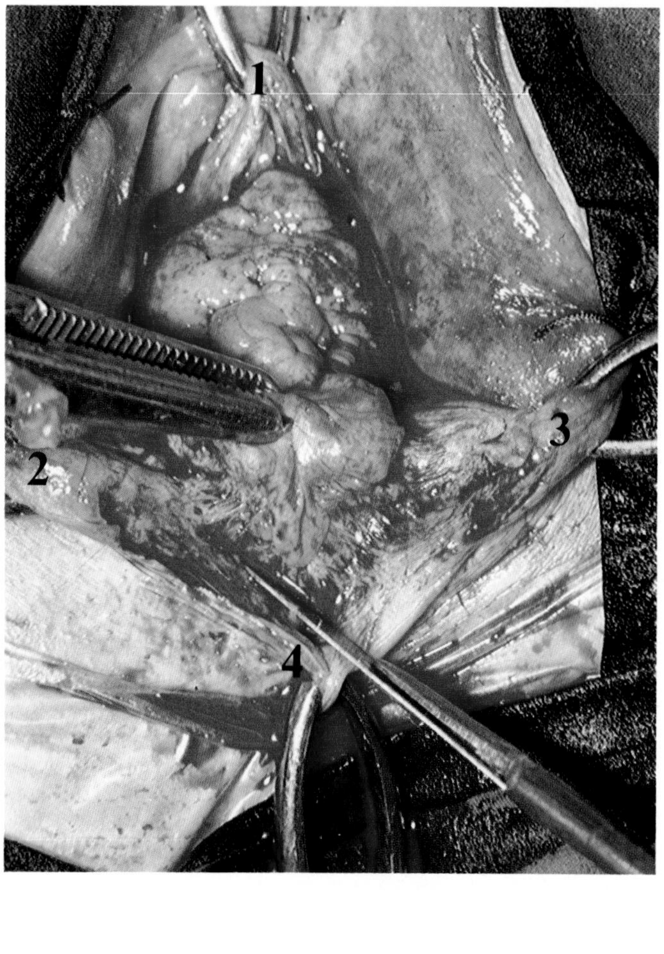

54 Posterior vaginal wall incision (left)

An incision is made on the patient's left side from (1) to (3), cutting quite boldly through skin and underlying attached layers of pre-rectal or para-rectal fascia. The rectum is loosely supported and falls away from the line of incision so that there is little danger of damage to it. Note the two layers of tissue: the outer is the vaginal skin edge, the inner the pre-rectal fascia.

55 Posterior vaginal wall incision (right)

A similar incision is made on the patient's right side. The two layers are again obvious. They are arrowed as in **54**.

56 Perineal skin incision

Points (2) and (3) are the starting points of the two limbs of a shallow V over the deficient perineum. The apex is at (4), and the outlining incision has just been made towards the forceps attached at this point.

57A

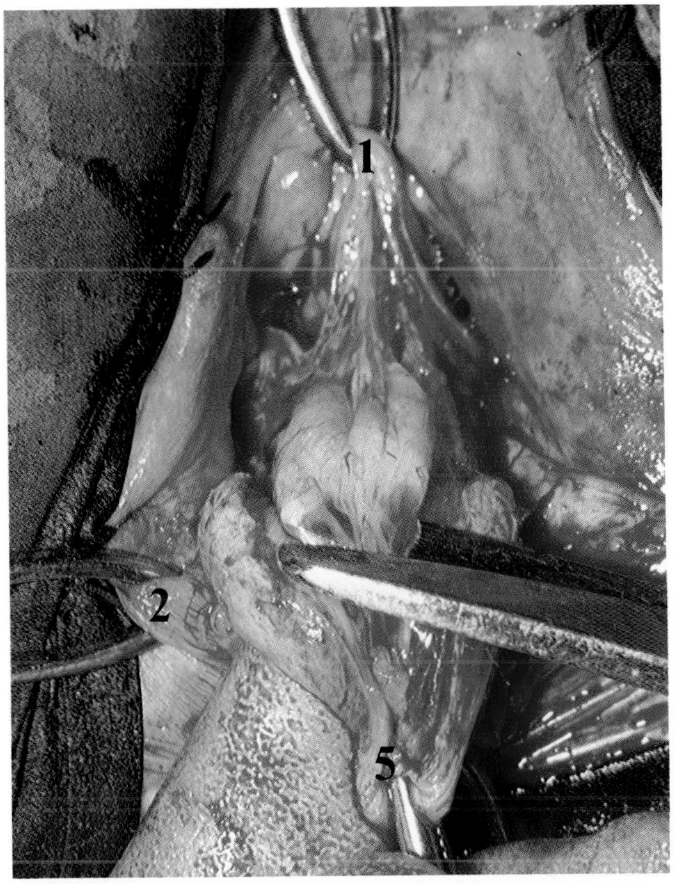

57B

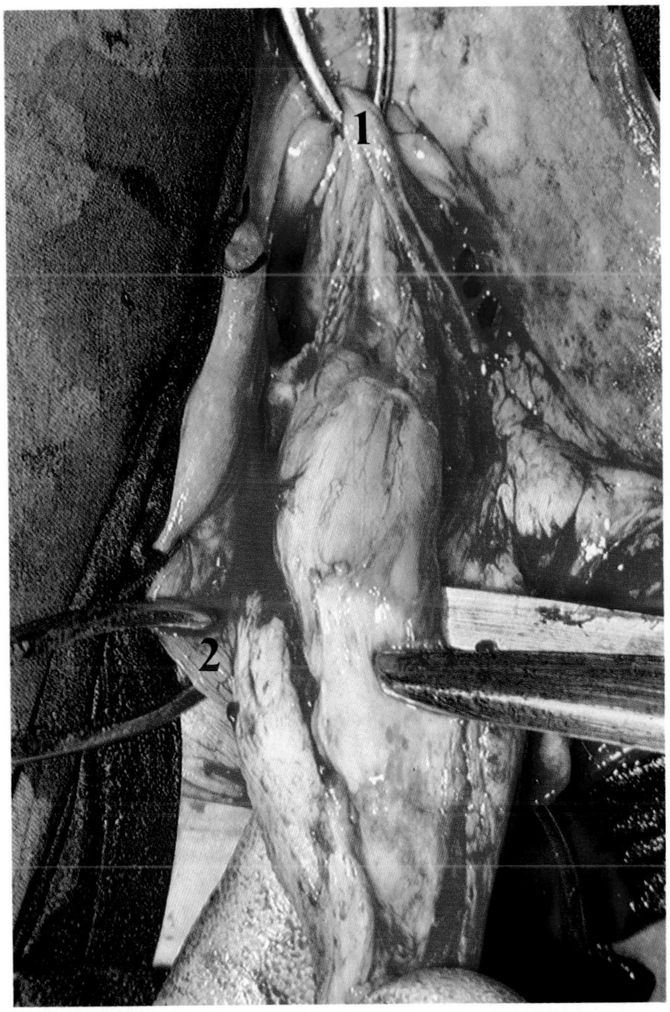

57C

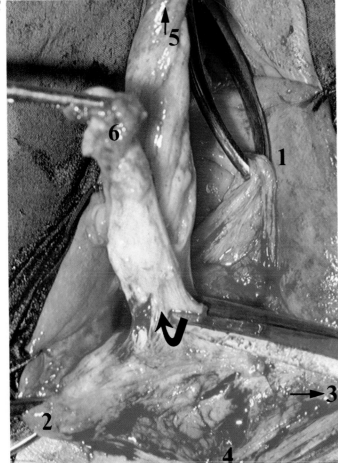

57A–57C Removal of excess skin (i)

57A shows the initial stage of separation starting from above. The skin flap is held taut by another pair of forceps (5) over the left forefinger and freed from the adherent pre-rectal fat by scissors. In **57B** the process has been carried a stage further and in **57C** the inverted perineal skin triangle held up by forceps (6) at its apex is dissected up off the external sphincter and perineal body (as arrowed).

58

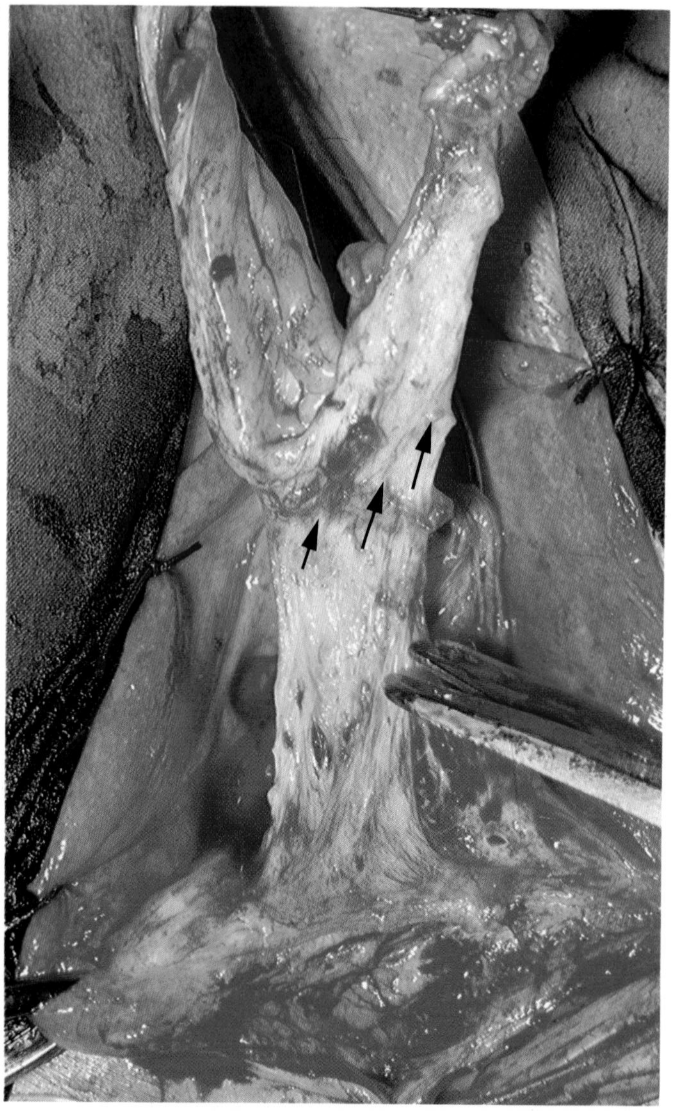

59

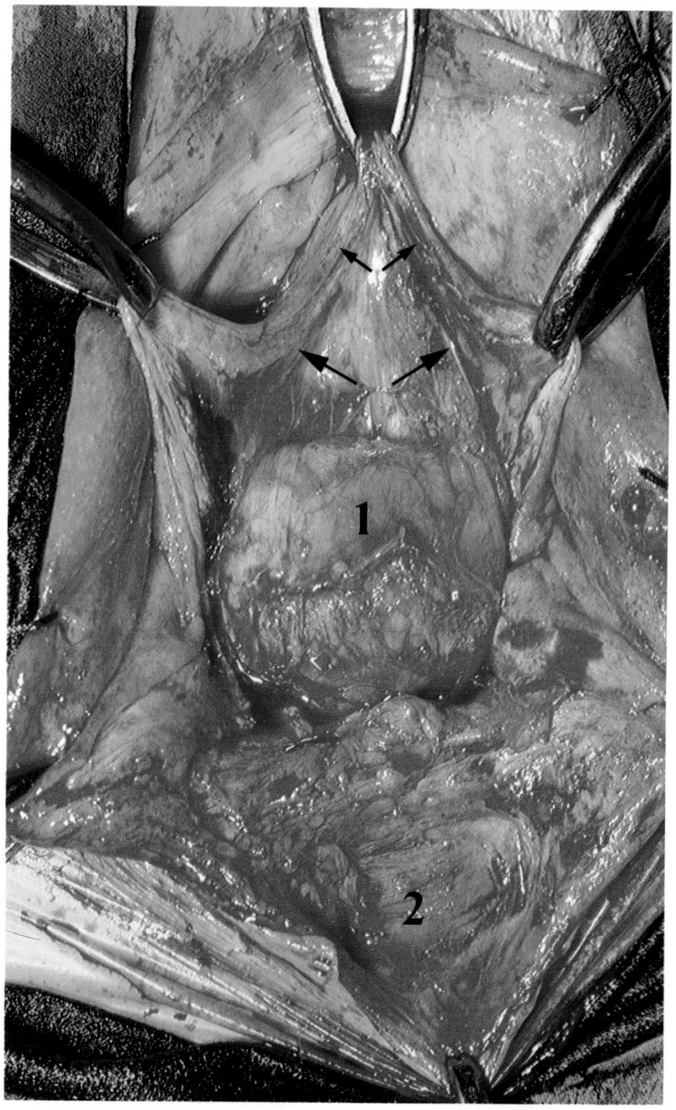

58 Removal of excess skin (ii)

The whole skin flap is ready to be detached and the scissors are being used to divide the remaining strands of pre-rectal fascia as arrowed. It is advisable to keep close to the skin layer to avoid any risk of opening into the rectum which might be pulled up in the 'pedicle'. In the photograph the scissors would not be used to cut at the level shown; they however mark the upper level of the rectum. The proper line of incision is as arrowed.

59 Removal of excess skin completed

The denuded area over the rectocele and deficient anterior perineum reveals the rectum uncovered above and with practically no anterior support as far down as the anal canal and the visible fibres of the external sphincter. The rectum is labelled 1, and the external sphincter 2. Strands of pre-rectal fascia are arrowed.

60

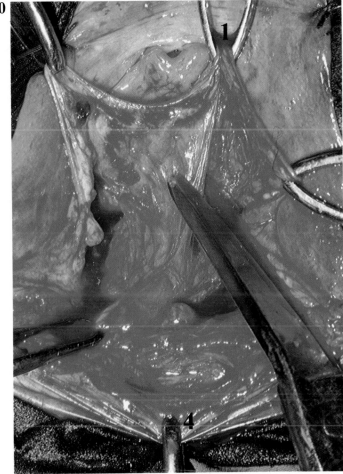

61

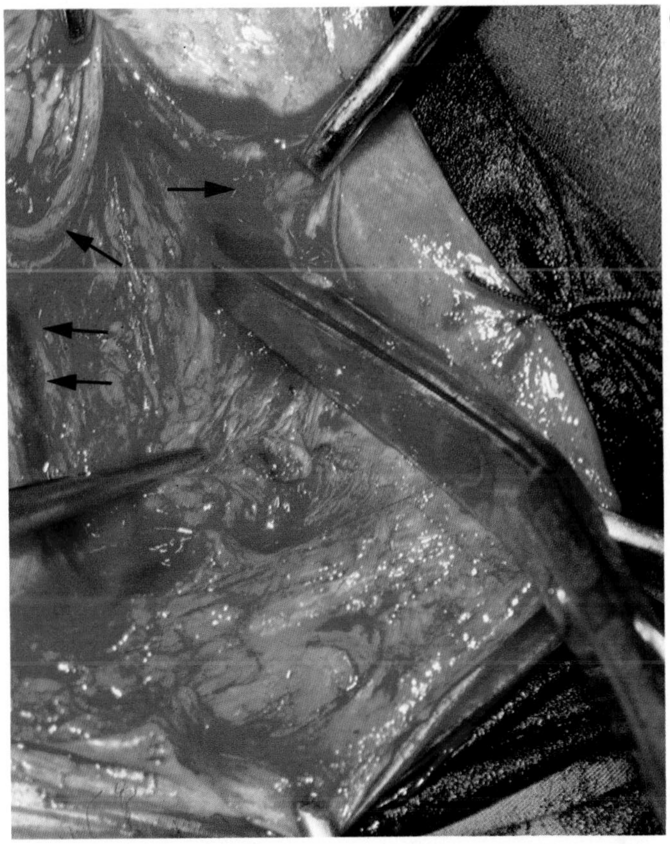

62

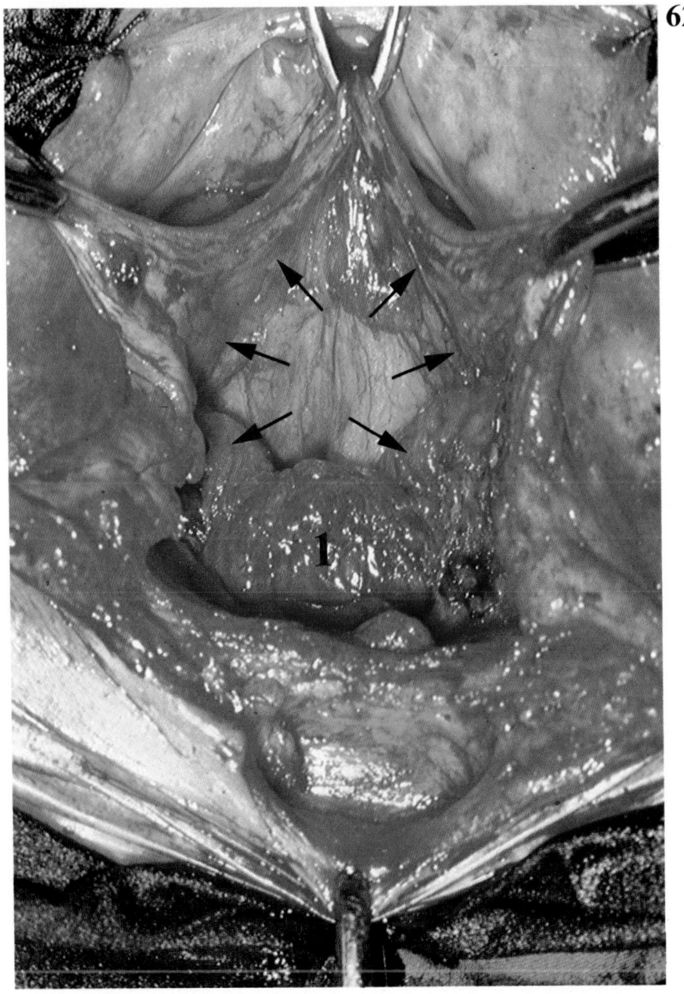

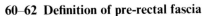

60–62 Definition of pre-rectal fascia

The vaginal skin is carefully separated from the underiying pre-rectal fascial layer. Sharp dissection is commenced in the mid-line in **60** to find the tissue planes and the space between is opened up by blunt dissection and carried well laterally. The fascial layer becomes thicker and better established away from the mid-line where it is thinned out and largely removed with the triangle of skin. The forceps (1) indicate the apex of the bare posterior wall triangle and are in the mid-line. The fibres of the external anal sphincter are just above forceps (4). Separation has been completed on the patient's right side where arrowed in **61** and a similar separation is now being carried out on the patient's left (arrowed). The fascial layer is becoming more distinct as the dissection proceeds laterally. The rectum (1) has been fully exposed anteriorly and freed from the posterior vaginal wall in **62**. The edges of the pre-rectal fascial layer are clearly visible on each side and are ready to be stitched together in the mid-line. They are marked with arrows.

63

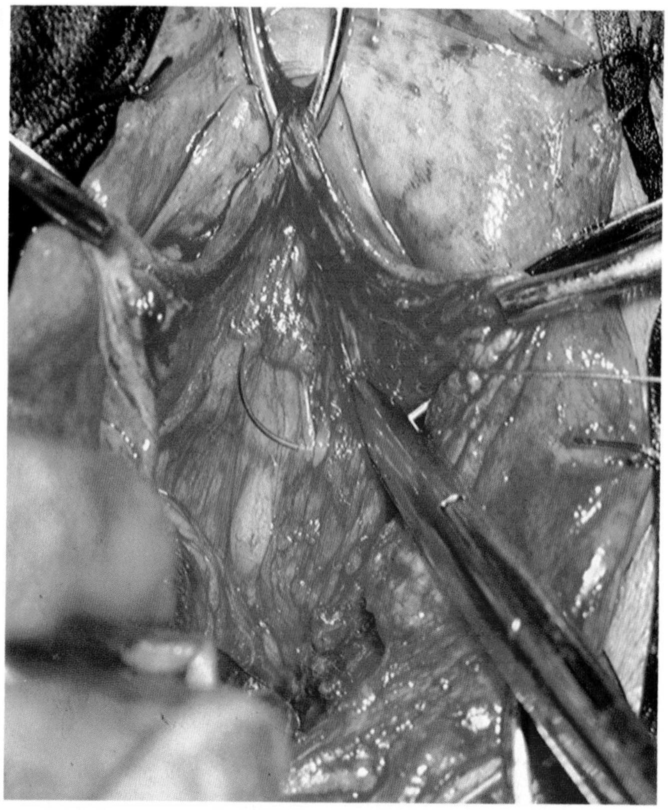

64

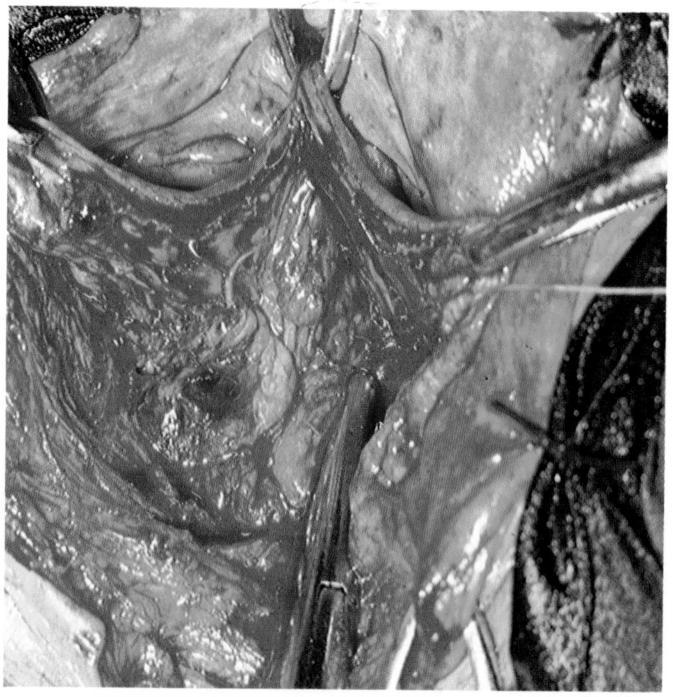

65A

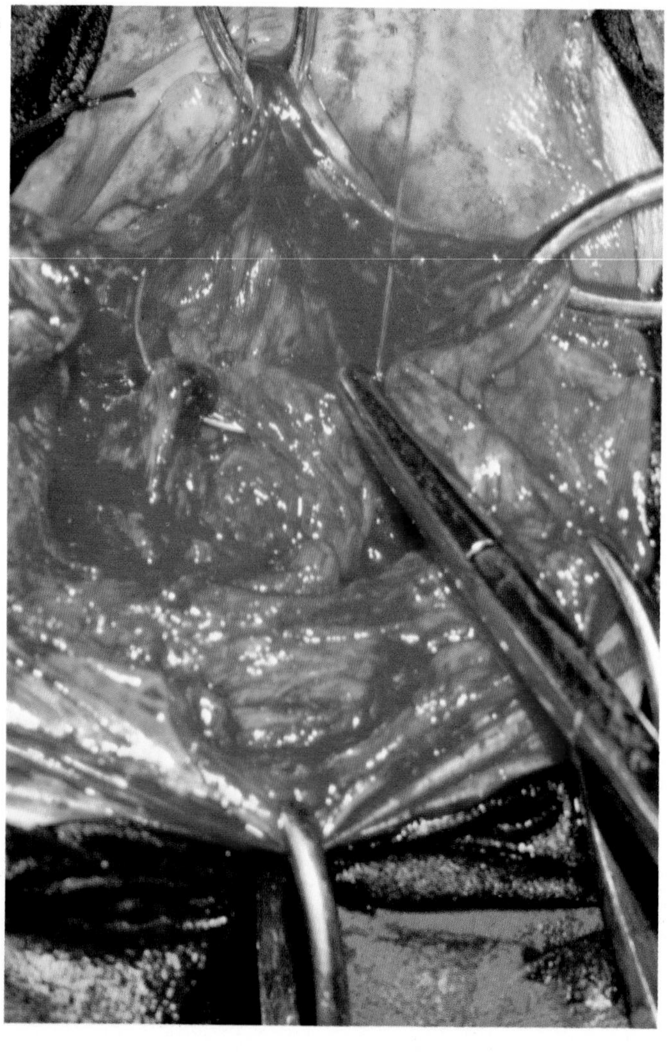

65B

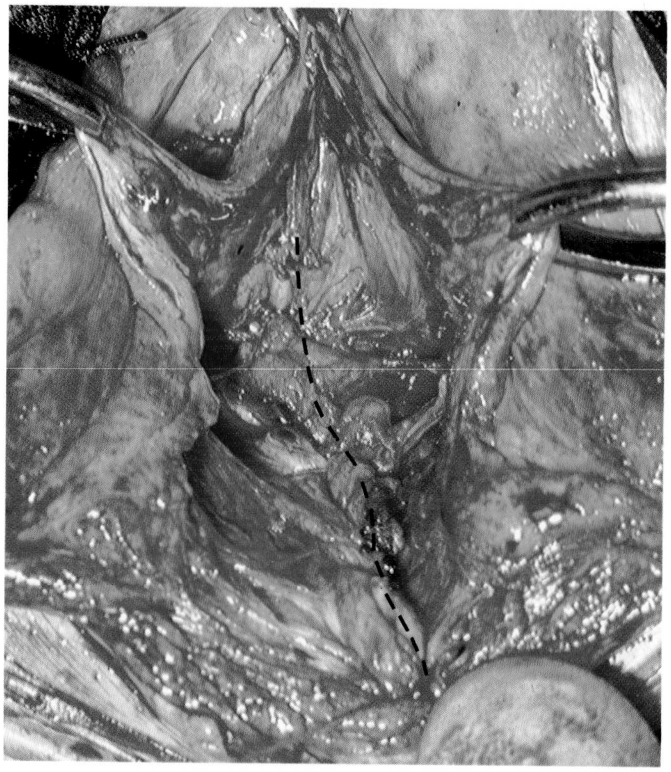

63–65B Repair of pre-rectal fascia

Displacing the rectum posteriorly with the left forefinger in **63**, the left leaf of the pre-rectal fascia is picked up ready to start its approximation. The needle carries a PGA No. 00 suture. In **64** the right leaf is included in the suture which then fixes them together in the mid-line. A further stage of the repair of the fascia is seen in **65A** and in **65B** the completed continuous suture is being tied off. The suture line is indicated by the interrupted tracing.

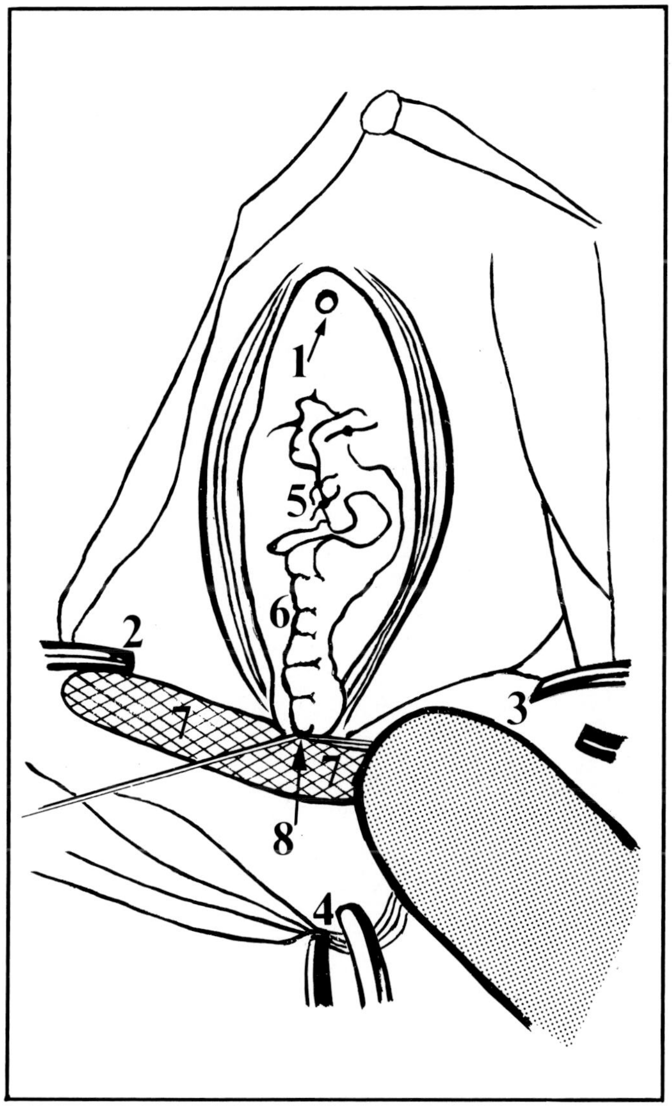

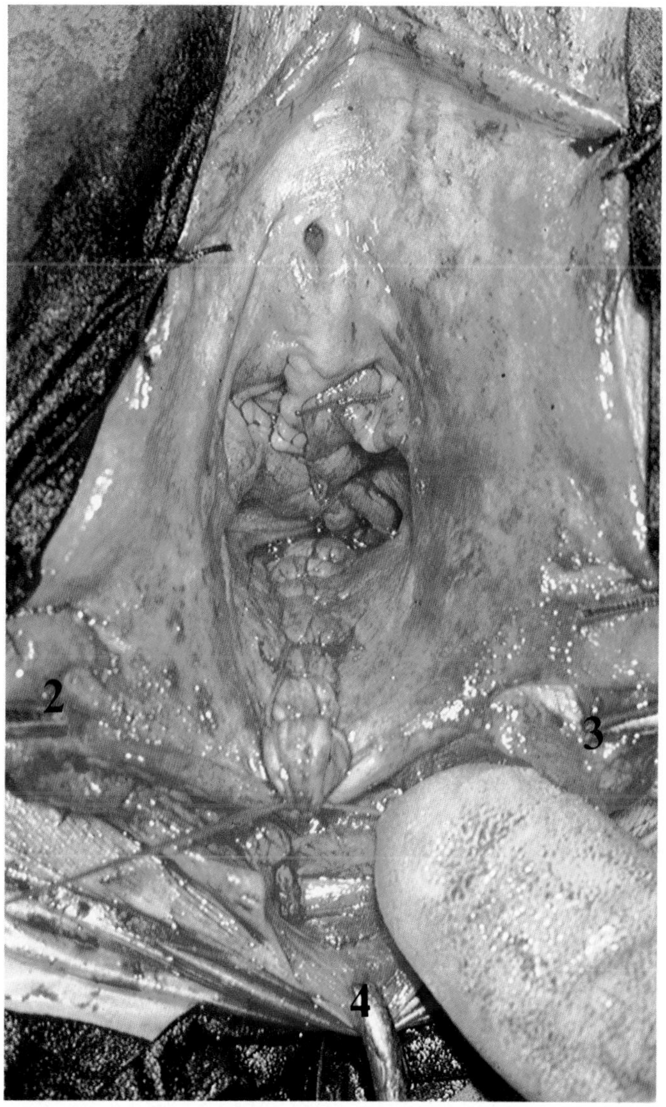

66

1 Urethra
2 and 3 Original Littlewood's forceps holding skin at vaginal introitus
4 Forceps holding skin anterior to anus
5 Anterior vaginal wall suture line
6 Posterior vaginal wall suture line (locking sutures)
7 Unrepaired perineal region
8 Posterior vaginal wall closure completed at level of introitus

66 Closure of posterior wall skin

The skin of the posterior vaginal wall is approximated by a continuous PGA No. 0 suture on an atraumatic needle. A locked stitch gives a neat and haemostatic effect and has been used here. It is tied off exactly at the level of the introitus and gentle traction on the Littlewood's forceps (2) and (3) indicates where it should be placed. The ends of the suture are left long. The forceps (2) and (3) are the original ones placed in position at the beginning of the repair.

Repair of perineum

The essential steps are to free the medial borders of the levator ani muscles from the overlying skin and superficial perineal muscles and then approximate them in the mid-line to reconstitute the perineal body. If the superficial perineal muscles present as worthwhile structures they are stitched together as a separate layer. They are generally thin and attenuated and it is only necessary to obtain a firm skin closure.

67

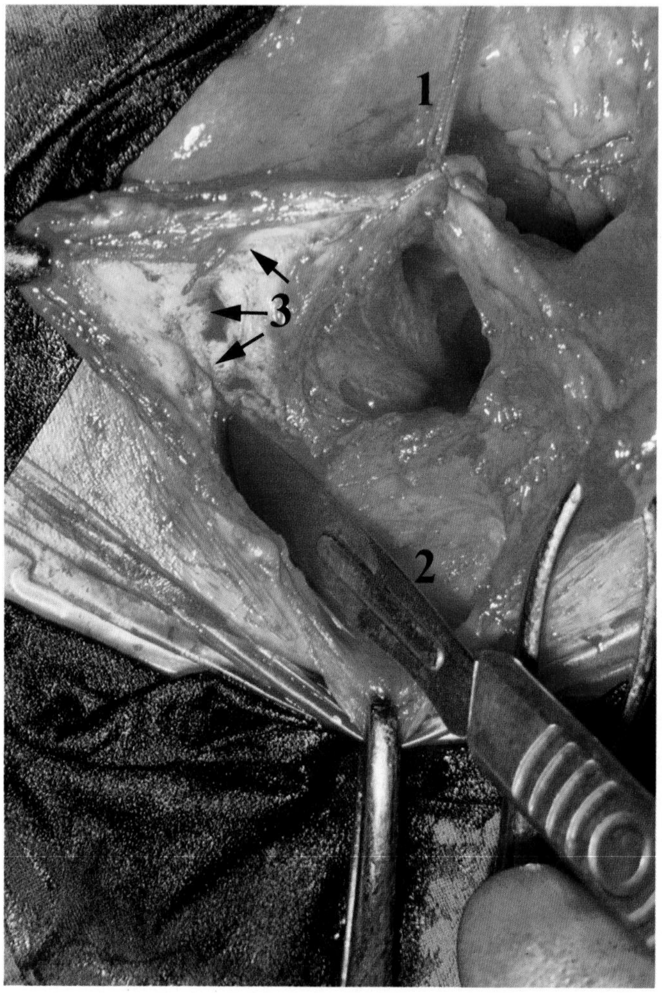

68

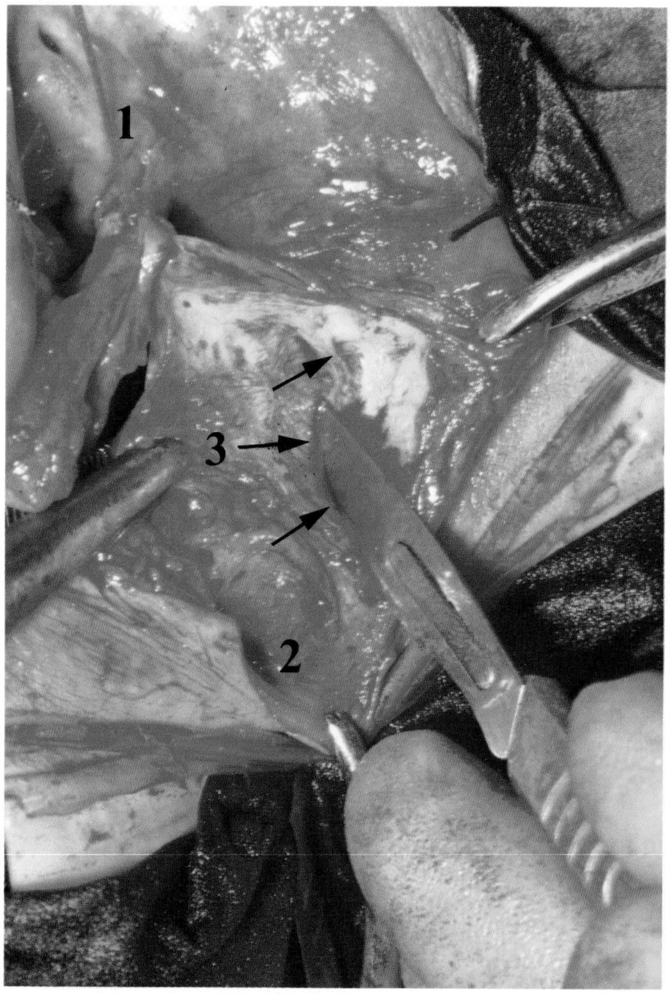

67 Definition of right levator muscle

The long ends of the suture are held up on a gentle stretch to display the perineum with the external sphincter visible posteriorly. The medial border of the levator ani muscle is freed from the skin with the scalpel and mobilised ready to cover the central defect. Number 1 indicates the long suture which closed the posterior vaginal skin; 2 indicates the external sphincter. Arrows show the plan of separation between skin and levator muscle which is indicated by 3.

68 Definition of left levator muscle

A similar procedure is carried out on the left side with the same numerals as used in **67** indicating similar structures. The plane of separation is again arrowed.

69

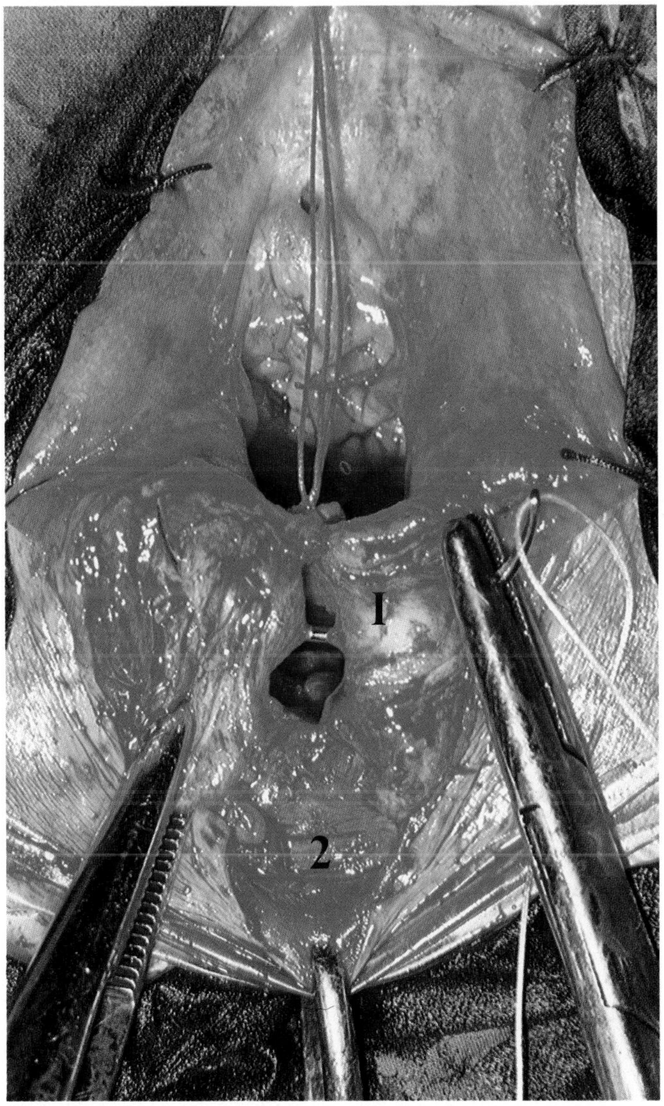

70

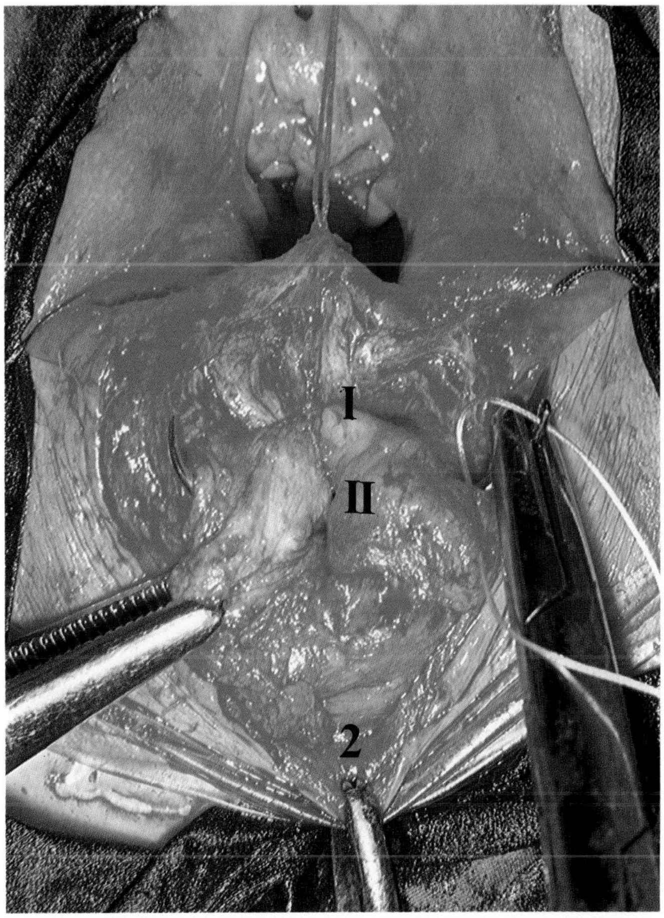

71

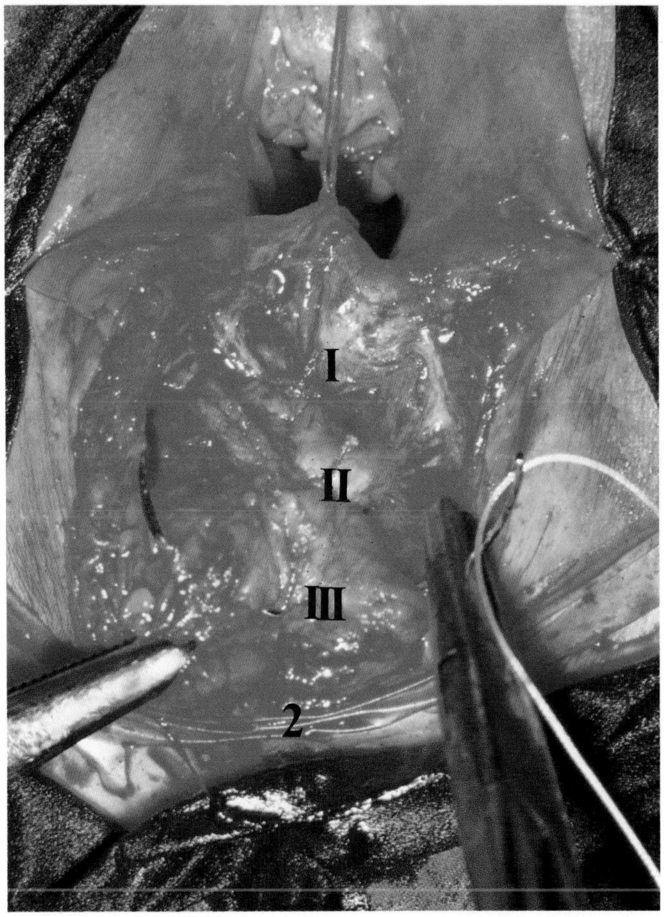

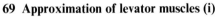

69 Approximation of levator muscles (i)

A round-bodied needle carrying a PGA No. 1 suture traverses the medial belly of each levator muscle 1 cm from its edge to approximate them in the mid-line. Note the external sphincter clearly defined posteriorly and numbered 2.

70 and 71 Approximation of levator muscles (ii)

These show further stages in approximation. In **70** a second stitch and in **71** a third stitch is being placed to give firm apposition of the muscles. Roman numerals I to III indicate the position of these three sutures.

Skin closure of perineum

We feel that the most satisfactory closure is by a subcutaneous rather than a subcuticular PGA No. 00 stitch on a straight triangular pointed needle. The sensitive skin nerve endings are undisturbed, the numerous vulnerable skin vessels are avoided and there are no stitches to catch on dressings or underclothing. There is minimal post-operative swelling or discomfort and little reflex disturbance of the bladder (i.e. urinary retention).

72A

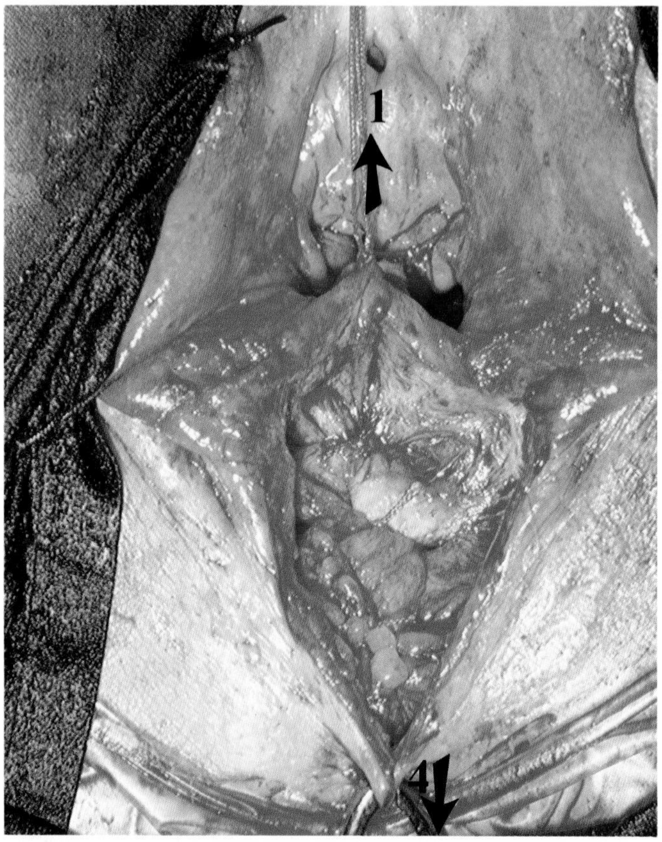

72B

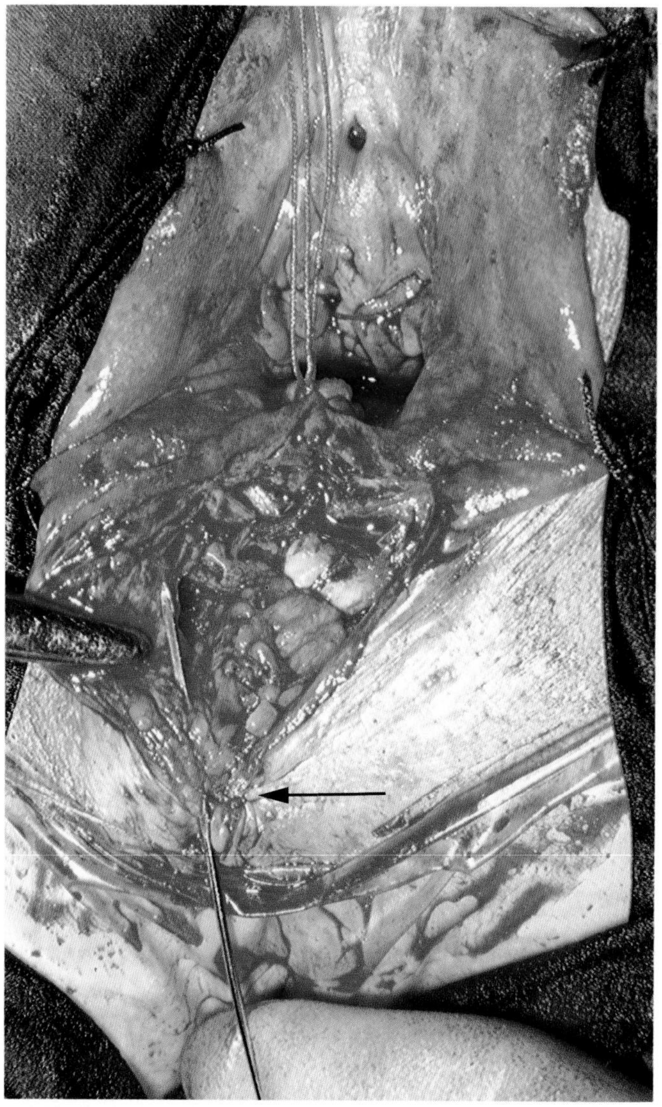

72C

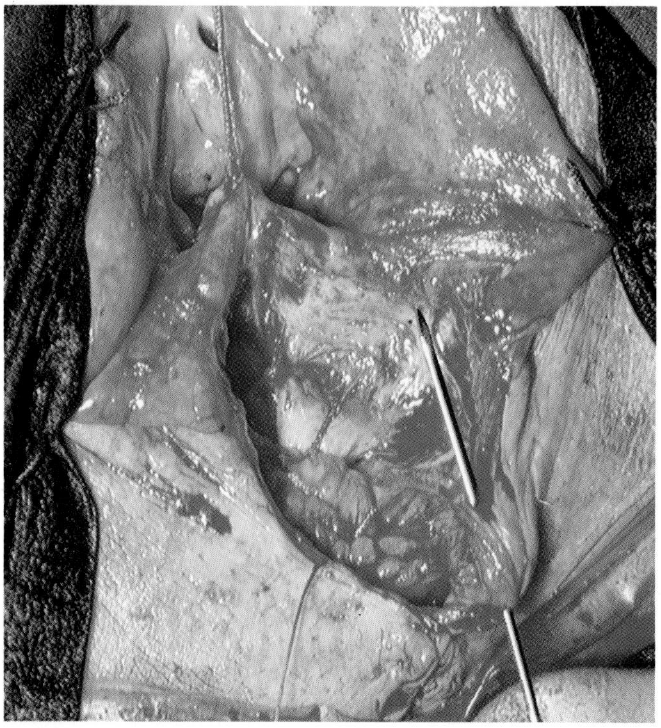

72A–72C Skin closure (i)

The lateral forceps are removed in **72A** and by pulling up the long ends of the vaginal skin stitch (1) and slight counter-traction on the forceps (4) which lie anterior to the anus, the skin layers are thrown into relief. Progressive steps in placing the subcutaneous stitch are then shown. In **72B** a slight puckering can be seen posteriorly where the end of the suture has been tied and cut short (arrowed), and the stitching proceeds in **72C**.

73A

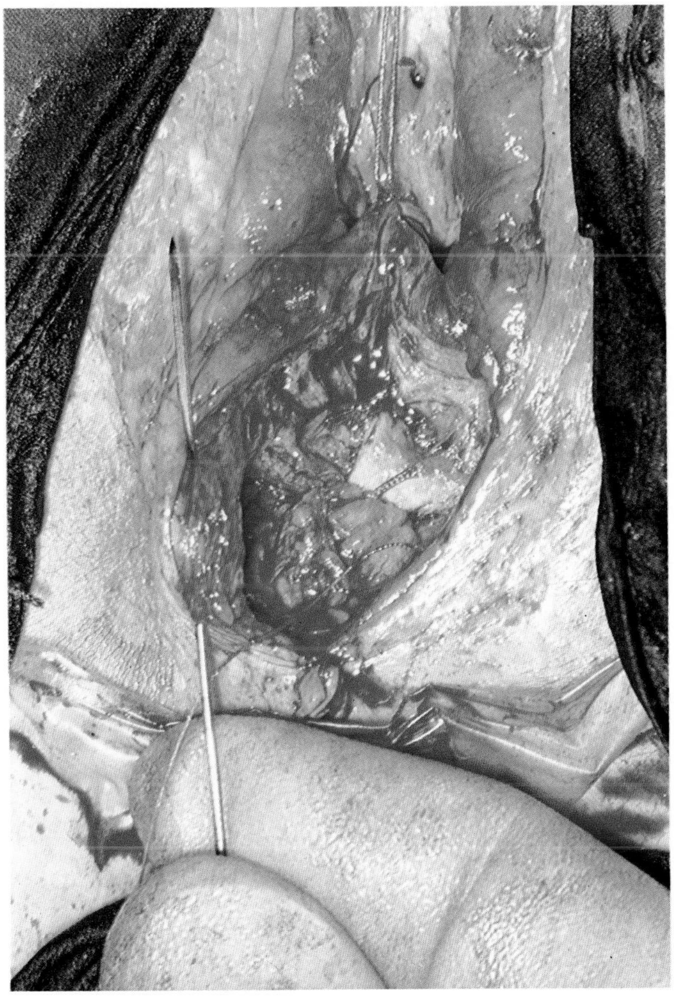

73B

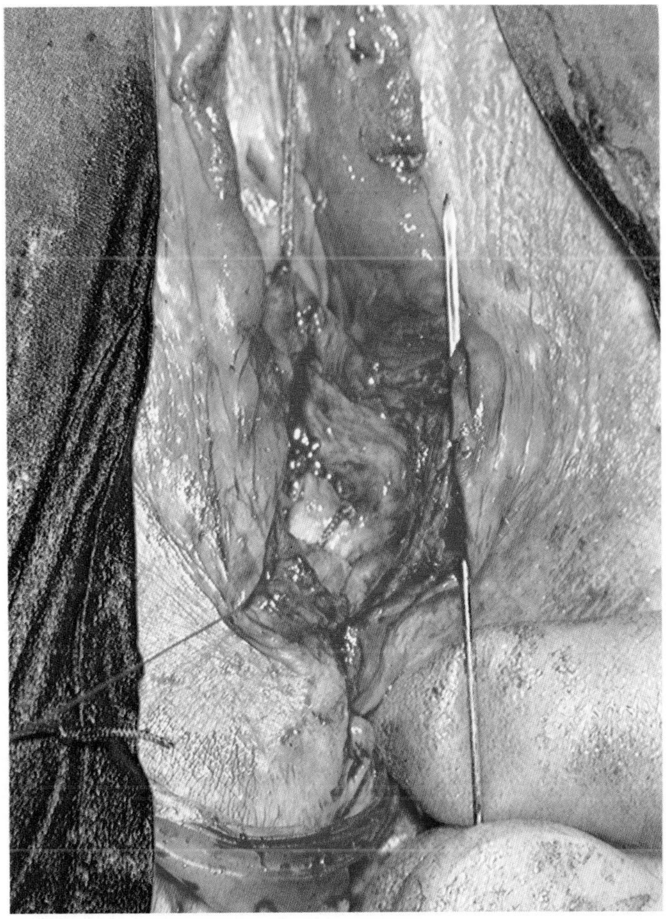

73C

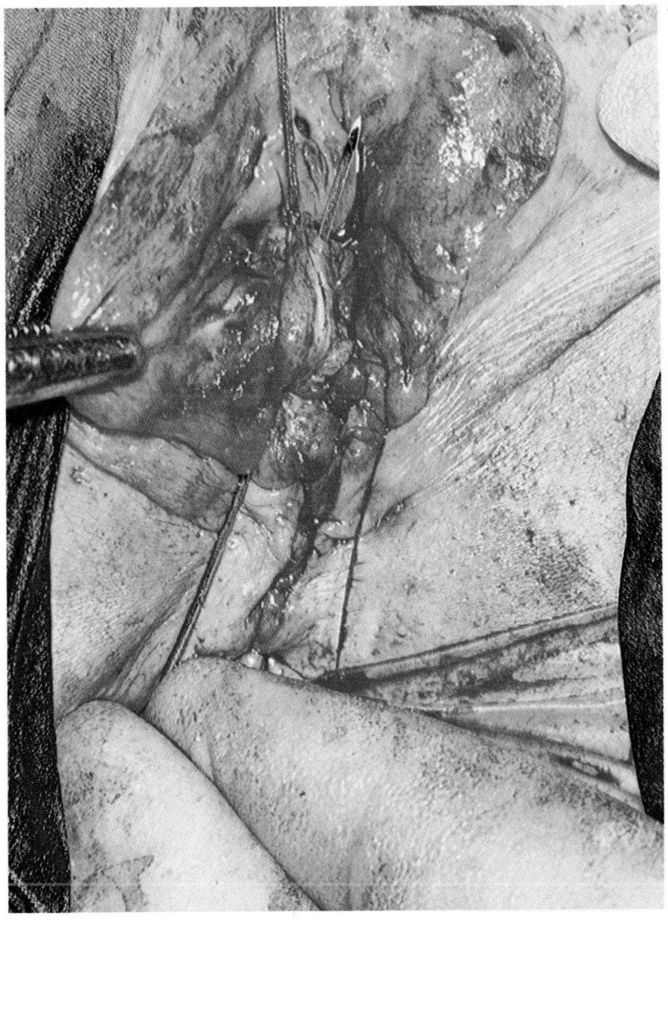

73A–73C Skin closure (ii)

The subcutaneous tissue is picked up in progression on each side in **73A** and **73B** and in **73C** the suture is emerging through the skin to be tied at an intra-vaginal level where it is clear of sensitive perineal nerves.

74

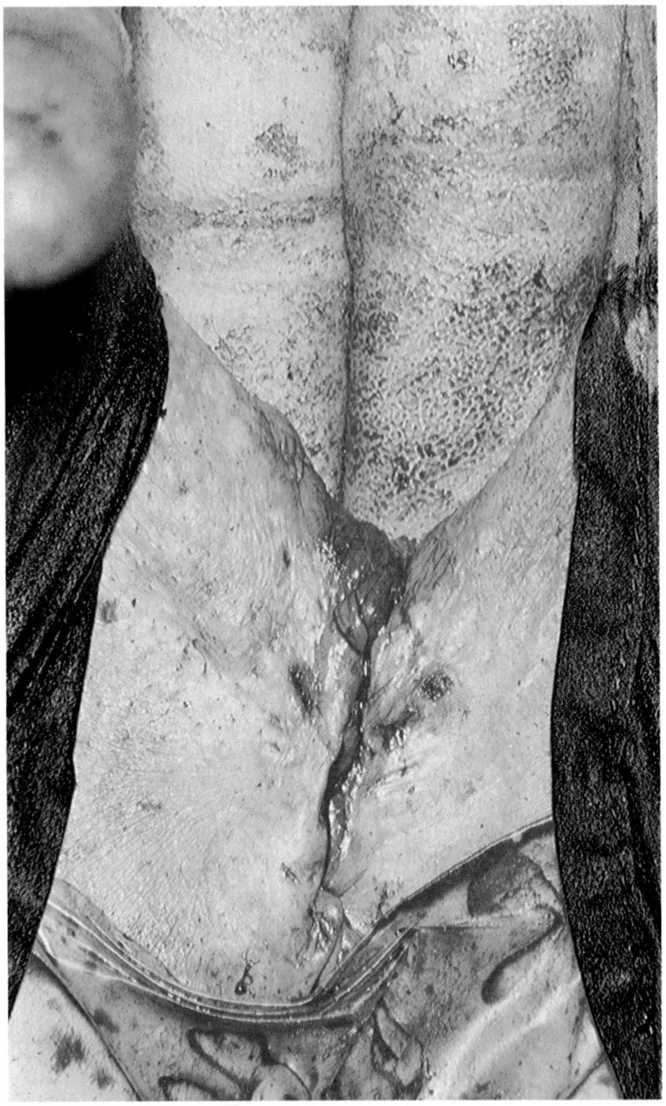

74 Checking the operative result

With the skin suture completed and cut short the lumen of the vagina is estimated by its capacity to take 2 fingers. It should be of uniform calibre and the suture lines should be quite dry. If there is persistent bleeding through either the anterior or posterior suture line, which is obviously not coming from the skin edge, then it is recommended that the suture line be reopened.

6: Repair of enterocele

Enterocele is rather different from the other elements of utero-vaginal prolapse, being in some ways more akin to a true hernia. A peritoneal sac develops to cover intra-abdominal structures attempting to escape through a potential hernial orifice in the abdominal parietes. The weak point is the floor of the pouch of Douglas between the utero-sacral ligaments. The enterocele generally has its origins in obstetrical trauma although this is also the prolapse that results from heavy lifting and particularly affects nullipara. In Britain it seems to have a predeliction for spinsters nursing and lifting heavy relatives and parents. There is usually a degree of enterocele associated with prolapse of any severity and it is by far the commonest type of recurrent prolapse.

When undertaking vaginal surgery it is important to remember the possible occurrence of enterocele and particularly in doing a vaginal hysterectomy and repair or a Manchester repair. In the former it is essential to remove the excess peritoneum in the pouch of Douglas and approximate the utero-sacral ligaments. In a Manchester repair the pouch of Douglas should be definitively opened, any excess peritoneum excised and the utero-sacral ligaments stitched together to obliterate the pouch.

The description which follows here particularly concerns recurrent enterocele but the operation is essentially the same. As in recurrent prolapse of all types there is an apparent excess or redundancy of vaginal skin but none should be removed until the operation is nearly complete and the true needs become obvious.

Stage 1: Definition and closure of sac

As this is essentially an operation for hernia it falls into two parts, or stages. The first requirement is to elevate, dissect out, open, transfix and tie off the sac as high as possible. These steps are shown in the following illustrations.

1

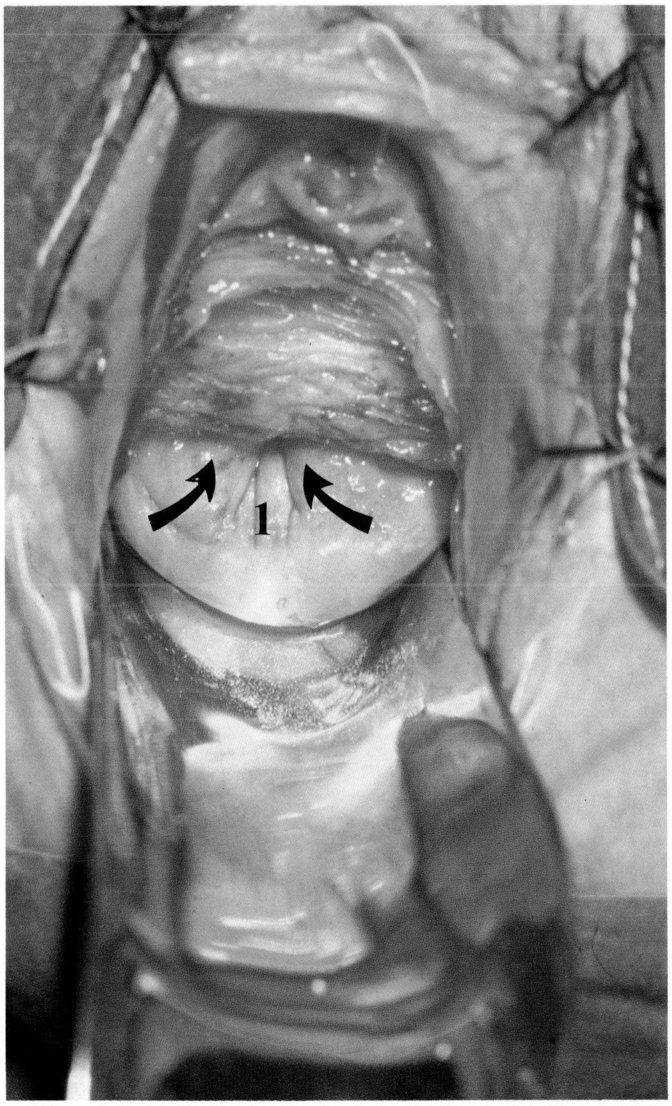

2

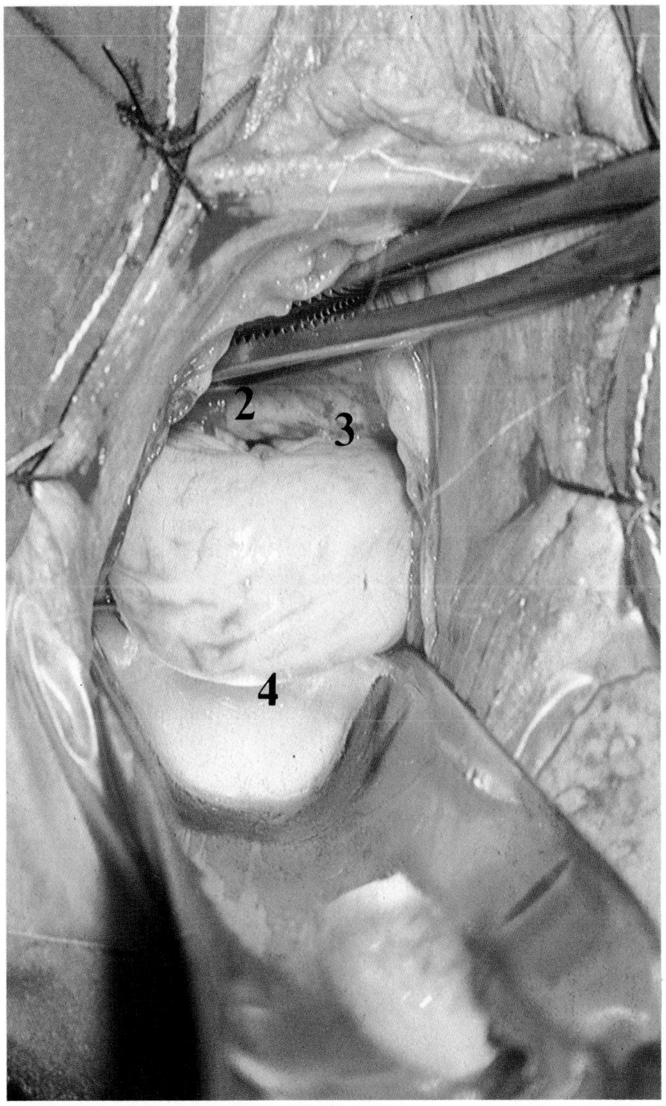

1 General view pre-operatively (i)

The appearances are typical of a recurrent prolapse in the form of enterocele. The posterior pouch hangs down like a tongue (1) which is seen on examination with a speculum. The anterior vaginal wall is quite well supported and there is no rectocele or perineal deficiency to speak of. The vault indicated by arrows is well supported and the recurrent prolapse is well localised.

2 General view pre-operatively (ii)

When the patient strains the enterocele sac fills up with intestine or omentum and bulges downwards towards the vulva. Even with straining this photograph shows that the anterior wall (2) and the vault (3) are adequately supported. The cervix is not seen in this photograph but lies behind the enterocele in the area 3 to 4. Note the thickening of the vaginal skin over the enterocele indicating that it has been subject to friction and pressure.

3

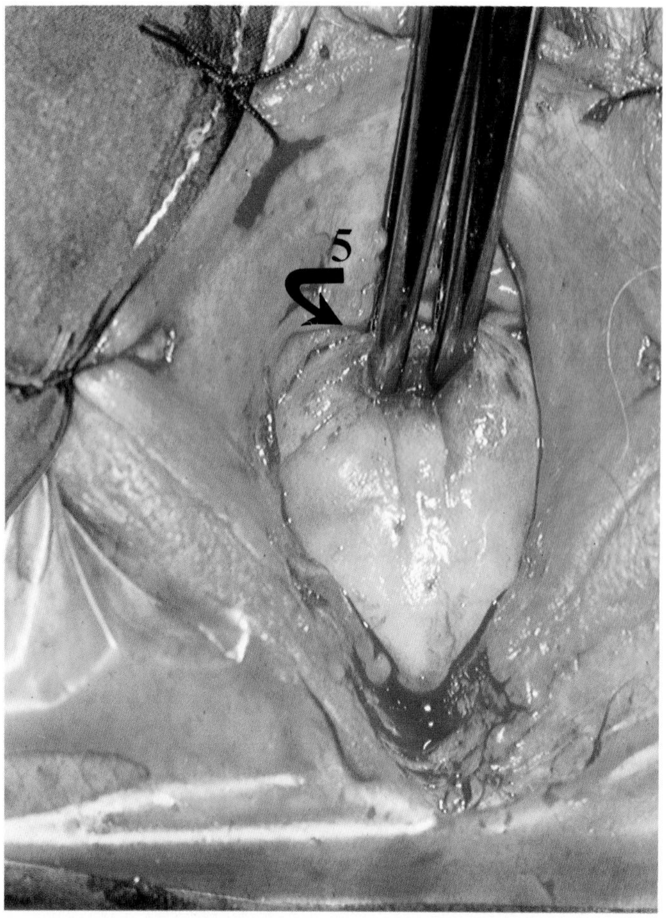

4

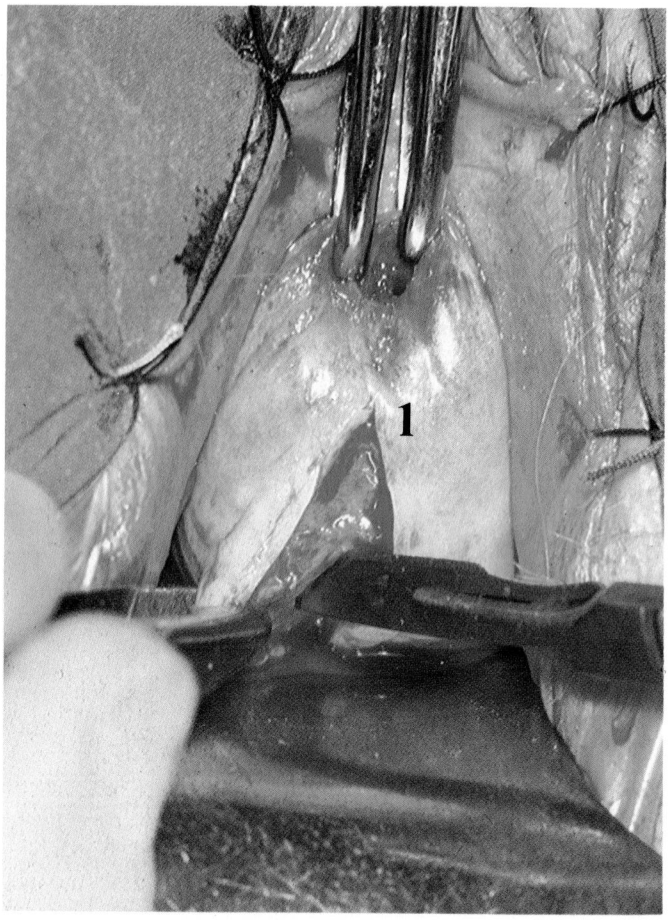

5

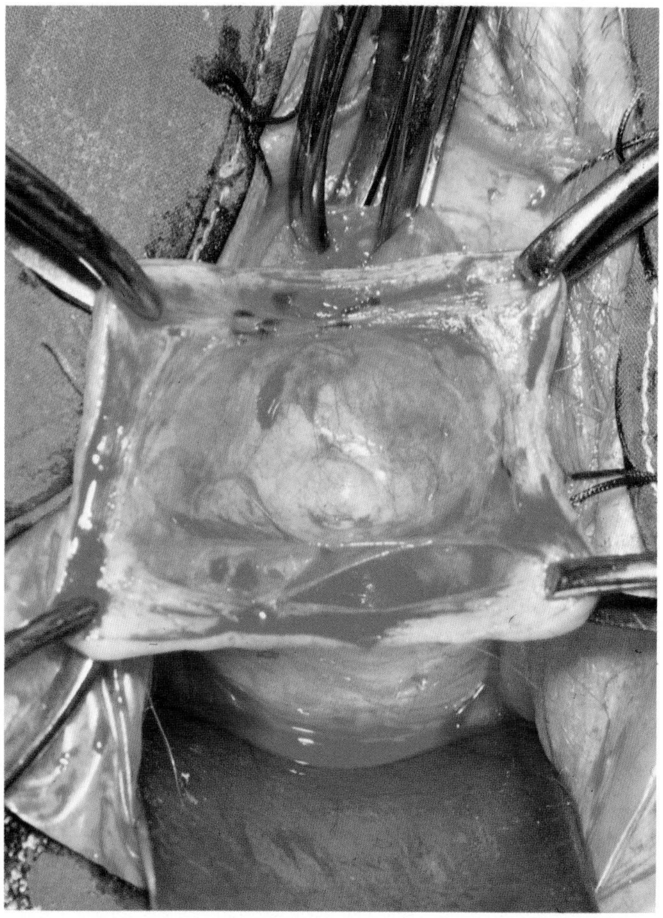

3 Preparation for repair of enterocele

The labia are stitched back to give wide access and a mid-line episiotomy also adds to accessibility. The cervical stump is held by the two pairs of forceps just in front of point (5).

4 Incision of posterior vaginal wall

The incision is made longitudinally in the mid-line in a direction to suit the surgeon's hand. It commences at point (1), divides the skin and just enters the lax subcutaneous tissue plane. There is no question of excising skin at this stage because one cannot judge how much will be required. Generally speaking there will be no excess at this level of the vagina.

5 Exposure of enterocele

The skin edges are retracted by two pairs of Littlewood's forceps on each side and the enterocele is clearly seen with all the appearance of a hernial sac. This illustration shows the lower posterior vaginal wall and there is no rectocele to be seen.

6

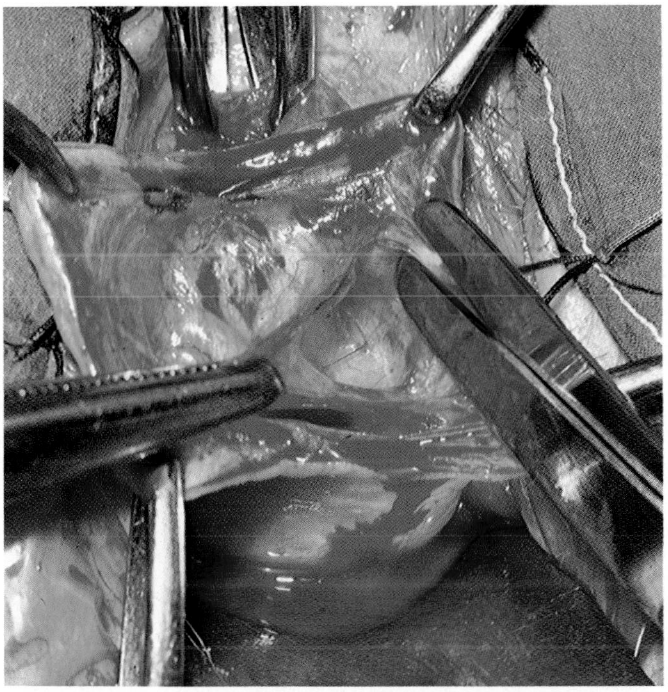

8

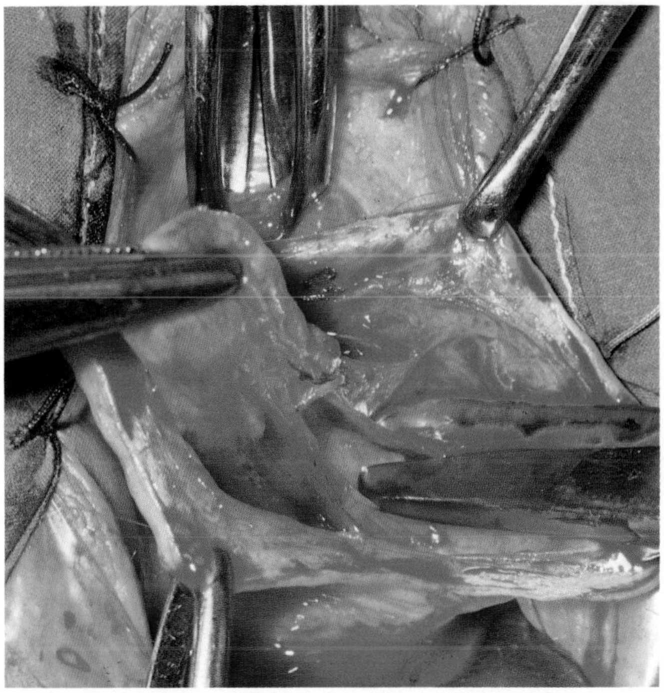

7

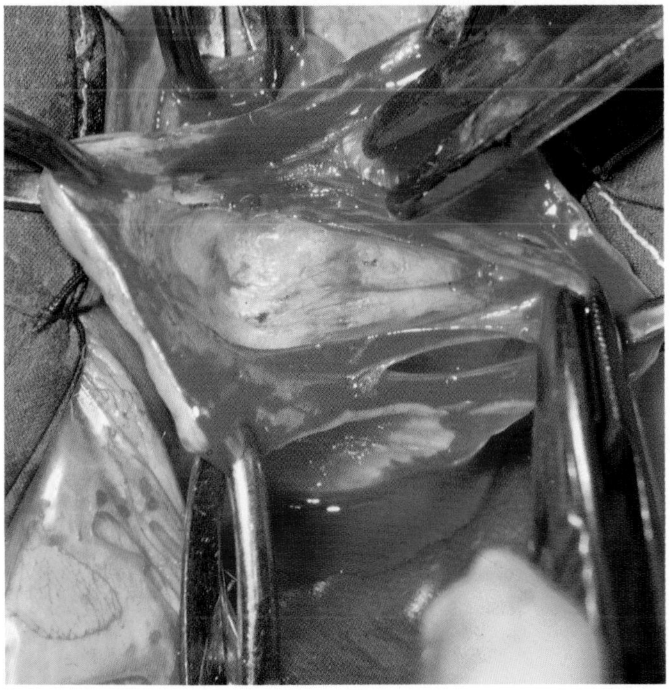

9

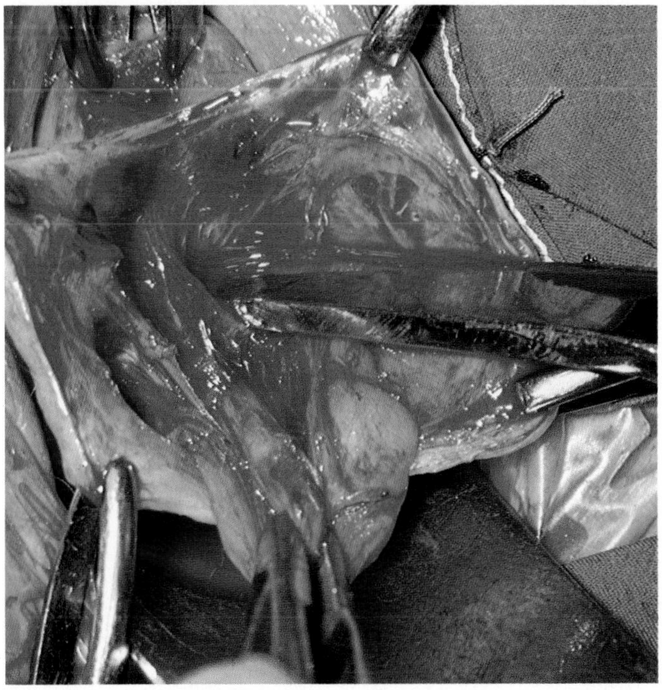

6 and 7 Reflection of vaginal skin

The vaginal skin must be reflected laterally on each side to give adequate access to the enterocele so that the sac can be defined. In **6** the left skin margin is being freed by scissors snips and pushed laterally and posteriorly. In **7** the same procedure is being followed on the right side and in this photograph the bands of fascial tissue held in the dissecting forceps are being pulled medially and divided. It will be seen that the tissues are loose and areolar and dissection is blunt and largely by pressure.

8 and 9 Definition of enterocele sac

The sac of the enterocele has a wide mouth and is empty when the patient is lying flat. It is dissected out like any other hernia. It is helpful to remember that it is bounded in front by the cervix and on each side by the medial border of the utero-sacral ligament so that its location is central and immediately adjacent to the vault. Figure **8** shows the sac held in the tip of the dissecting forceps and pulled to the patient's right while the scissors divide the anchoring fascial bands. In **9** the sac, now pulled down by the dissecting forceps posteriorly, is being freed from the fascia anteriorly and on the patient's right side.

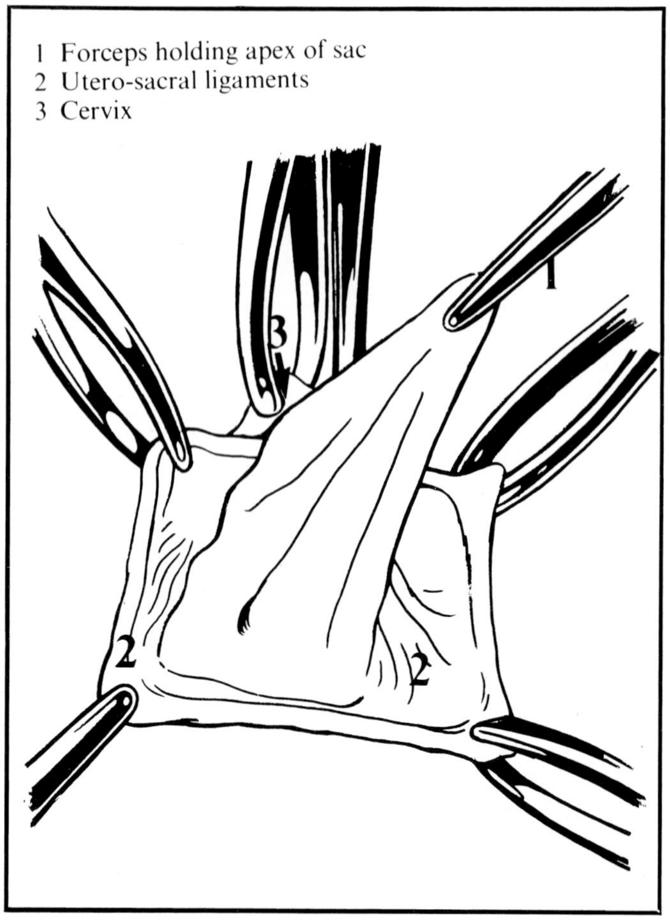

10

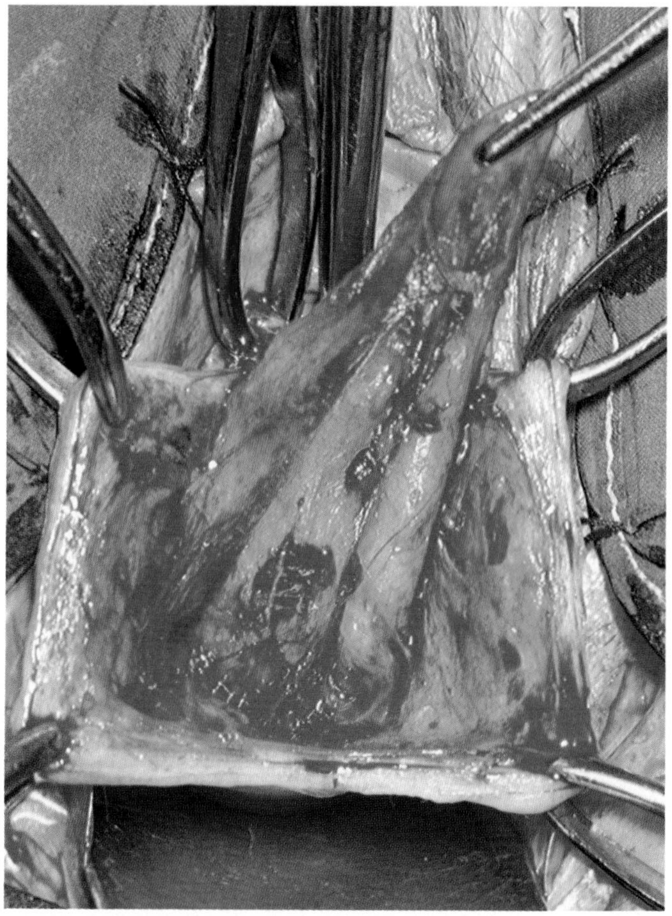

11

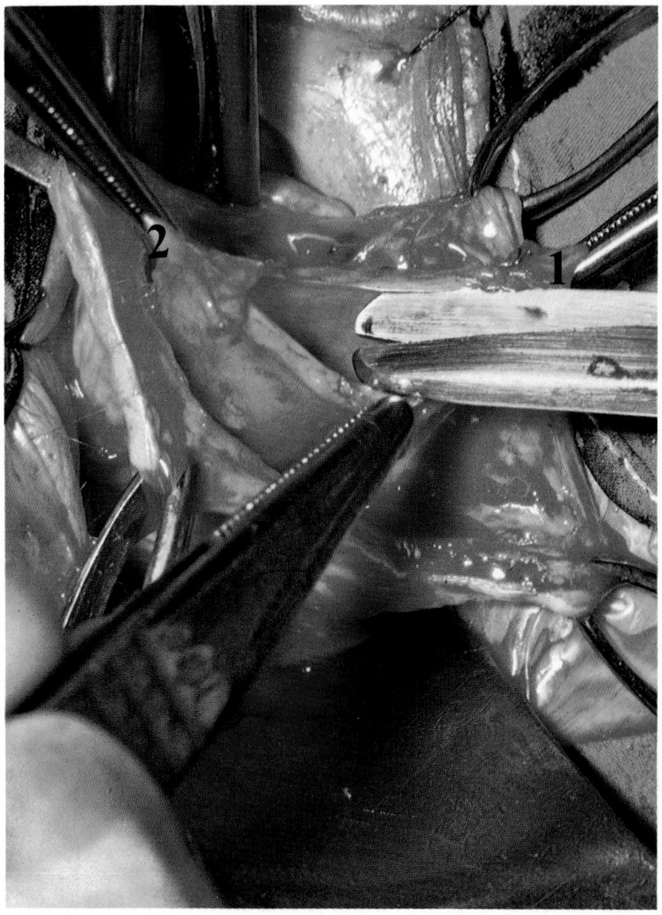

10 and 11 Opening enterocele sac

The sac is covered by fat and areolar tissue and is seen to be quite capacious. It has a broad base and the medial borders of the utero-sacral ligaments are pushed well laterally as indicated in the diagram. In **10** the sac has been grasped at its left apex by tissue forceps (1). In **11** the right apex of the sac has been grasped by tissue forceps (2). With these forceps in place and demarcating the apex of the sac an incision is made into it by scissors. This incision has been enlarged in the photograph. The dissecting forceps hold the sac open by its posterior margin.

1 to 4 Holding forceps on edge of sac
5 Left utero-sacral ligament outlined
6 Vaginal skin edge

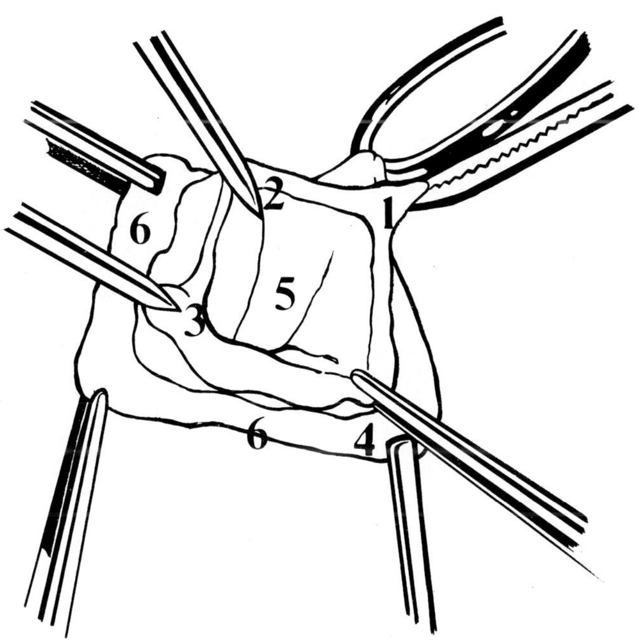

12

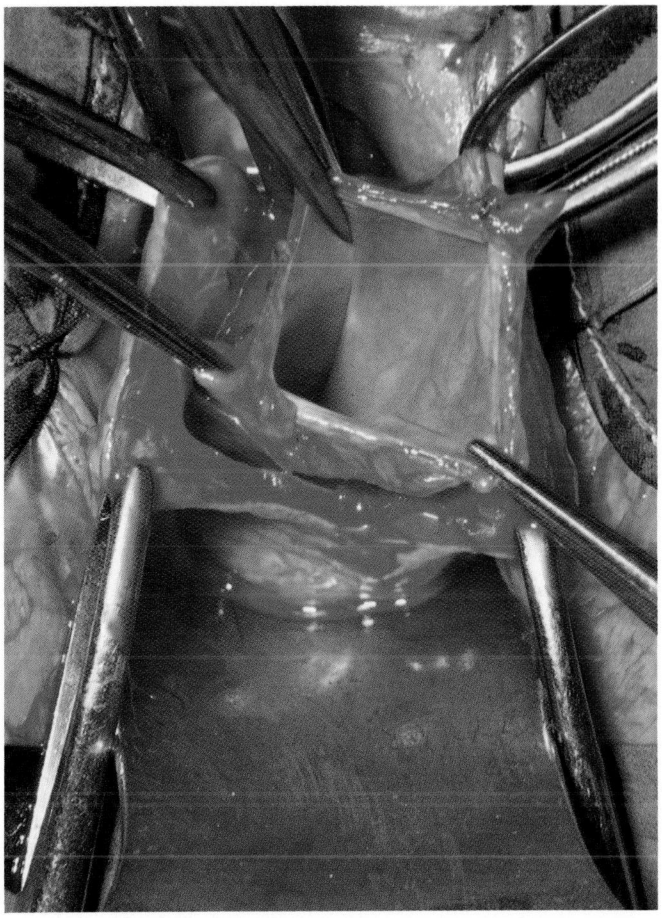

13

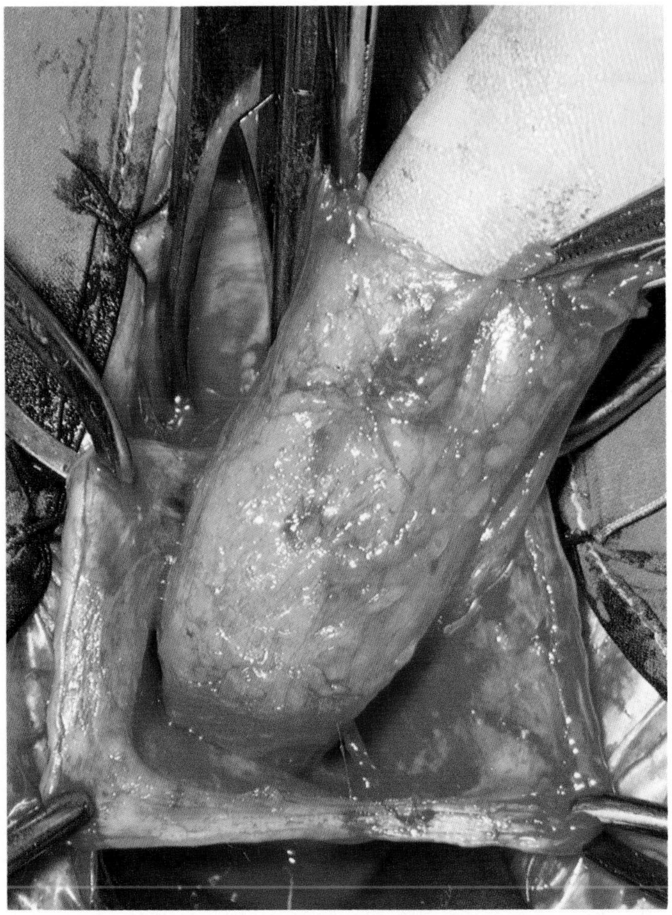

12 Interior view of sac

The margins of the opened hernial sac are now held by four tissue forceps (1), (2), (3) and (4) and the peritoneum is seen clearly. The contents have fallen back into the peritoneal cavity and the width of the neck of the sac is apparent. The left utero-sacral ligament can actually be seen as a ridge under the peritoneal surface.

13 Isolation of enterocele sac

In all herniae it is very important that the peritoneal sac be isolated as high as possible so that when ligated there is no dimple or pouch internally to serve as the leading point of a further protrusion. General surgeons believe that this aspect is really more important than subsequently closing the hernial orifice. In the photograph, the right index finger is inserted into the opened sac as into a glove and dissection is continued upwards against the finger. The adherent fine extraperitoneal fat is clearly seen on the sac.

14

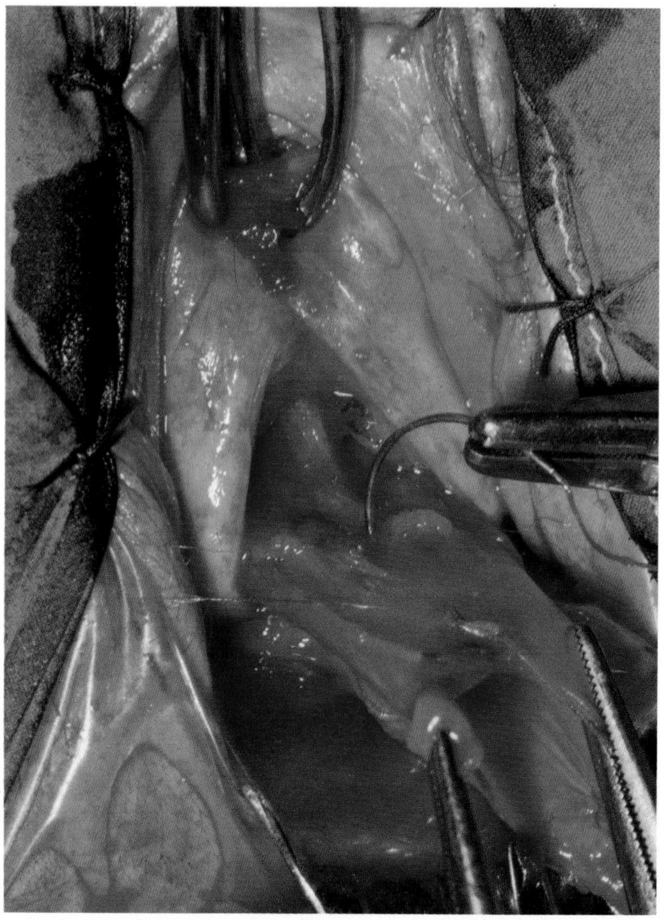

15

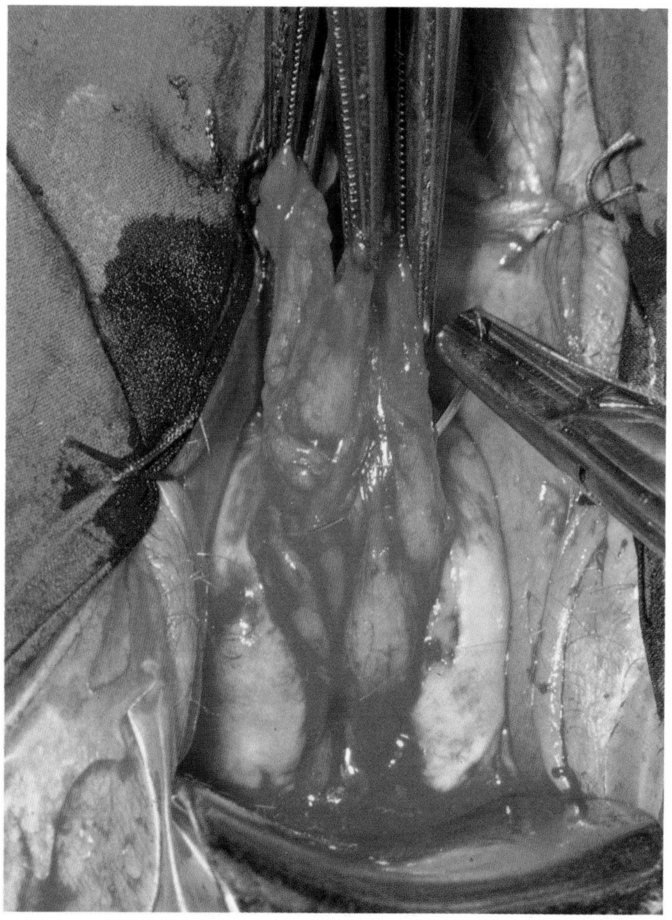

16

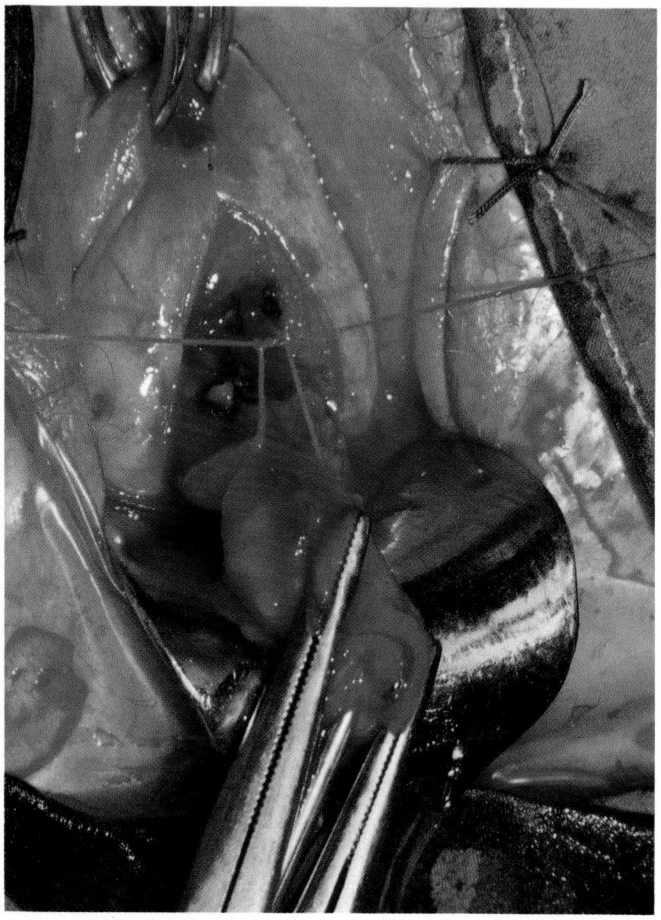

14 and 15 Transfixion of enterocele sac

The mouth of the sac is held open by the assistant using the attached forceps and under direct vision the surgeon transfixes the sac at its neck or as high up as possible and making sure that no abdominal contents are caught up or endangered. In **14** a round-bodied needle carrying a PGA No. 0 suture is piercing the sac from the anterior aspect and in **15** it is seen emerging posteriorly.

16 and 17 Ligation of enterocele sac

The first hitch tied anteriorly closes half the area of the opening and as the ends are brought round and tied posteriorly, this closes the gap completely. The two steps are shown in figures **16** and **17** respectively.

17

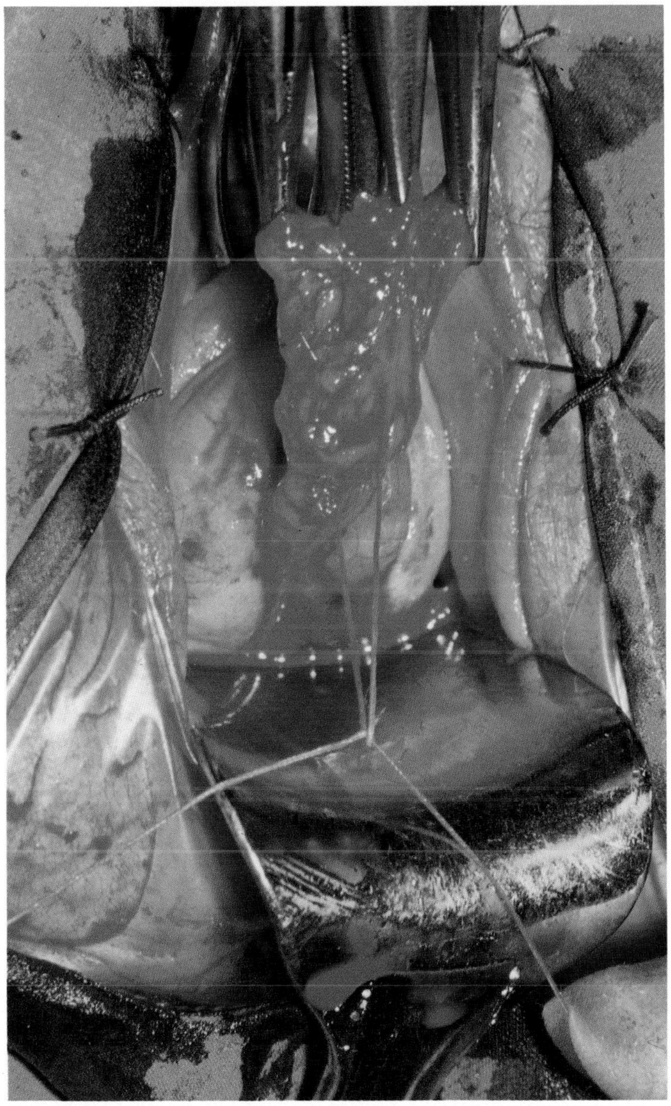

18

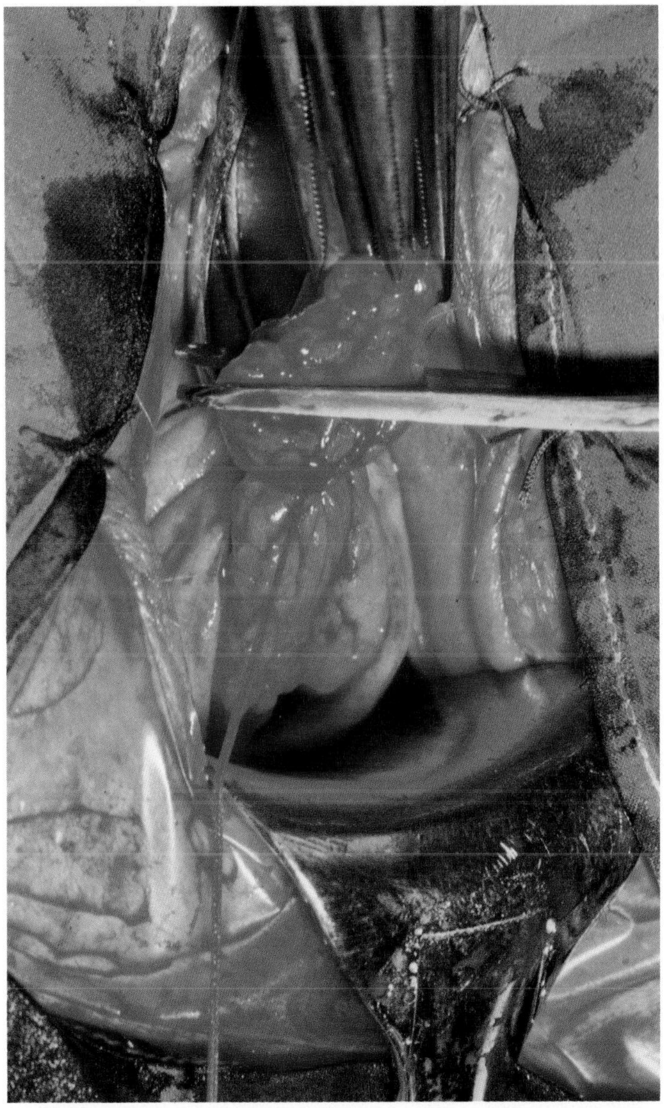

18 and 19 Trimming and replacing the enterocele sac

The excess tissue beyond the ligature is seen being trimmed off with scissors in **18**. The stump should not be too short in case the ligature should slip off. With this done and the ligating suture cut short, the sac is pushed up into the pelvis between the utero-sacral ligaments with forceps (1) as shown in **19**.

19

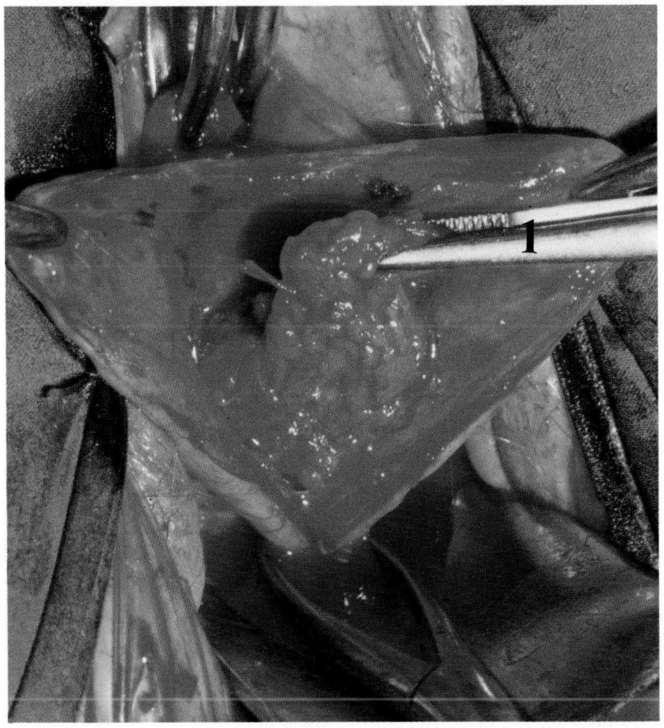

Stage 2: Closure of vault defect

Attention is now directed towards repairing or closing the hernial defect – in this case the pouch of Douglas or space between the utero-sacral ligaments. As the sac is dissected up and tied off, the medial borders of the utero-sacral ligaments are recognised on each side. They are lying too far laterally and are lax, although intact and composed of strong fibrous and muscular tissue. The main requirement at this stage of the operation is to stitch them together over the closed enterocele sac to give good vault support and prevent recurrence.

20

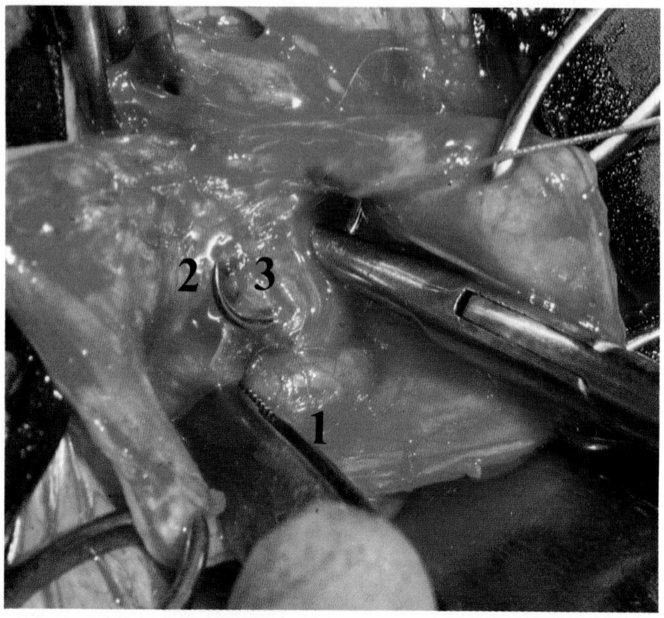

22

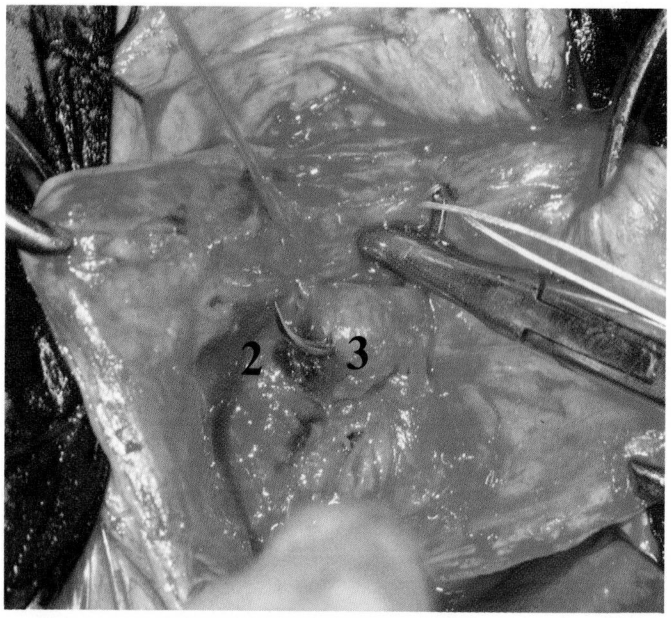

21

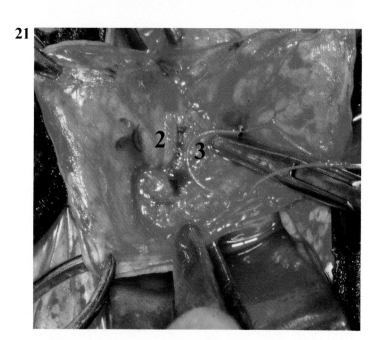

23

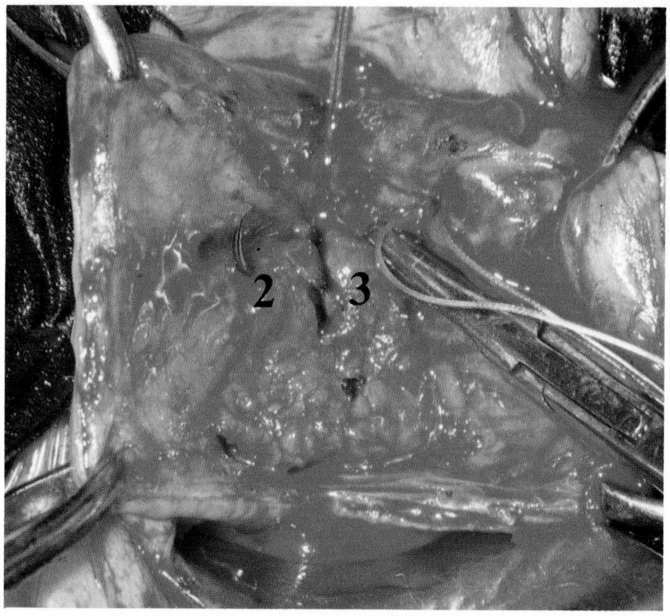

20 and 21 Approximation of utero-sacral ligaments (i)
The first stitch in this approximation is shown being placed. A short, rather stubby round-bodied needle carries PGA No. 1 suture and a series of interrupted stitches are inserted. In **20**, the dissecting forceps (1) hold the stump of the sac and pushes it up into the pelvis between the utero-sacral ligaments (2) and (3), whilst the needle picks up the left ligament with a good deep bite of tissue. In **21** the stump has now disappeared above the approximated ligaments and the right utero-sacral ligament has also been caught in the needle.

22 and 23 Approximation of utero-sacral ligaments (ii)
The process continues with the insertion of the second stitch, whilst the long ends of the first suture are held up. In **22** the left utero-sacral ligament is caught up on the needle and in **23** the right one. The tied off sac is almost directly beneath this second stitch and the edges of the utero-sacral ligaments are seen standing out quite clearly.

24

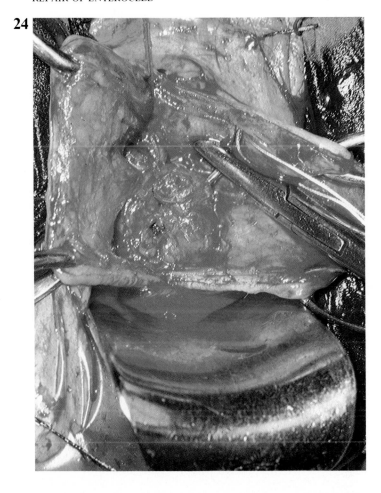

25

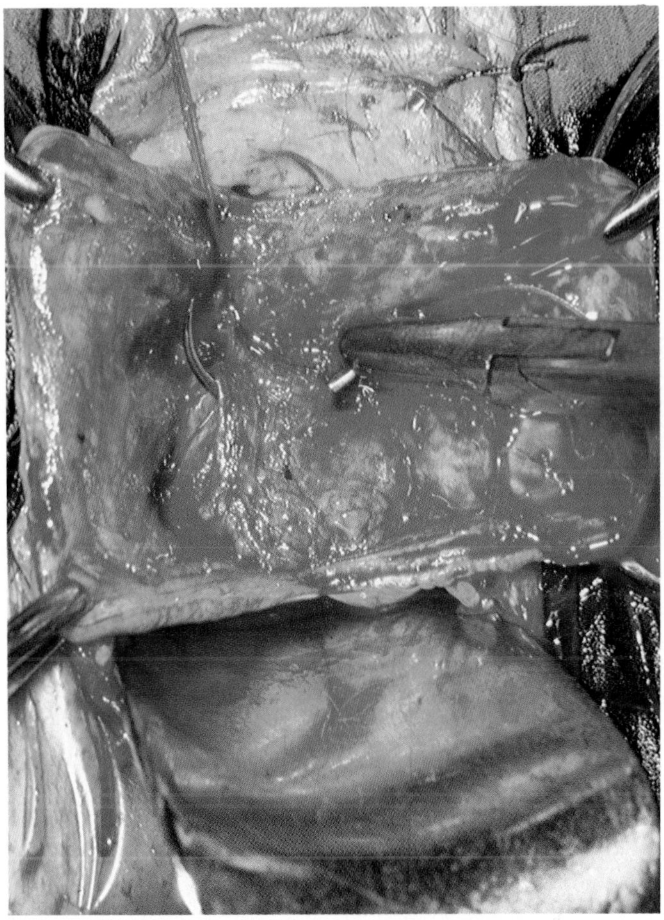

26

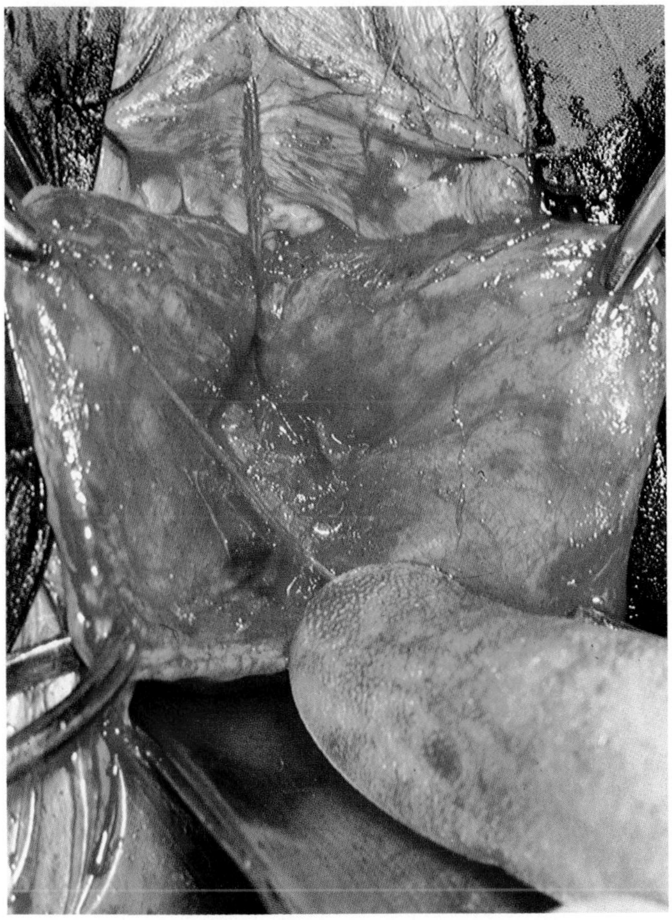

24 and 25 Approximation of utero-sacral ligaments (iii)

A further stage of approximation is shown with the left (**24**) and then the right utero-sacral ligament (**25**) transfixed. Three or four such sutures are usually required.

26 Approximation of utero-sacral ligaments completed

The final suture is seen being tied and any defect or opening between the utero-sacral ligaments has now been closed. The amount of skin looks excessive at this stage but it must be remembered that the upper vagina is very capacious and the appearance alters dramatically when the posterior vaginal wall retracts upwards and backwards to its natural position.

27

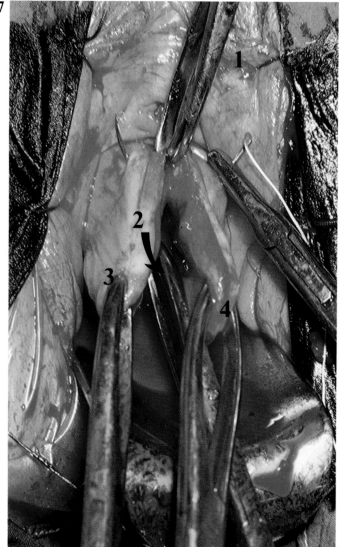

28

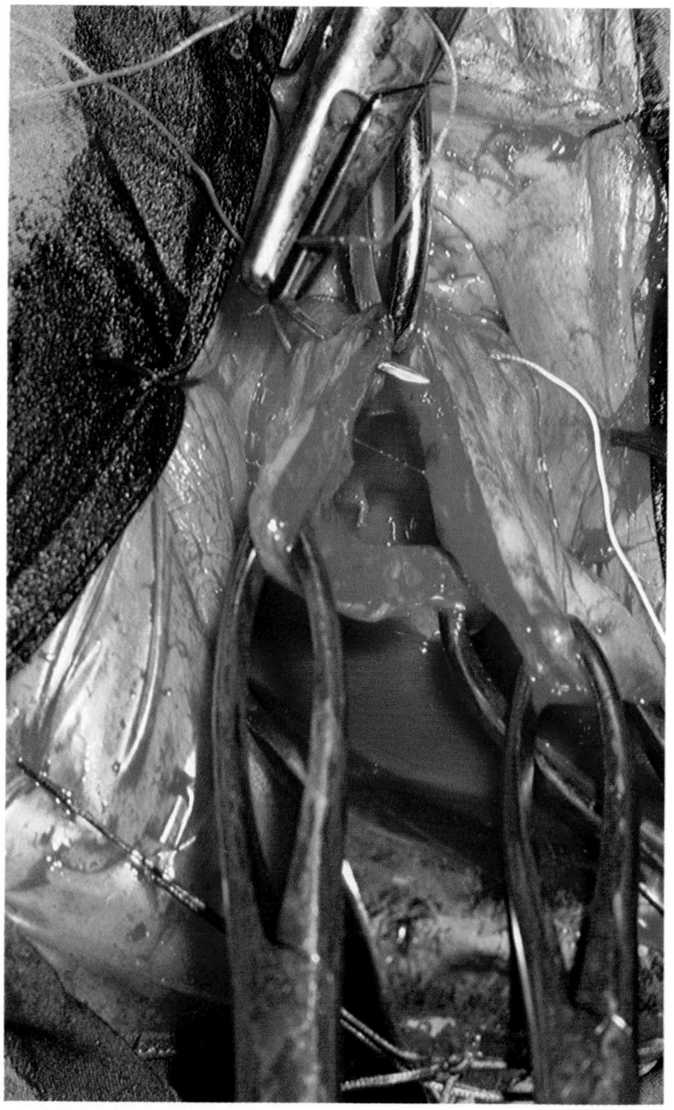

27 Closure of vaginal skin (i)

The upper end of the vertical incision is held in forceps (1), the lower end by forceps (2) and each lateral skin edge by forceps (3) and (4). The first stitch is being placed, and placed deeply to absorb some of the lax skin and to obliterate underlying dead space over the approximated utero-sacral ligaments.

28 Closure of vaginal skin (ii)

Vertical mattress sutures are used routinely for such cases and the needle is seen negotiating the skin edges. Note how the skin flaps are already receding into the upper posterior vault and closing up to the utero-sacral ligaments seen just underneath.

29

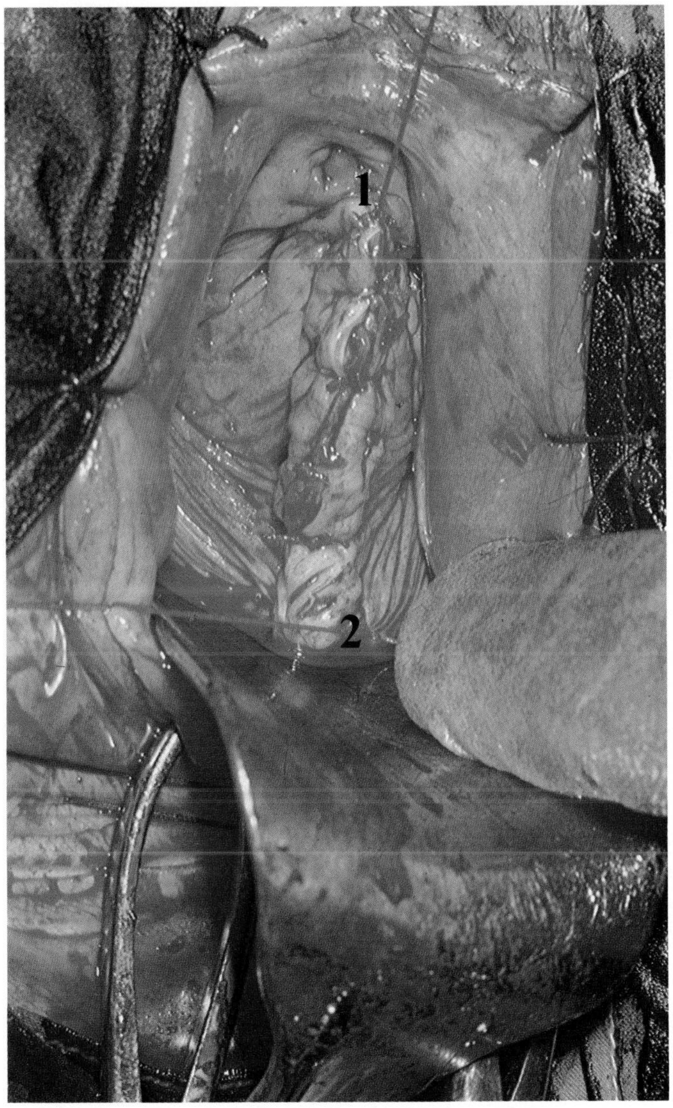

30

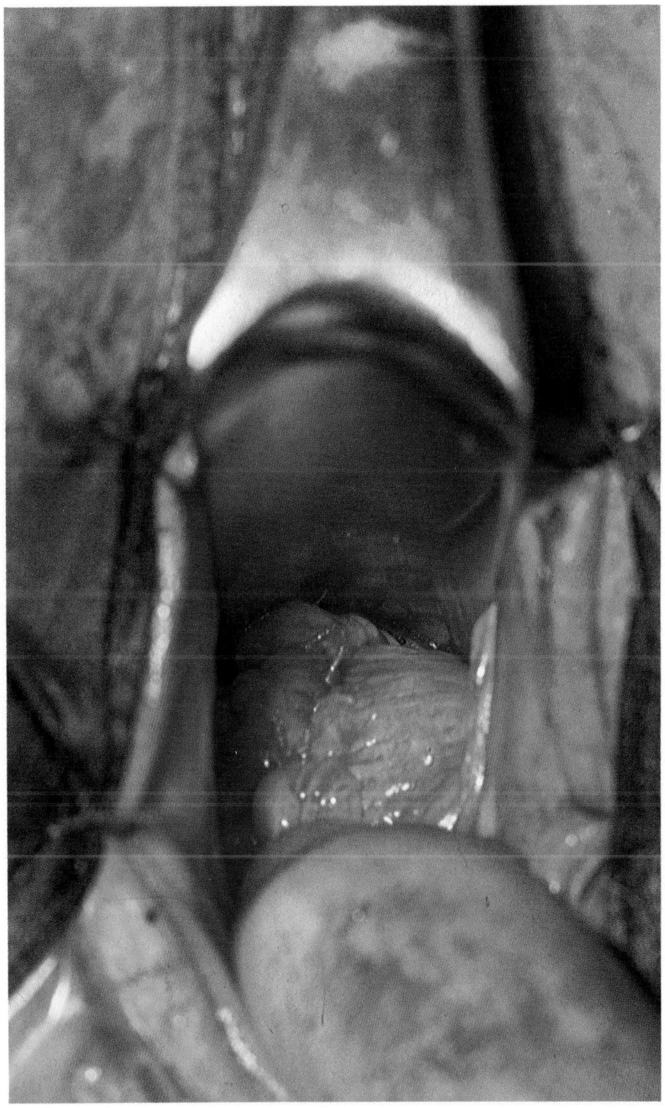

29 Closure of vaginal skin completed

The final stitch is being tied and the line of the incision is made prominent between the first stitch (1) and that being tied (2). When the sutures are cut the whole posterior wall will fall back into place revealing an adequate vault space with the skin closely applied to the underlying structures. No skin has been removed, emphasising again that to have done so would have resulted in a cone-shaped vault space.

30 General appearance post-operatively

The episiotomy has been repaired, the anterior vaginal wall is retracted from above and the flat upper posterior vaginal wall covering the obliterated enterocele is seen above the forefinger, which is retracting the perineum.

7: Repair of rectocele

Rectocele is an almost invariable concomitant of cystocele and vault prolapse and a plastic repair operation is generally assumed to include a posterior colpo-perineorrhaphy. This latter is not particularly easy and unless anatomical considerations are carefully observed there is a distinct tendency for the bulging rectum to reassert itself, although generally concealed behind a narrowed introitus which itself may cause coital difficulties and dyspareunia. Because such developments sometimes occur the need for a posterior repair in the first place has been questioned by some authors. The mere mention of such doubts has unfortunately led to the procedure being omitted in many cases where it should have been done. For these reasons one frequently sees patients, many of them overweight, with severe low rectocele. Some are straightforward cases of recurrent rectocele following operation; others did not have the benefit of a posterior repair when the operation was done.

The principles of treatment are based on the anatomy of the area. The rectum is invested anteriorly and laterally by a continuous layer of fascia described as the pre-rectal fascia. This layer corresponds to the pubocervical fascia anteriorly and in the same way it is found to be disrupted and deficient where there is a major degree of rectocele. Away from the mid-line the layer is continuous and intact and especially where it supports the rectum laterally as the para-rectal fascia. Just as a cystocele is covered only by anterior vaginal wall skin so is rectocele covered only by posterior vaginal wall skin. It is necessary to incise and reflect the vaginal skin so that the pre-rectal fascia can be recognised and followed laterally till an intact edge is displayed on each side. The two edges of the fascia are then approximated in the mid-line to support the rectum and the skin is subsequently closed over it. The rectocele may be accompanied by a deficiency of the perineum or if recurrent by a thin barrier of skin with no underlying muscle support in the area of the fourchette. In either case the defect should be dealt with when repairing the rectocele.

There is one other important matter when operating on these cases. The appearances suggest a considerable excess of skin and this can be misleading. The mistake of removing too much is irremediable so that it is essential to leave such decisions until closure of the Skin layer is imminent. This point is discussed in detail in the text.

1

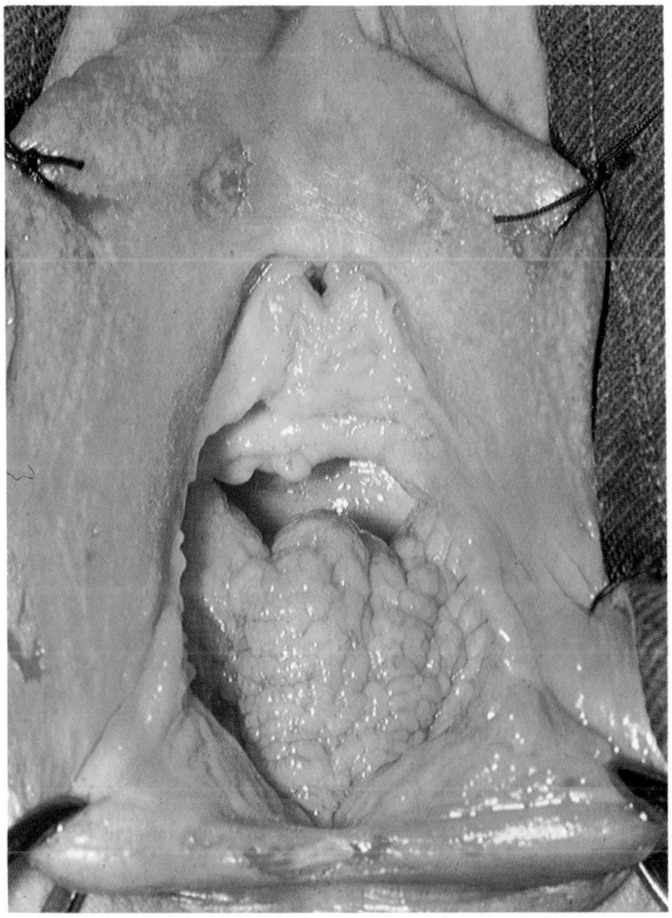

2

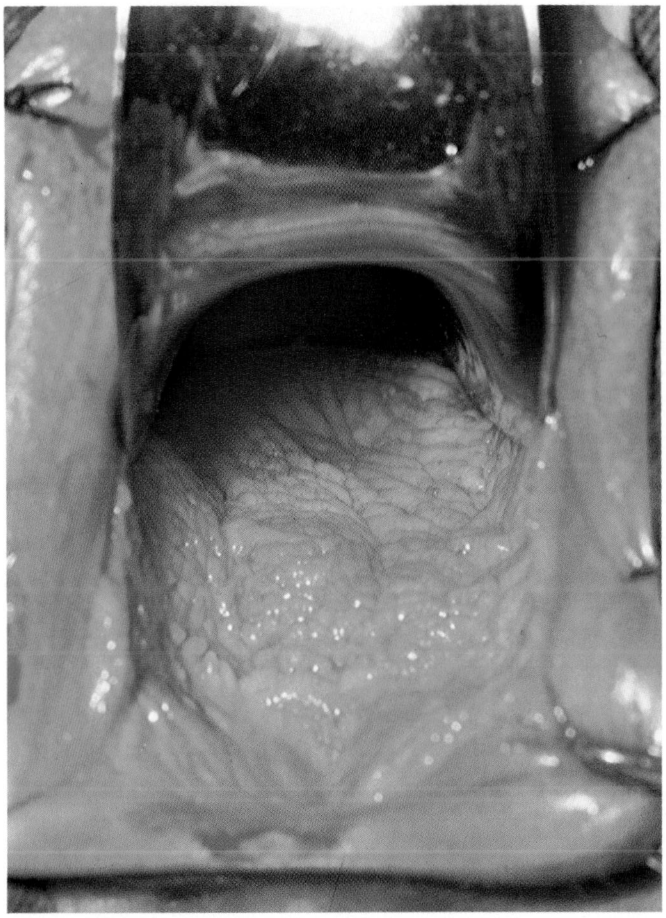

3

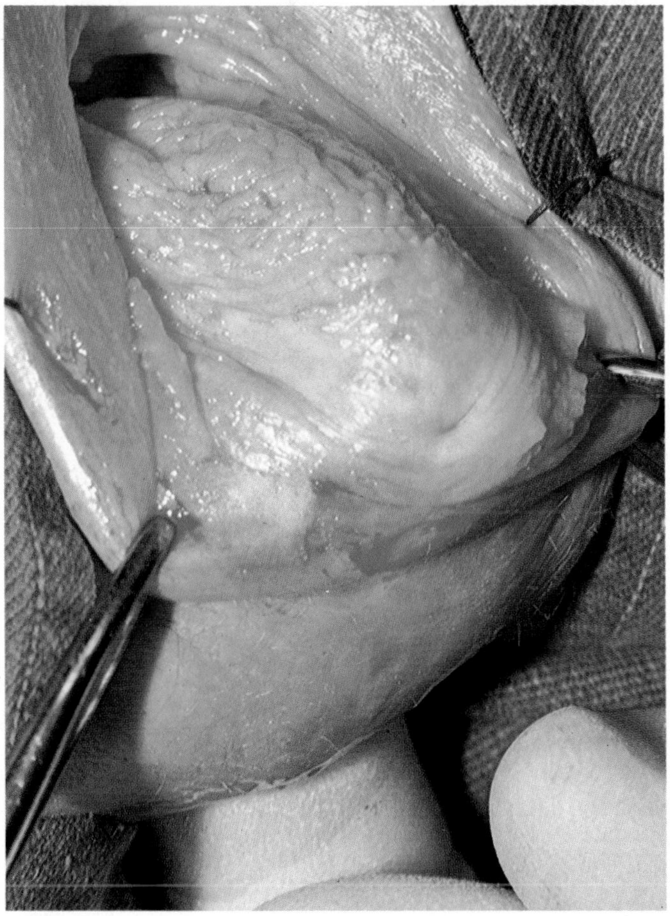

1–3 General appearance pre-operatively

In **1** and **2** the lax posterior vaginal wall is obvious and also the accompanying perineal deficiency. In **3** the finger has been put in the rectum and when pushed forward the defect is very obvious.

Stage 1: Definition of defect (pre-rectal fascia)

4

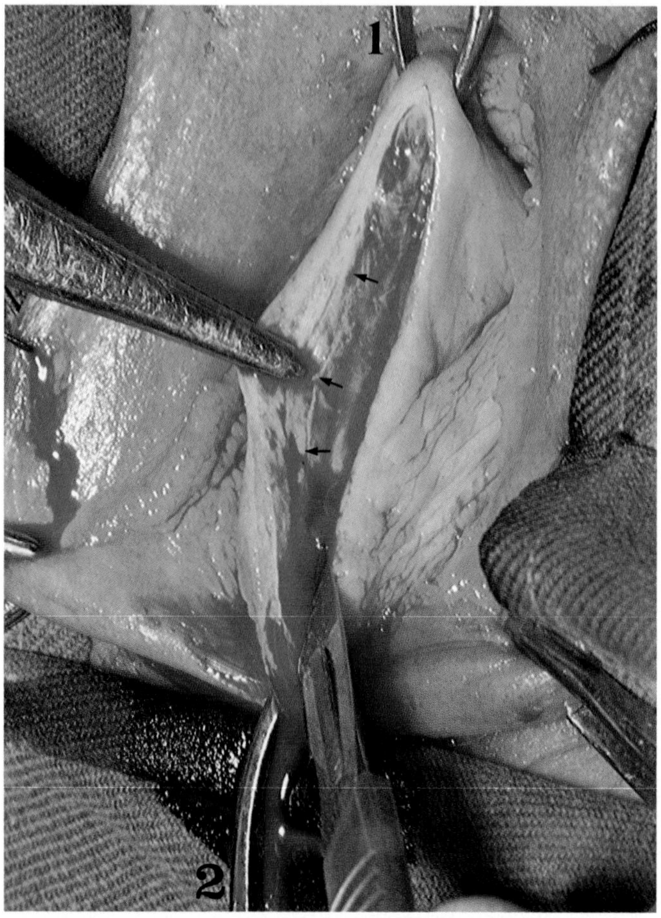

5

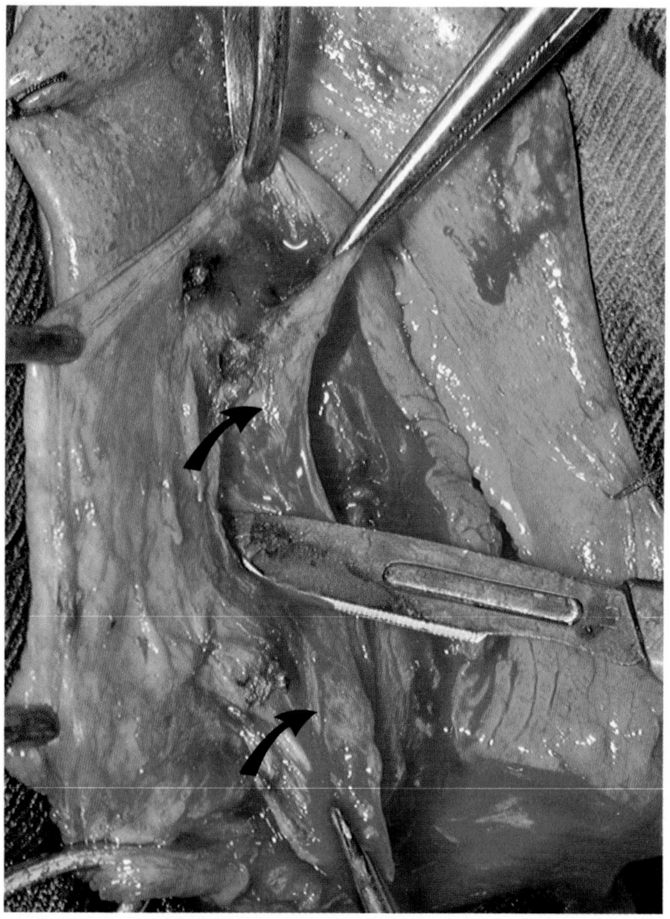

6

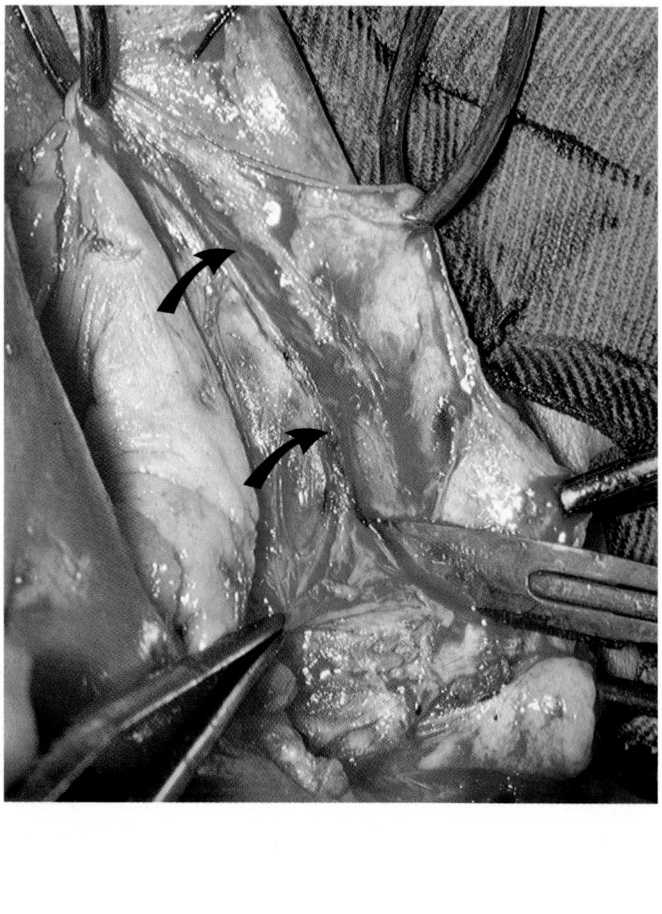

4 Posterior vaginal wall incision

It is wise to make a mid-line incision in these cases because it is not possible to predict how much excess skin there will be. The incision goes through the skin and into the thin pre-rectal fascia beneath. The vaginal wall is held up by the Littlewood's forceps (1) and (2) and there is no fear of cutting the rectum as it is loosely attached and falls away from the stretched skin.

The small arrows indicate the attenuated pre-rectal fascia.

5 Dissection of pre-rectal fascia (right side)

The thin layer of pre-rectal fascia is separated off the vaginal skin by sharp dissection in the first place because they are closely adherent. As dissection proceeds laterally a tissue space is found between them and blunt dissection becomes possible. In the photograph this stage has just been reached and the developing fascial plane can be seen, as arrowed.

The vaginal skin is held back laterally by two Littlewood's forceps.

6 Dissection of pre-rectal fascia (left side)

The same procedure is followed as on the right side. In this instance the fascial planes are more apparent and dissection is easier. Arrows again indicate the fascial edge.

7

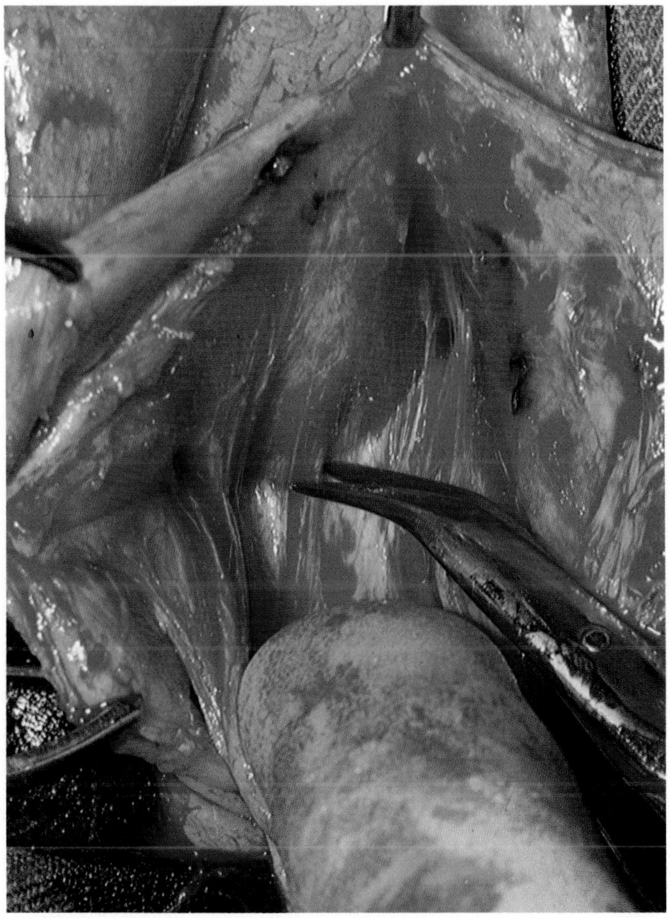

8

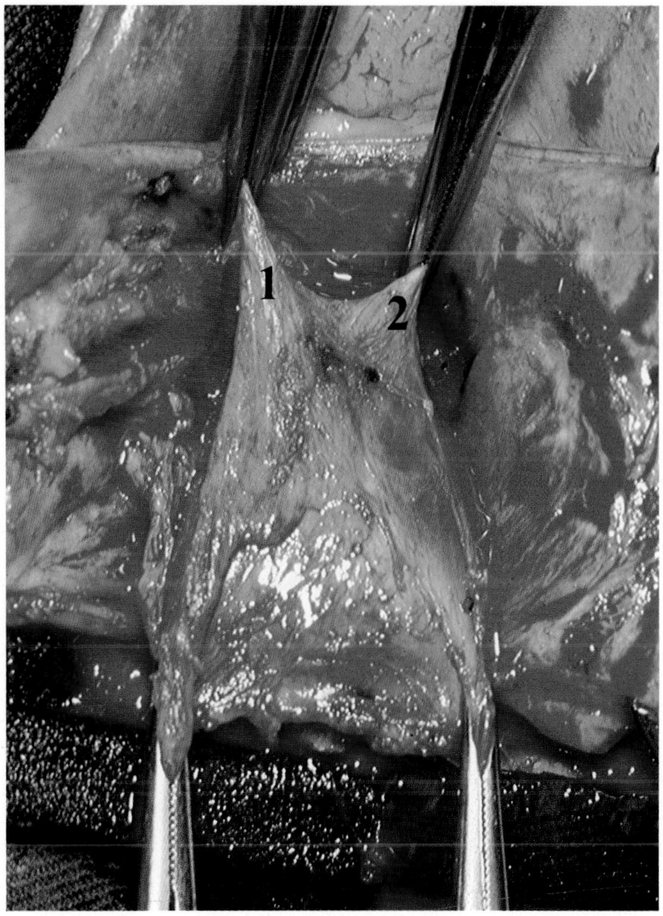

9

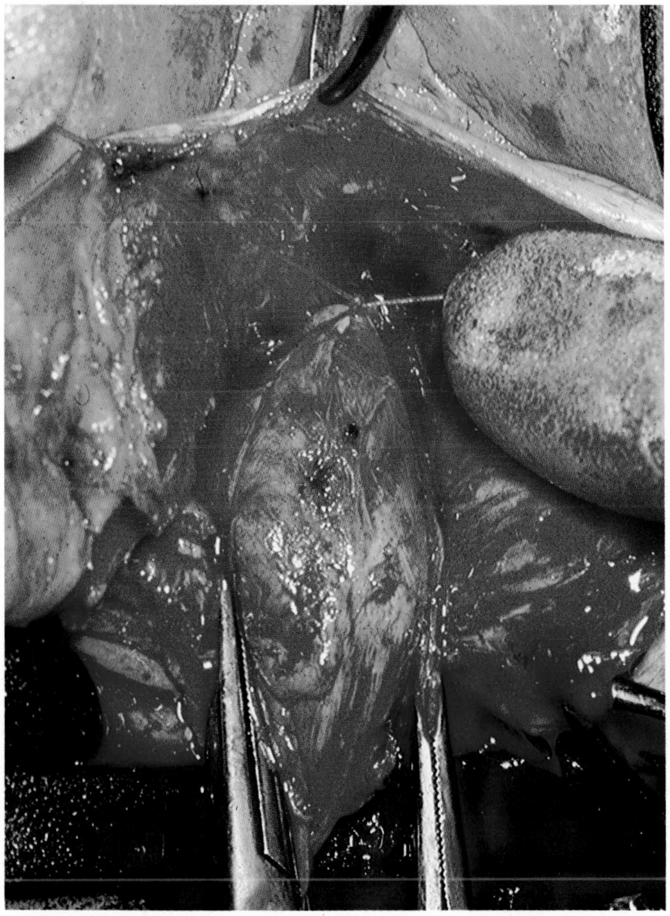

7 Freeing rectum from posterior vaginal wall

Having defined the layers of pre-rectal fascia the next step is to ensure that the rectum itself is dissected clear and able to be retroposed in preparation for the stitching together of the pre-rectal fascia. The scissors are being used to divide the loose attachments towards this end.

8 Demonstration of pre-rectal fascia

The relationship of the pre-rectal fascia on each side to the rectum medially and to the surrounding structures is shown. Each layer is held taut between two pairs of forceps. The next step of the operation will be to approximate the pre-rectal fascial edges over the rectum. Numbers (1) and (2) indicate the points at which the needle will pick up the two edges of fascia.

Stage 2: Repair of defect

9 Approximation of pre-rectal fascia layers (i)

The suturing together of the edges of the two layers has commenced and the first stitch is being tied.

10

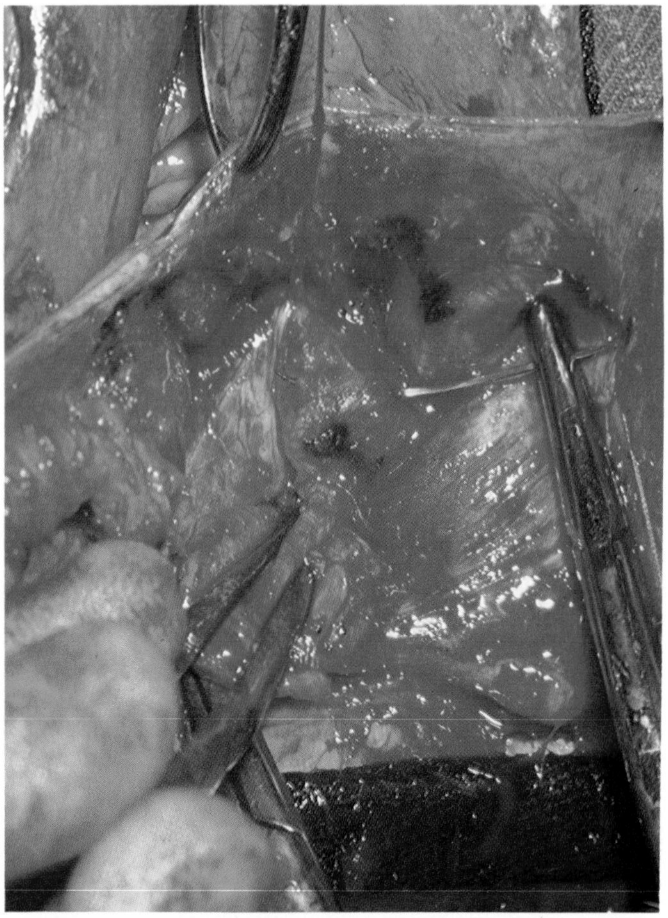

11

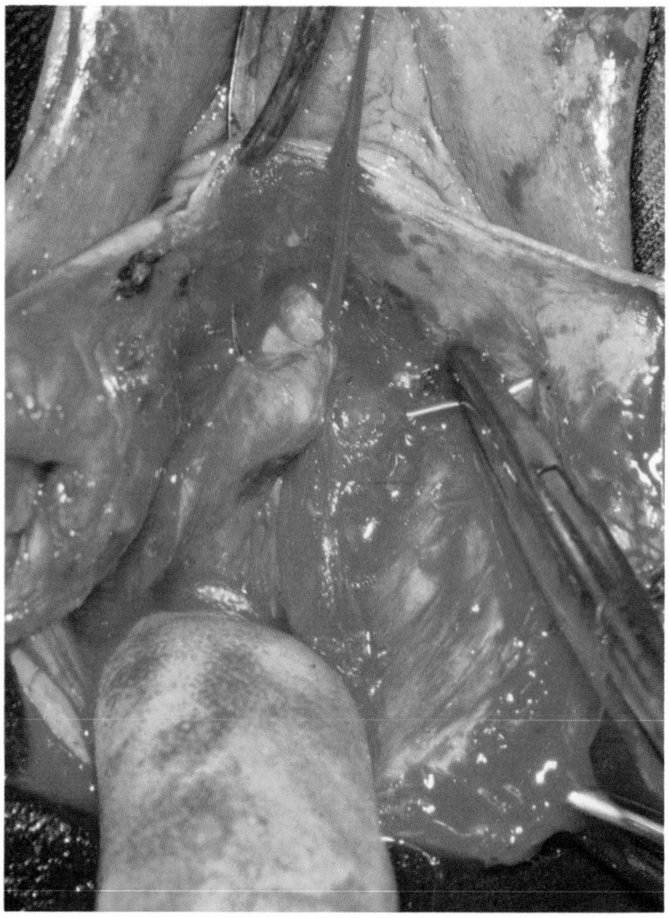

12

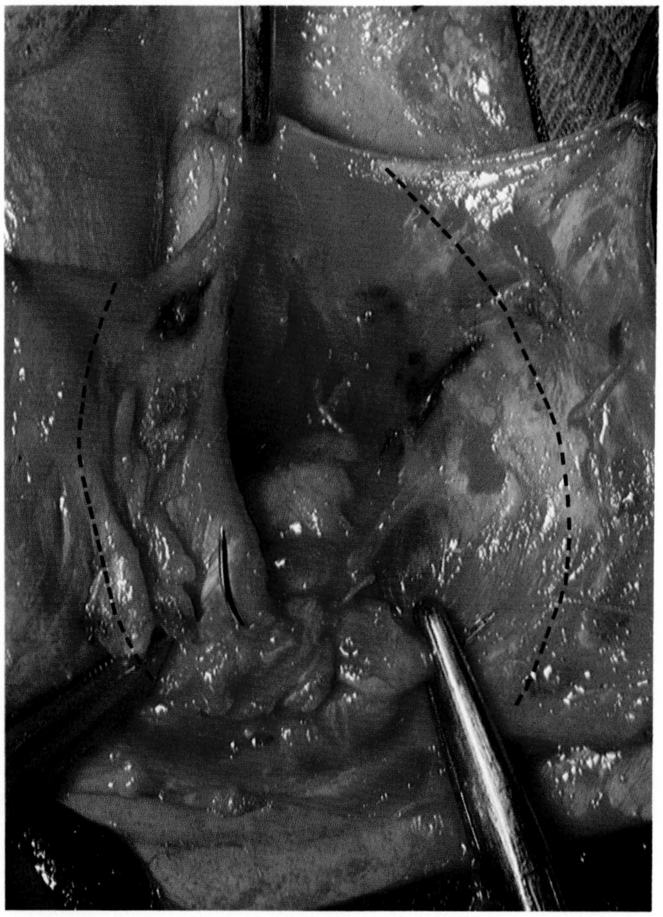

10 and 11 Approximation of pre-rectal fascial layers (ii)

In **10** the edge of the pre-rectal fascial layer on the left side has been picked up on the needle, and in **11** the needle is emerging from the right pre-rectal fascial layer.

12 Approximation of pre-rectal fascia completed

Here the fourth stitch joining the pre-rectal fascial layers is being inserted and the rectum is seen to be well supported anteriorly. The next stage will be to close the skin layer, but there is obvious redundancy and an area of skin will have to be removed from each side. The dotted lines indicate the line of incision which may be made either with the scissors or a scalpel. This is seen in the following illustration.

13

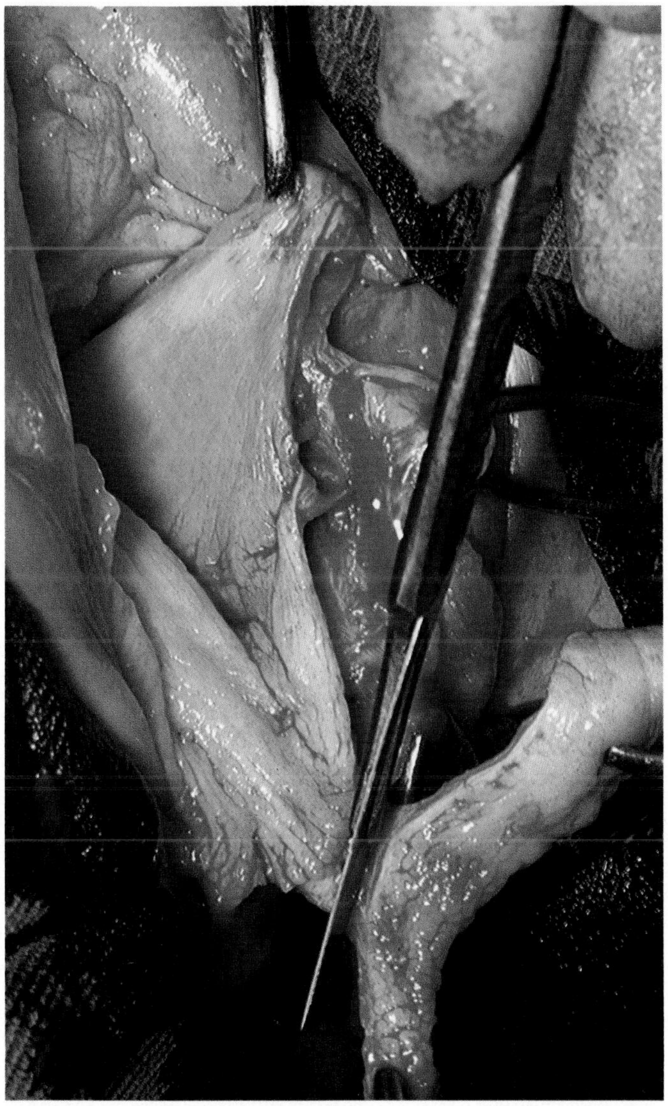

14

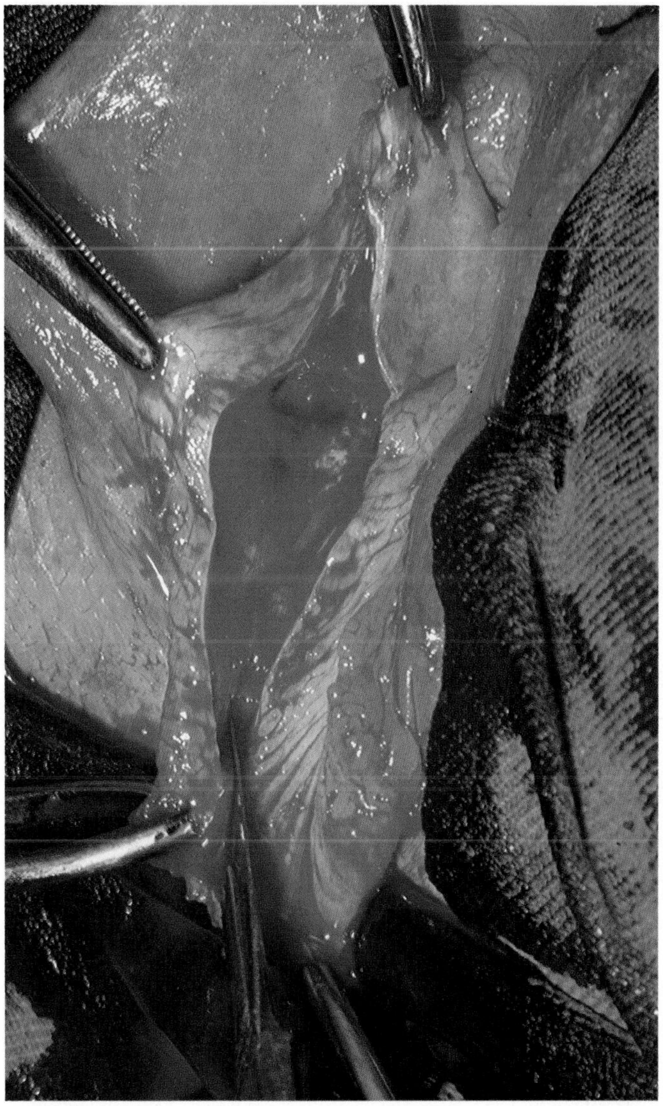

13 and 14 Excision of excess posterior vaginal wall skin

As indicated in the introduction the surgeon has to be careful not to remove too much skin and the decision is best left till this stage. With the rectum supported it is now possible to assess exactly how much skin to remove by bringing the two layers together and actually measuring the excess. In **13** the excess is being removed from the right flap with the scalpel and in **14** the same procedure is being followed on the left. It will be seen that the amount of skin removed on each side is considerably smaller than one would have expected.

15

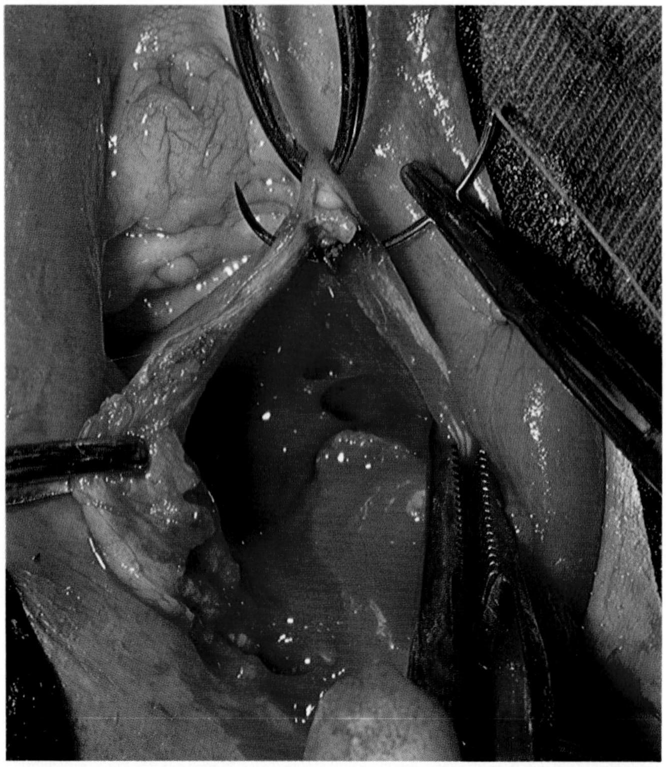

16

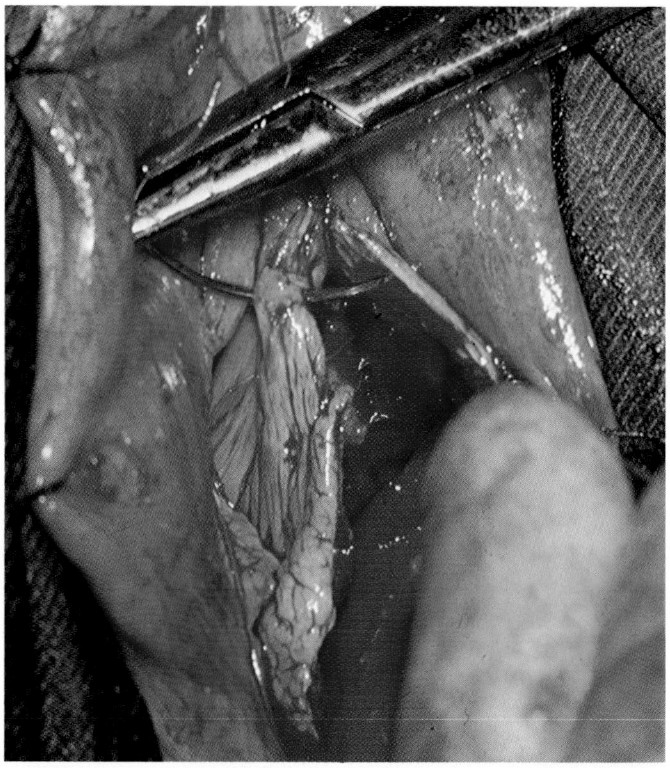

17

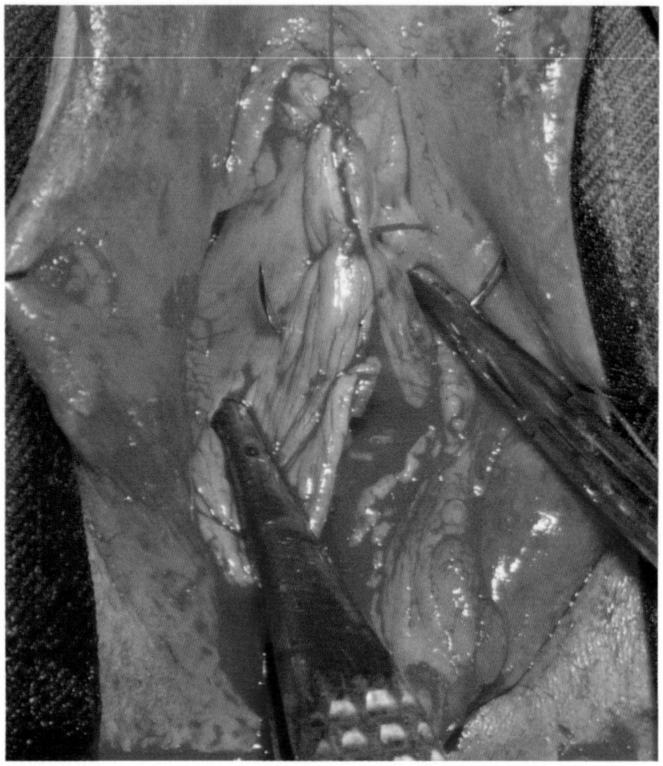

18

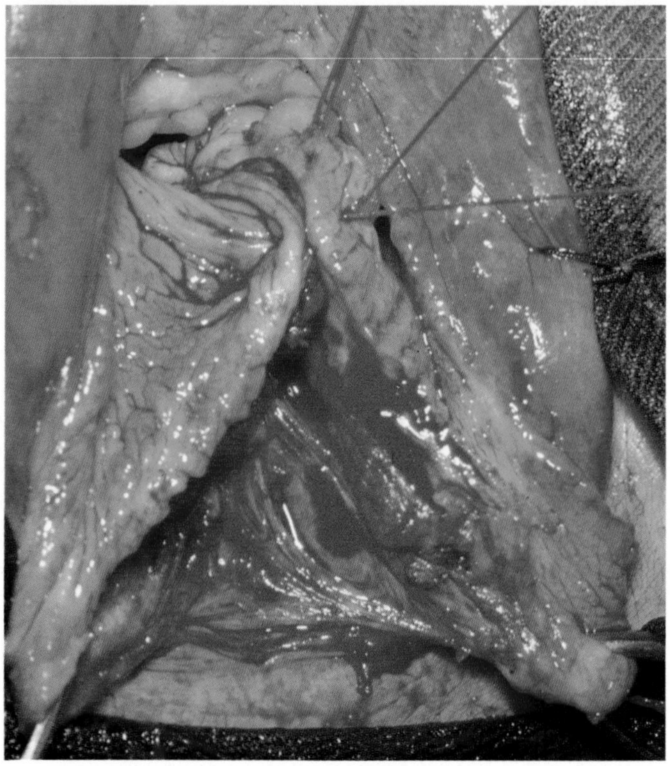

15–18 Closure of skin of posterior vaginal wall

Interrupted sutures are preferred in a case such as this and **15–18** show stages of the posterior wall closure. This has already been described in posterior colporrhaphy following the Manchester repair operation. vertical mattress sutures are used routinely. Approximately five are required and the final stitch is inserted just below the hymeneal ring.

19

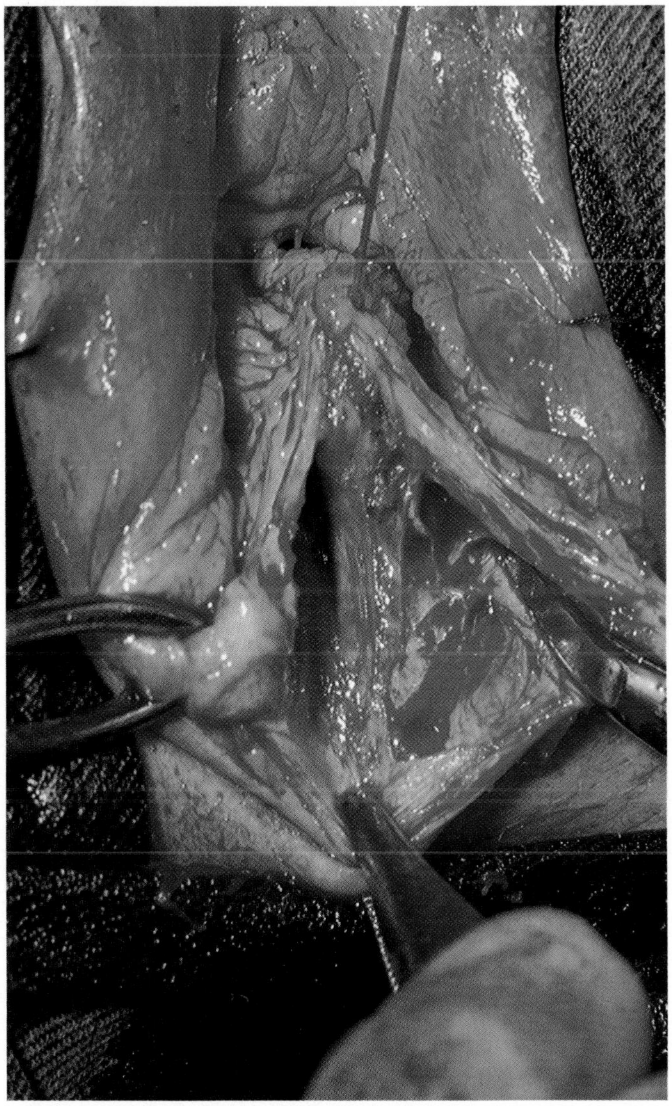

20

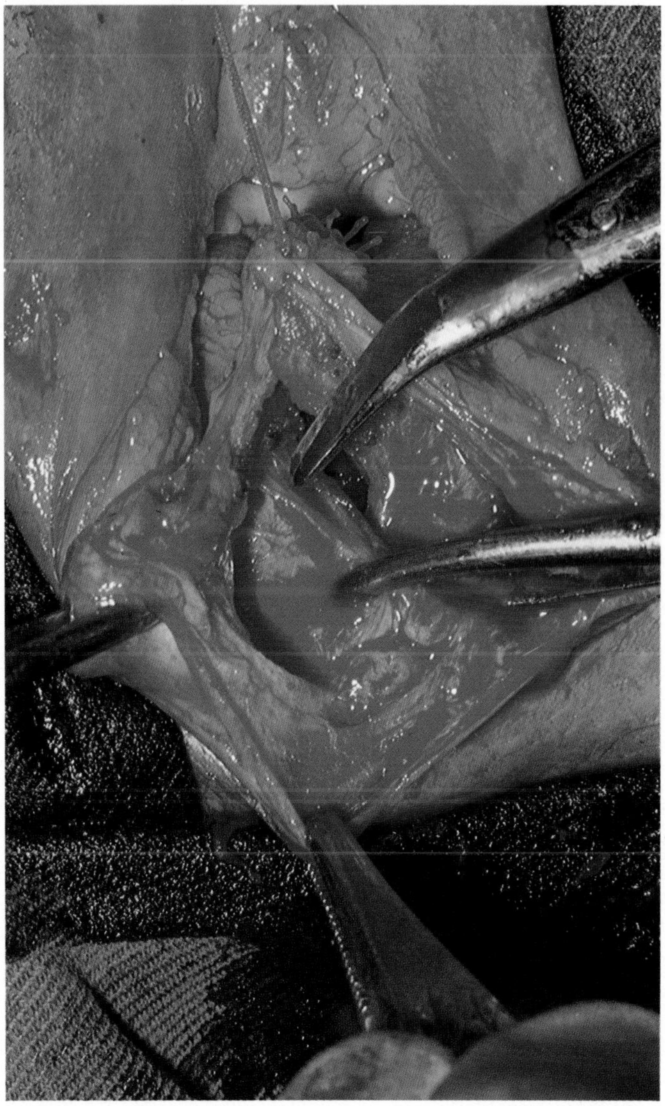

19 and 20 Definition of levator ani muscles

As explained in the introduction there is clearly always a degree of perineal deficiency due to separation of the levator muscles and the condition was quite marked in this case. In **19** the levator muscle is being separated from the overlying skin and the same procedure is being carried out on the opposite side in **20**. The separation is effected partially by sharp and partially by blunt dissection. Further details of this step are described under posterior colporrhaphy in the Manchester repair operation.

Stage 3: Perineorrhaphy

21
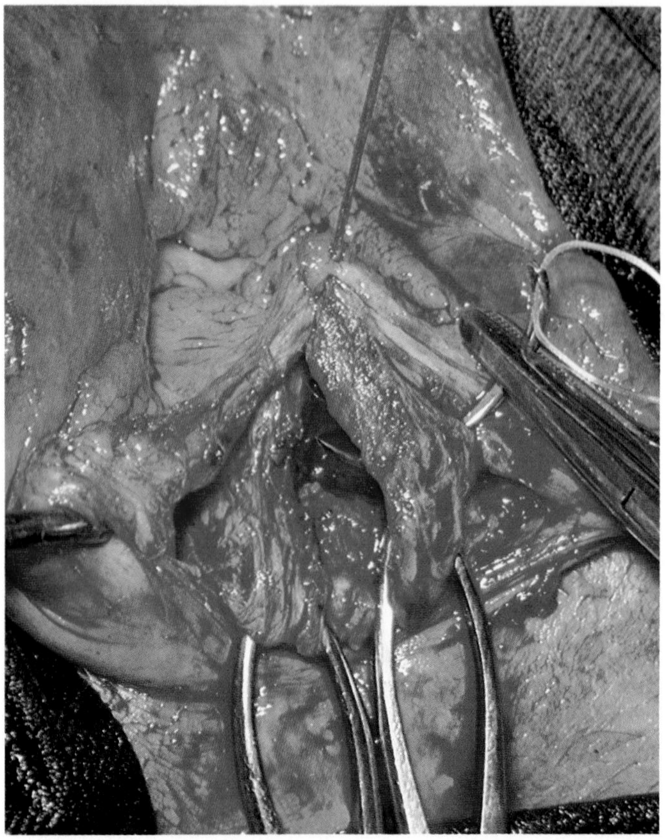

22
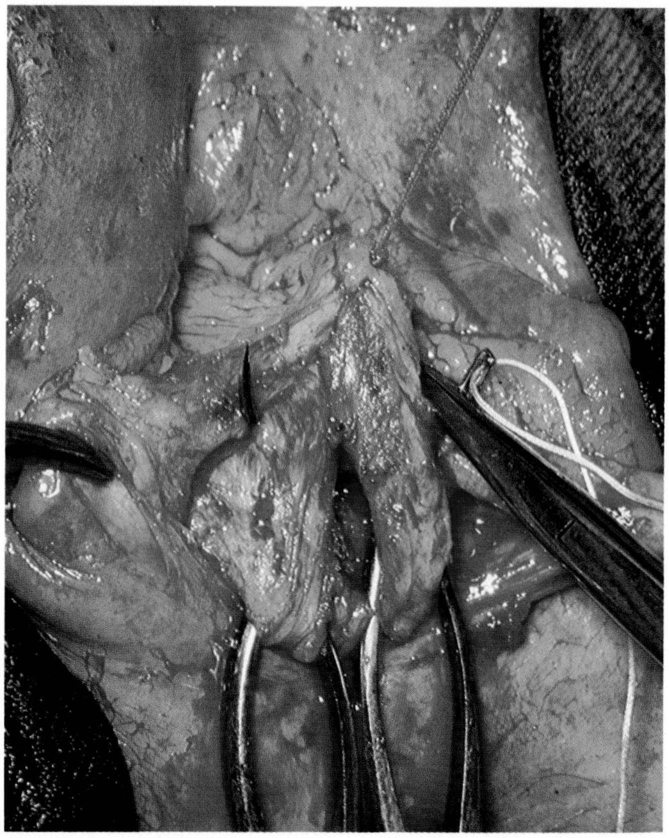

23
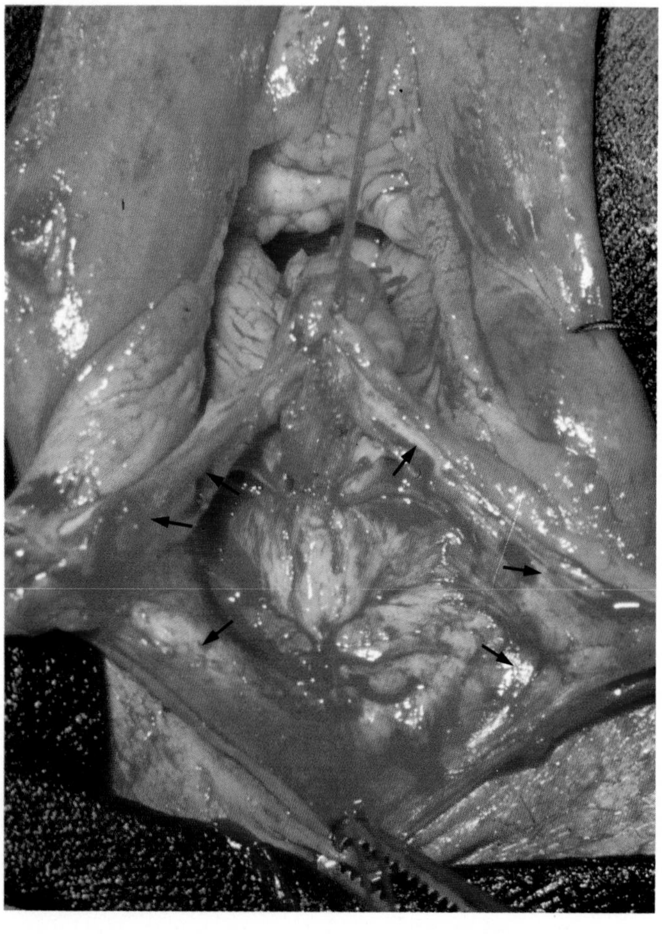

21 and 22 Approximation of levator muscles
The muscles are stitched together using PGA No. 1 suture carried on a round-bodied needle and a good bite of each levator belly is picked up by the needle.

23 Approximation of levator muscles completed
This photograph shows the muscles approximated in this case by two fairly deep sutures. Occasionally it is advisable to approximate the superficial perineal muscles over the levators (as indicated by arrows in the diagram) but that step was not considered necessary in this case.

24

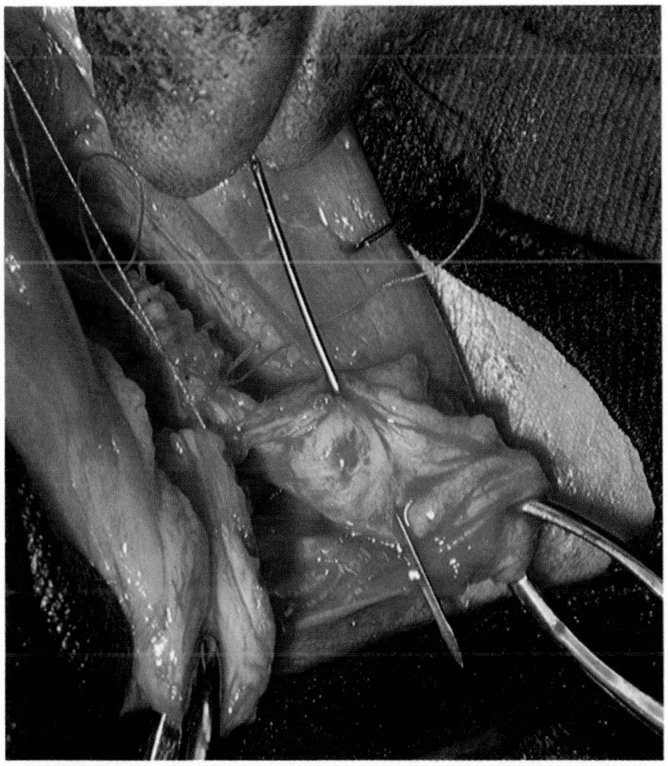

25

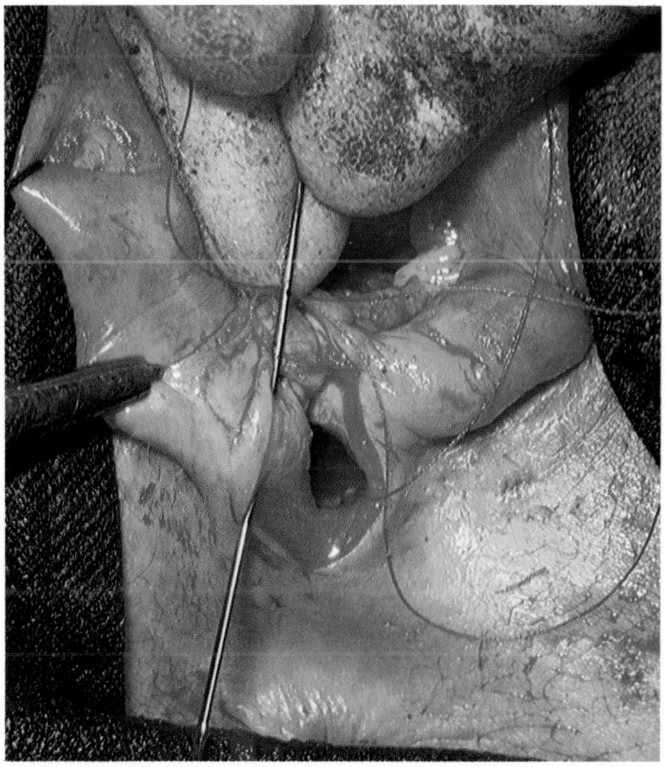

26

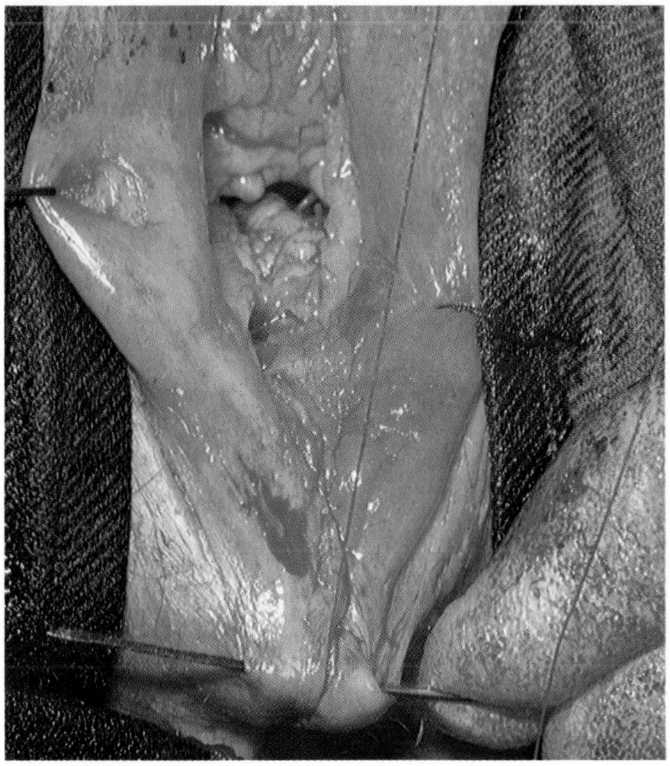

27

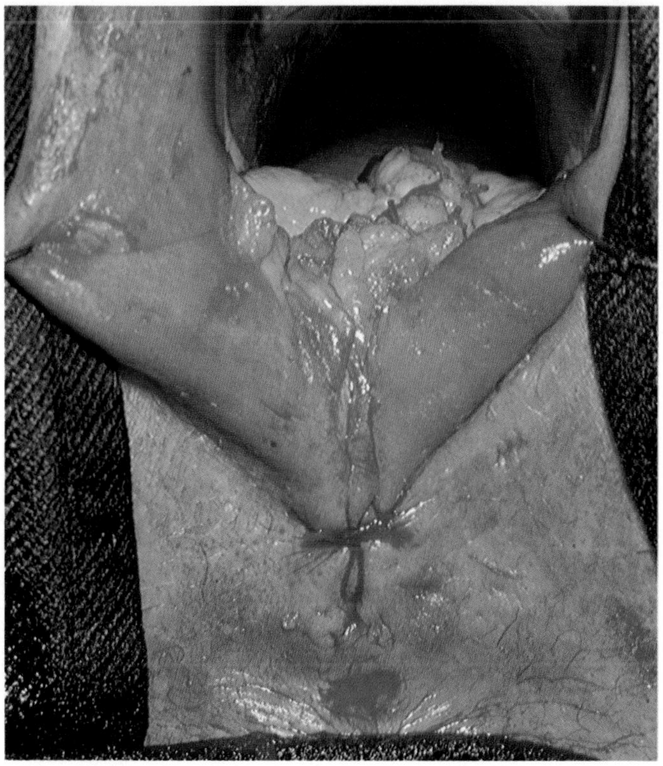

24–26 Closure of perineal skin

Three stages in the closure of the skin are shown and illustrate that the stitch is really a subcutaneous rather than a subcuticular one. With this type of skin closure there is less need to stitch the superficial perineal muscles as mentioned in the commentary to figure **23**.

27 Appearance at completion of operation

The lumen of the vagina is narrowed but is adequate, uniform, and functionally satisfactory. The perineum is shown to be well supported and skin apposition is neat and without tension.

8: Vaginal hysterectomy

Vaginal hysterectomy should be the ideal operation when hysterectomy is necessary or advisable and where there is a significant degree of utero-vaginal prolapse. It should not be used unless every possibility of malignancy in any of the pelvic organs has been excluded. It is not the method of choice if the uterus is larger than 8 to 10 weeks gestational size, or if there is any significant evidence of pelvic endometriosis. With these reservations it is the appropriate operation in a very large number of cases.

The indications have increased enormously in recent years. For instance, the younger woman who has completed her family and is seeking sterilisation frequently has a degree of utero-vaginal prolapse. She may also have heavy periods related to dysfunctional uterine bleeding which has been masked by the oral contraceptive steriods, or a uterine enlargement due to small fibroids. Women in early middle age with cervical dyskaryosis (in whom clinical cervical cancer has been excluded) or hyperplastic endometrium and some laxity of the vaginal vault are also natural candidates for the operation.

There may indeed be the risk of over-enthusiasm amongst those skilled in this form of hysterectomy, but that is counterbalanced by a sizeable proportion of gynaecologists who do not like the operation or its reputation.

It is only right to consider the latter point of view and its basis. Vaginal hysterectomy can be difficult unless selection is meticulous; bleeding can be a problem and injury to the lower urinary tract is always a possible hazard. The main criticism is the morbidity which has come to be associated with the procedure. This means pyrexia, bladder difficulties, and vault haematomata which become infected and cause a stormy post-operative course. Discharge of pus from the vaginal vault is followed up by rapid clinical recovery and all is assumed to be well, although follow-up shows that the operative support is invariably weakened where it is most needed – at the vault.

If we considered these objections valid we could not recommend the operation; in fact we do not think they are. The technical difficulties can be overcome by securing good access, using vaso-constrictive agents and following a properly planned procedure. Practically all post-operative problems and morbidity are related to inadequate haemostasis and the development of vault haematomata. Once it is recognised that the only safe control of the uterine pedicles is by definitive repeat ligation after they have had time to contract and decrease in volume, the problem is largely overcome. This will be discussed later. The use of thick catgut in considerable quantity in a limited space where the ends of the pedicles have lost their blood supply is a recipe for troubles. We have found during detailed clinical studies that the use of thin, inert, absorbable synthetic sutures reduces the risk of infection enormously.

There is rarely any indication for the routine use of antibiotics as recommended by some authors.

We shall describe the operation step by step, pointing out those areas in which post-operative and operative complications can arise and discussing points in operative technique which is used should avoid or certainly reduce their frequency.

Stage 1: Exposure of operation field

1

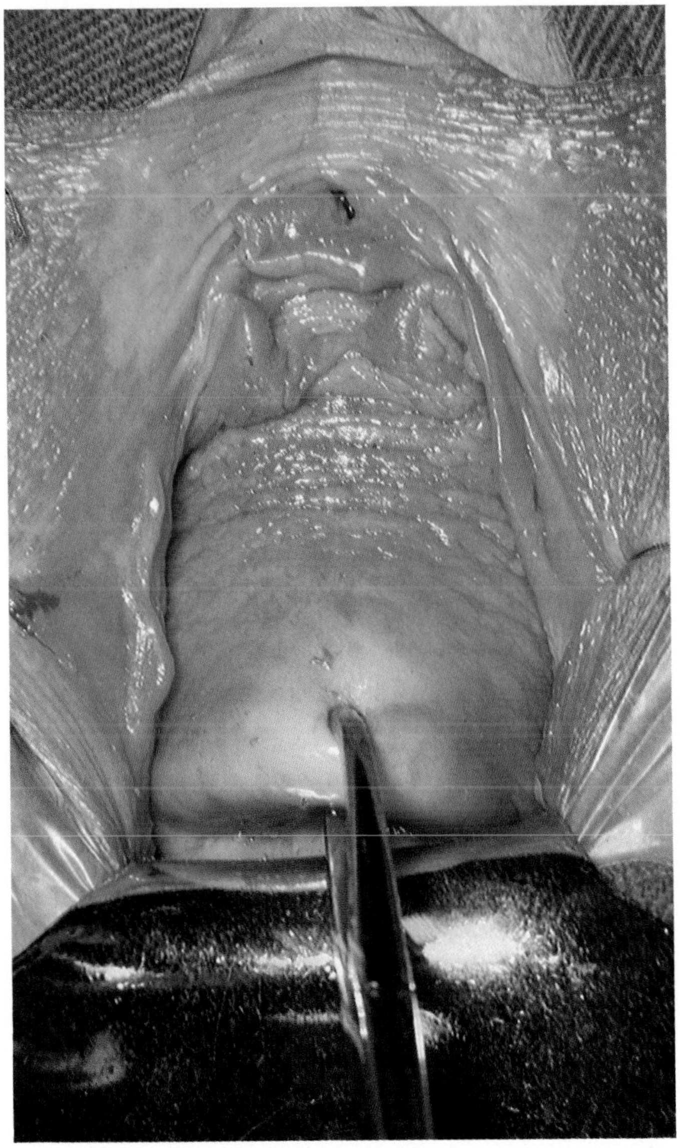

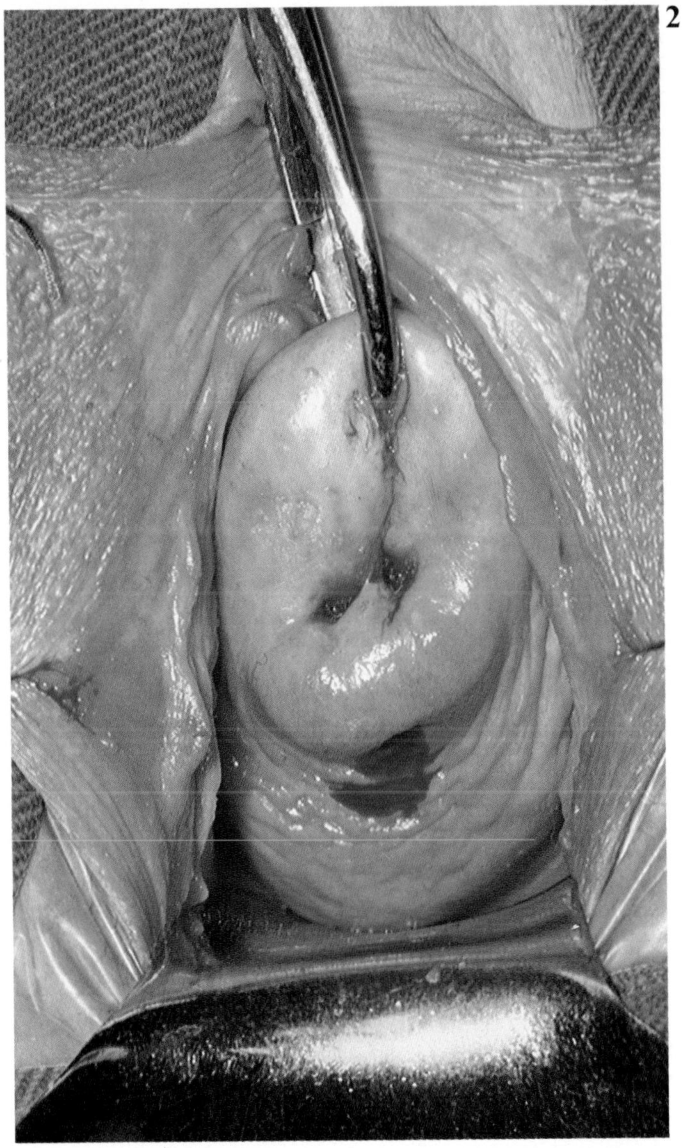

2

1 The general view (i)

This is the general view of the utero-vaginal prolapse as seen by the surgeon. The cervix, grasped by Littlewood's forceps, has drawn down the uterus to the level of the introitus, making it a second-degree prolapse. The manoeuvre exposes the bulge of anterior vaginal wall in which is incorporated the bladder, the appearance being that of a cystocele.

The operation is always conducted with the patient in lithotomy position. Occasionally in patients with previous lumbo-sacral disc pathology, or in those with arthritic conditions of the knee or hip joint, it is necessary to operate with the legs extended and in special supports.

Two assistants are ideally preferred, but where only one is available, it is usual for the operation (instrument) nurse to act as second assistant. The first assistant always stands on the patient's right side, his left hand over the patient's thigh and his right one below.

2 The general view (ii)

The cervix is lifted forwards to show a considerable degree of enterocele which merges into rectocele under the blade of the Auvard speculum. As will be seen in the subsequent illustrations there is also deficiency of the perineum.

The requirements in this case are therefore a vaginal hysterectomy with a complete pelvic floor repair.

3

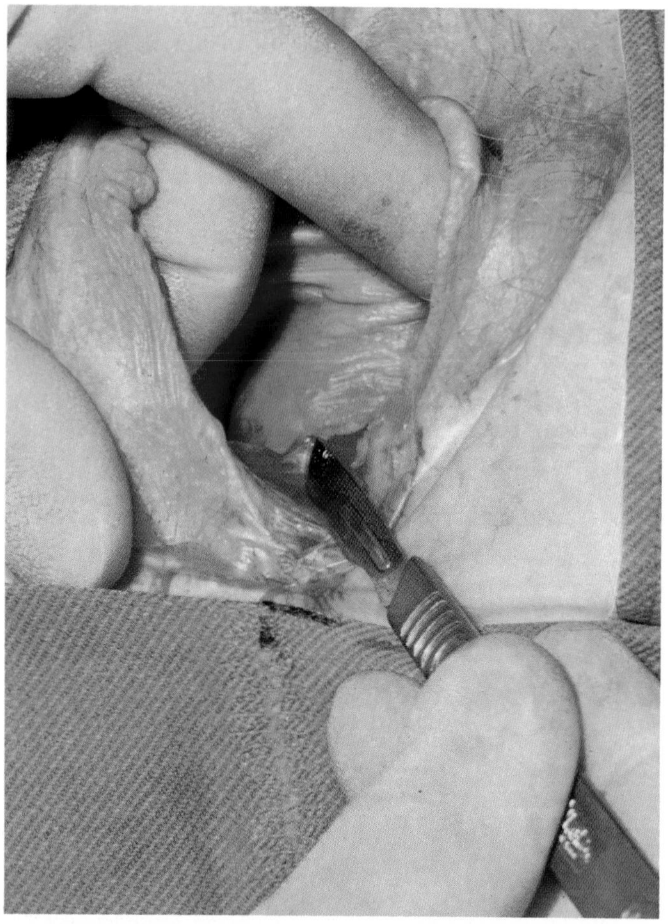

4

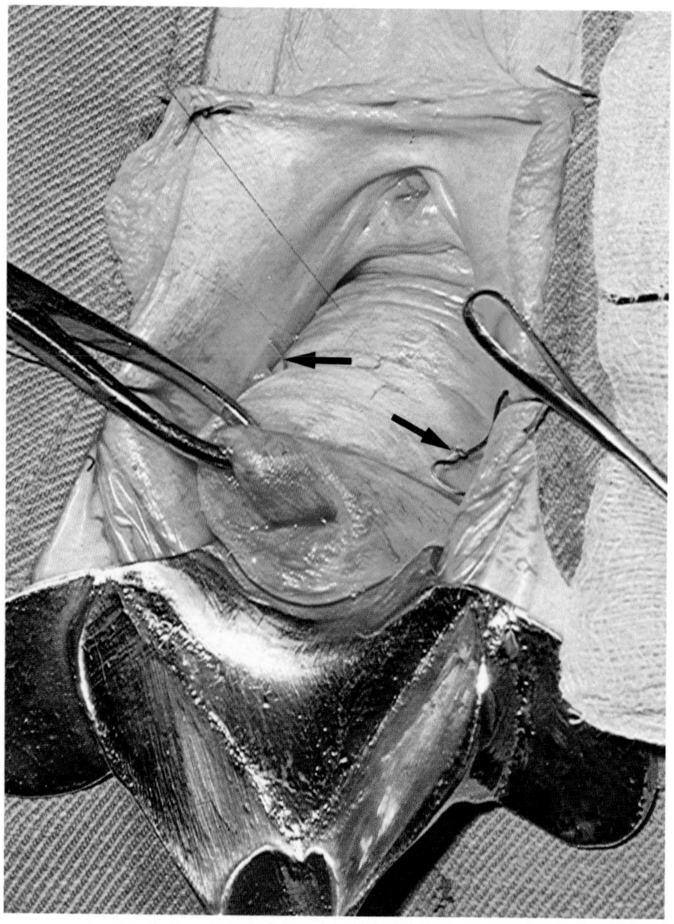

3 Mid-line episiotomy

As a preliminary to vaginal surgery, a mid-line episiotomy is routinely performed to give improved access. This is of particular importance in the post-menopausal woman, where minimal prolapse exists, or where a narrow sub-pubic angle impedes access to the anterior vaginal area.

Note in this case how anal contamination has been minimised by exclusion of the anus with an impermeable drape.

4 Increasing access and insertion of marking sutures

An essential part of vaginal hysterectomy is adequate access. Together with the mid-line episiotomy the labia are stitched back on each side both anteriorly and at the mid-point as marked. An Auvard speculum is inserted posteriorly and covers the mid-line episiotomy. This automatically extends the operative field of vision.

Curettage is an essential preliminary to the operation and is done routinely to exclude endometrial malignancy. Should clinical evidence of the latter exist by the appearance for example, of profuse and necrotic curettings, then this operation should not be continued with. Two marking sutures (arrowed) are inserted just laterally and anteriorly to the estimated reconstituted vault of the vagina, and are designed to ensure symmetry in closing of the anterior vaginal skin after the removal of the uterus.

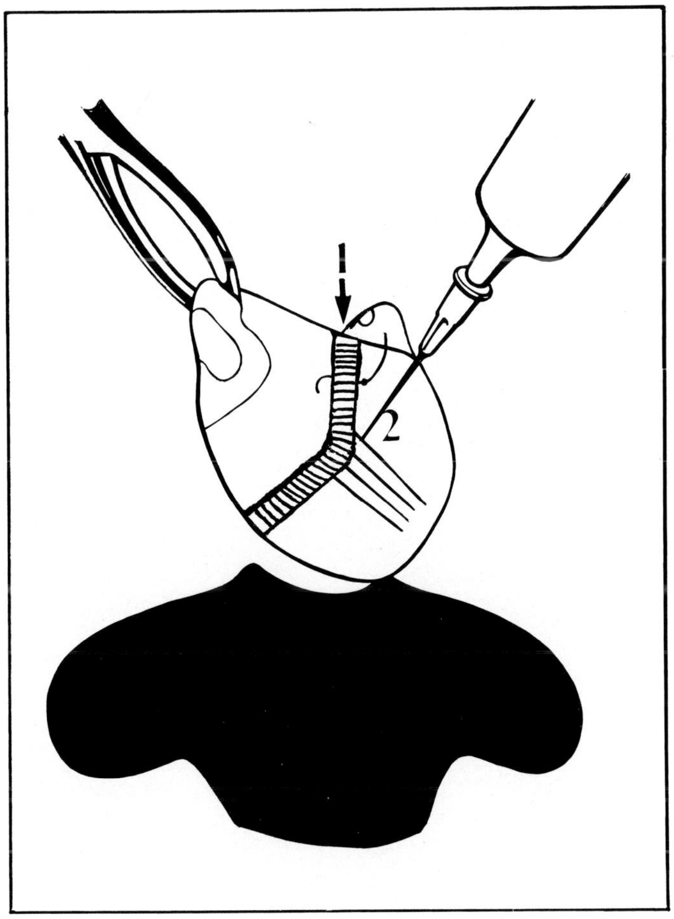

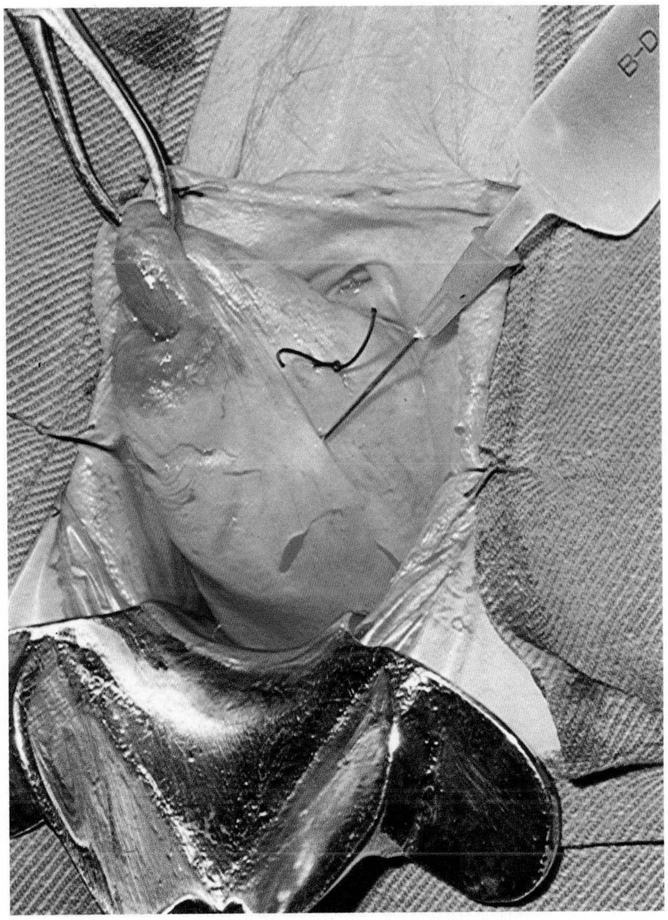

5

5 Local vaso-constrictive agents

Local vaso-constrictive agents are used in vaginal surgery, especially hysterectomy. They serve to minimise blood loss from the vascular superficial areas, as well as ensuring a relatively non-vascular field. It also results in the fascial layers becoming more easily seen and able to be accurately defined. A very weak solution of 1/240,000 adrenalin* and saline is generally used but some anaesthetists are happier with Phenylephrine† and their agreement is always sought before using these agents. If they are contraindicated it is possible to use saline alone, which is surprisingly haemostatic and also defines the tissue planes.

The points of insertion of these agents are:

1 In the line of the anterior wall incisions,
2 Posteriorly at the insertion of the utero-sacral ligaments to the uterus (as illustrated).

The skin blanches within a few seconds of its insertion. Care must be taken to exclude an intravascular injection of the solution. Approximately 25 ml are used.

* 0.25 ml of 1/1,000 adrenalin B.P. is mixed with 60 ml of normal saline solution.

† 1 ml of 1 per cent phenylephrine is mixed with 40 ml of normal saline solution.

Stage 2: Definition of urethra, bladder base and peritoneal pouches

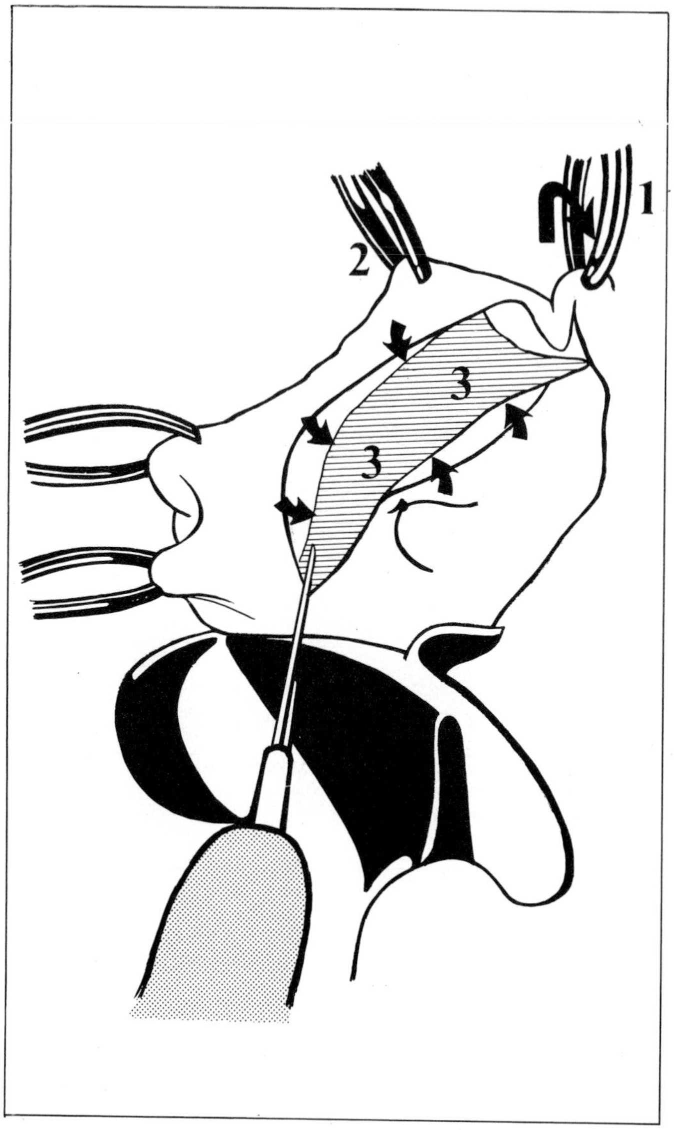

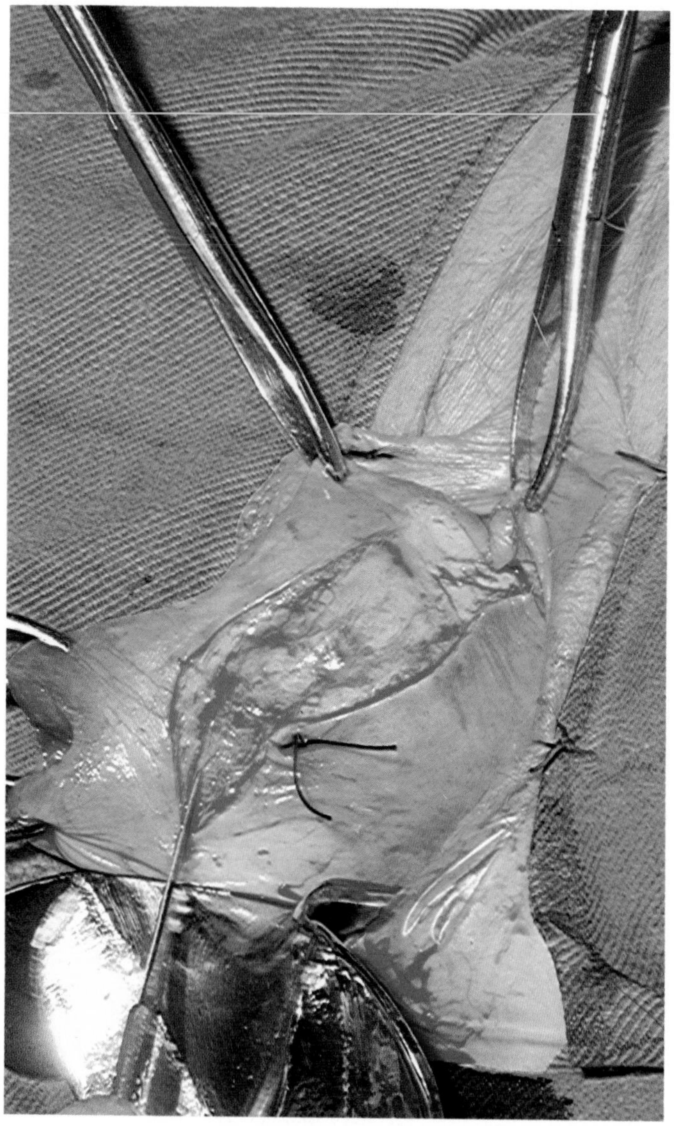

6

6 Anterior vaginal wall incision (i)

This incision commences just below the external urethral orifice (arrowed), the upper end of which is indicated by the Littlewood's forceps (1). Similar forceps hold up the redundant anterior vaginal skin at approximately mid-point (2).

The uterus is pulled over to the patient's right and the incision is carried down the anterior vaginal wall on the left side, slightly convex medially so as to curve round the cervix and at the same time keeping just within the marking sutures. After it reaches the posterior aspect of the cervix as shown here, the incision is carried downwards and medially to form one limb of a 'V' which lies over the pouch of Douglas.

Note the bloodless field provided by the adrenalin solution and the clear definition of the pubocervical fascia which is shaded, its margins arrowed, and marked 3.

7

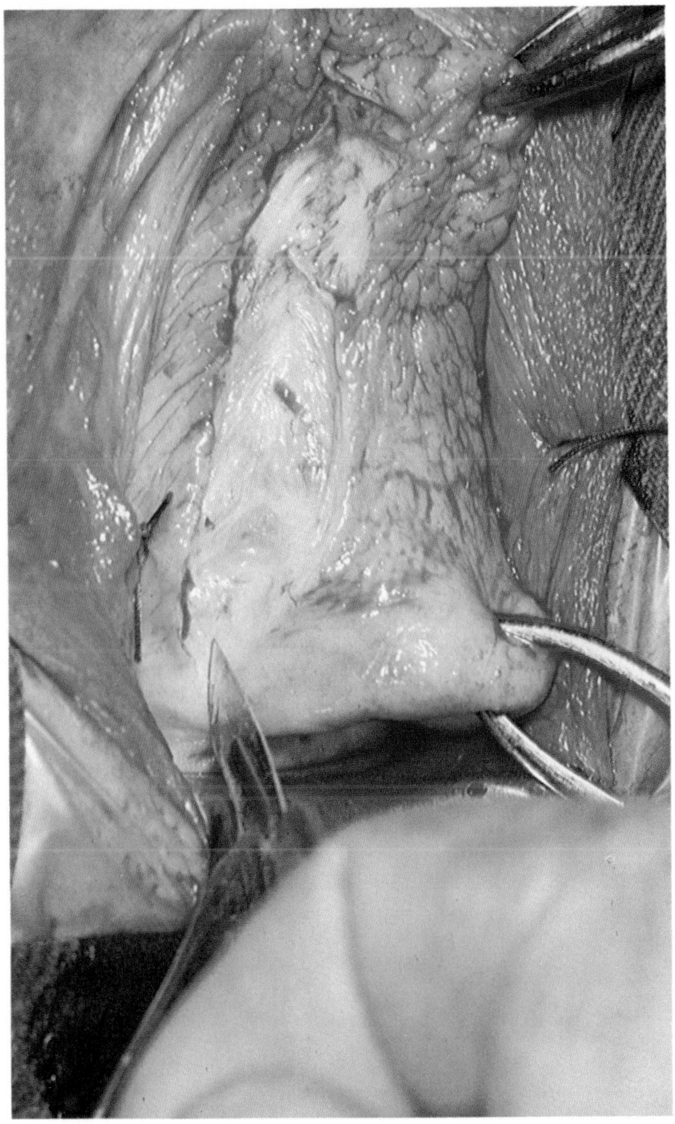

8

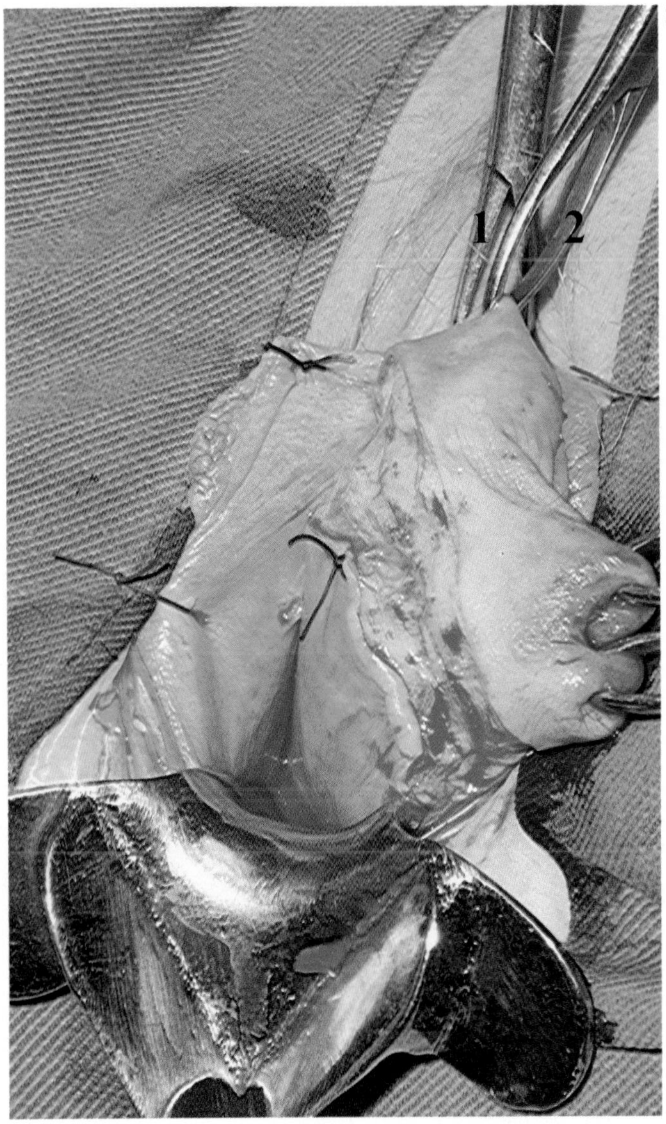

7 Anterior vaginal wall incision (ii)

A similar incision is now made on the patient's right side, the uterus having been drawn towards the patient's left side by the lower pair of Littlewood's forceps. The upper forceps are at the apex of the incision. This incision contributes the other limb to the 'V' posteriorly.

8 Completion of vaginal wall incision

With the cervix pulled to the left and upwards by the lower pair of forceps and keeping forceps 2 on tension, the incision on the right side of the patient is carried around the cervix and then downwards and inwards to contribute to the other limb of the 'V'-shaped incision that overlies the pouch of Douglas.

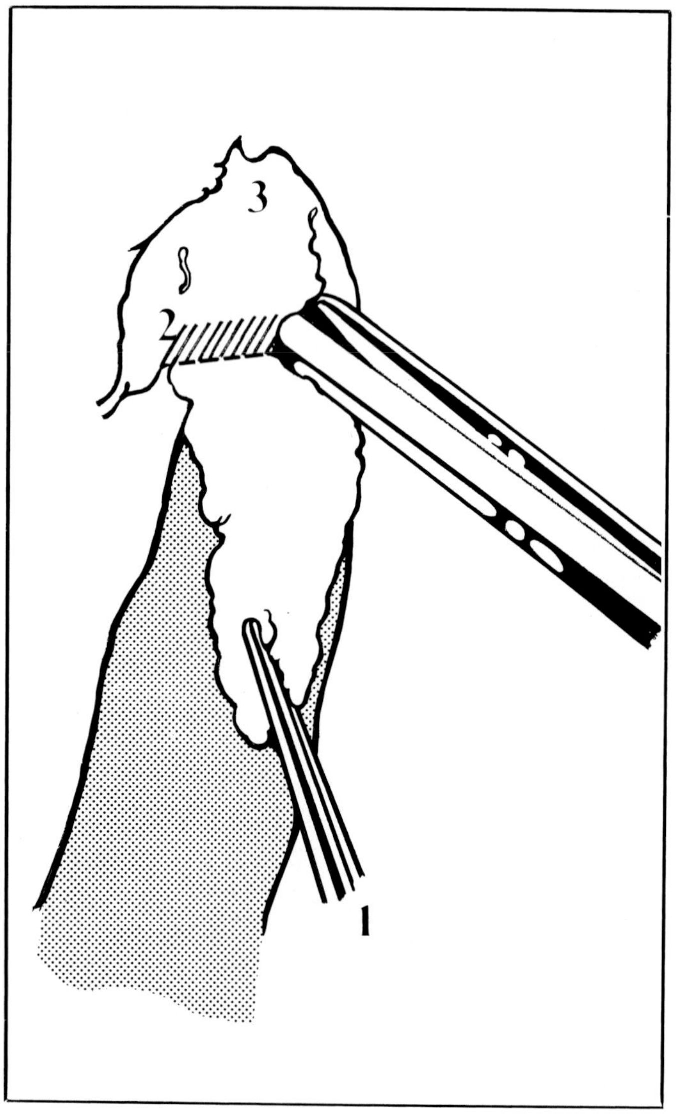

1 Kocher forceps attached to apex of triangle of vaginal skin
2 Level of bladder neck
3 Urethra

9

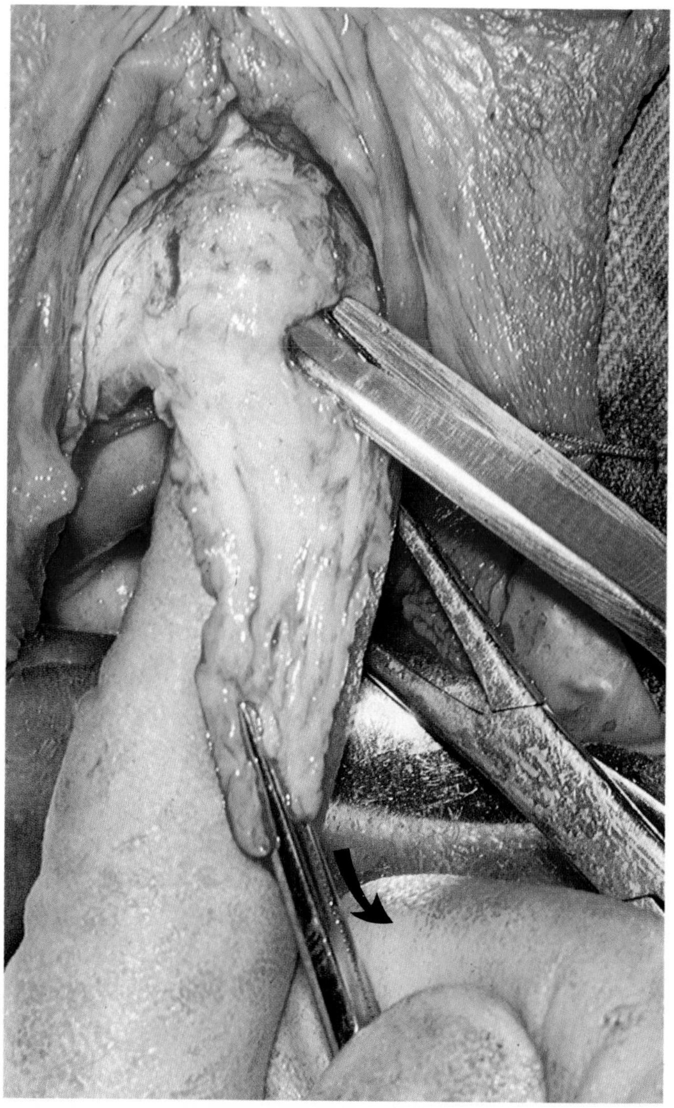

9 Removal of anterior vaginal wall skin (i)

This photograph shows the dissection and removal of the triangular flap of anterior vaginal wall skin. This removal has commenced at the apex of the triangle which is now grasped and held by a Kocher forceps; the flap being dissected down by a combination of a downward traction (arrowed) and snipping with scissors. It is helpful to support the skin flap on the left index finger and push up gently in the region of the bladder neck. This shows up the line of bladder attachment (indicated in diagram) and indicates where the plane of separation should be sought. The advantages of doing this are seen in this and the subsequent illustration.

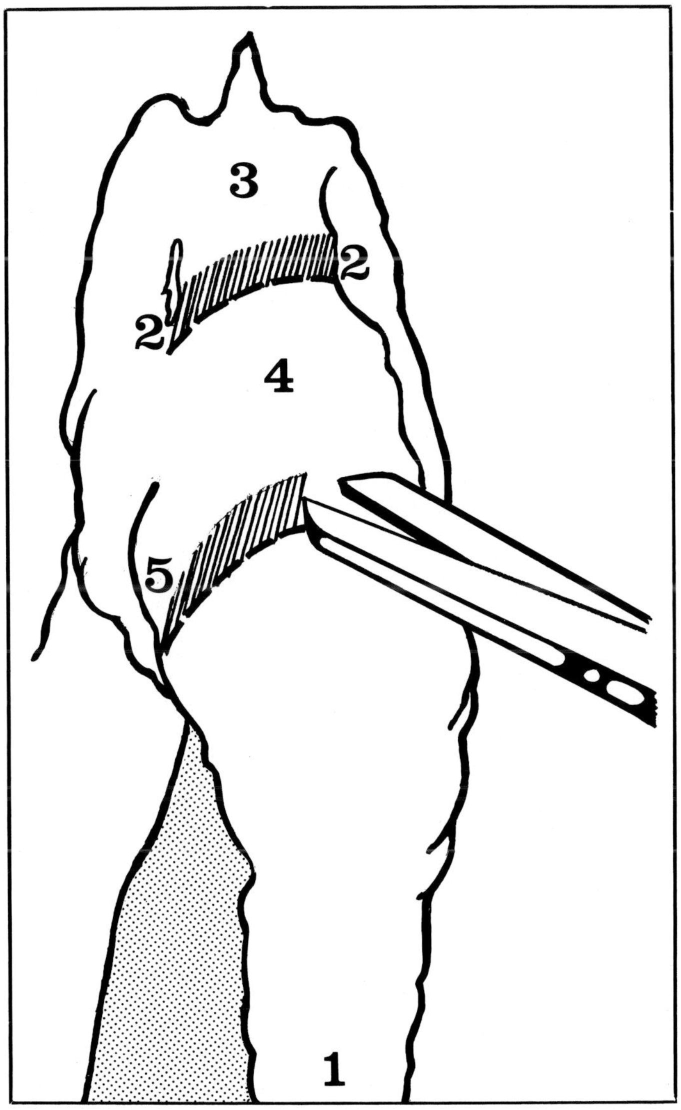

10

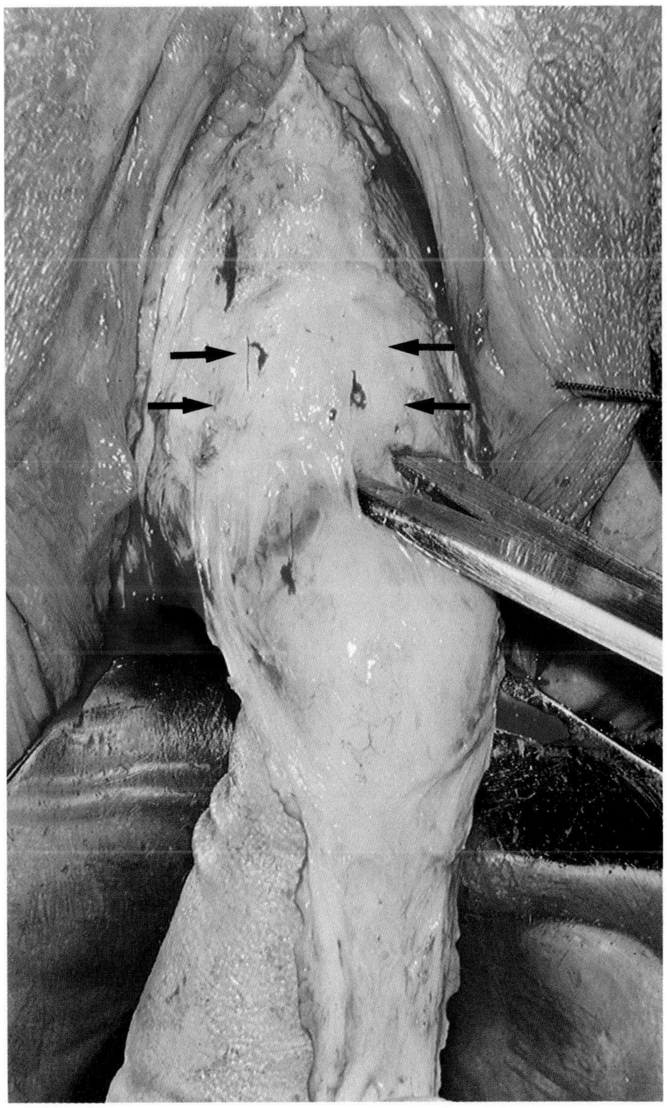

1 Triangle of vaginal skin
2 Bladder neck
3 Urethra
4 Bladder
5 Separation of vaginal skin from bladder base

10 Removal of anterior vaginal wall skin (ii)

When the triangular flap is clear of the urethra it is much more easily separated, and as a result of this manoeuvre there appears a natural plane of cleavage between the vaginal integument and the bladder. The vaginal skin carries with it the attenuated pubocervical fascia in the mid-line which is indicated (arrowed). Only occasional cuts with the scissors are required at this level, and the bladder strips off in almost bloodless fashion. Some surgeons use a gauze swab over the finger to strip off the bladder but we are not happy about this method of dissection. Unless dissection is proceeding in exactly the correct tissue plane it is very easy to tear the bladder.

11

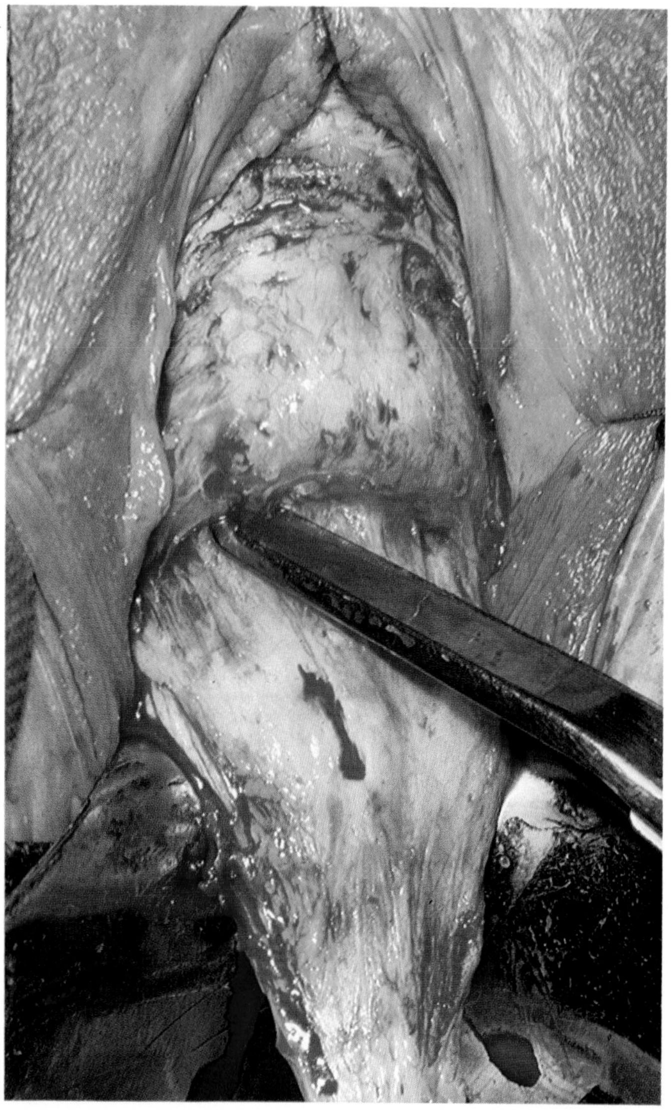

12

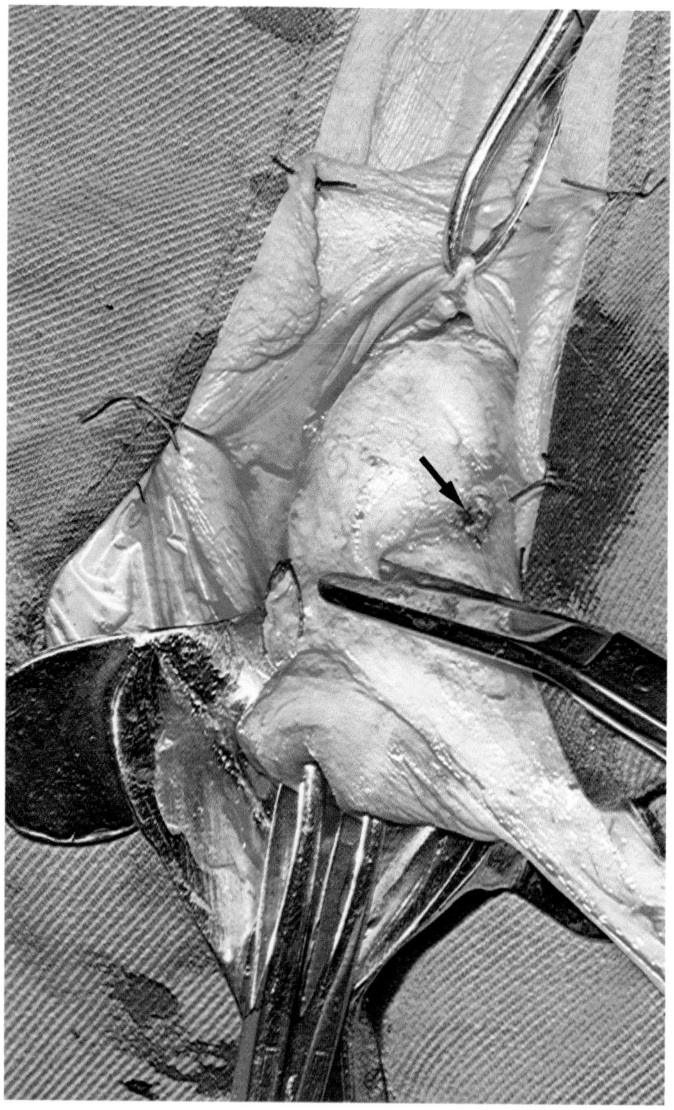

11 Mobilisation of bladder (i)

The anterior flap has now been carried down clear of the bladder. The bladder and its attachment to the cervix is being defined by the tip of the scissors. In the dissection it is useful if the partially closed scissor points are pulled downwards to complete dissection without actually cutting the tissue. Note the considerable amount of completely redundant vaginal skin that has been removed.

12 Mobilisation of bladder (ii)

The bladder pillars on the patient's right side are divided to allow access behind the bladder and to free the uterus. Some medium-sized blood vessels may be encountered at this stage and are generally suitable for diathermy coagulation as seen in the photograph (arrowed).

Diathermy coagulation is an ideal way of dealing with the bleeding that occurs during vaginal hysterectomy, especially from vaginal skin edges and in the dissection of vaginal skin. The vessels in these positions are not large, can be easily visualised, and the degree of coagulation need only be minimal. Used in this way we have not inflicted any damage to the lower urinary tract.

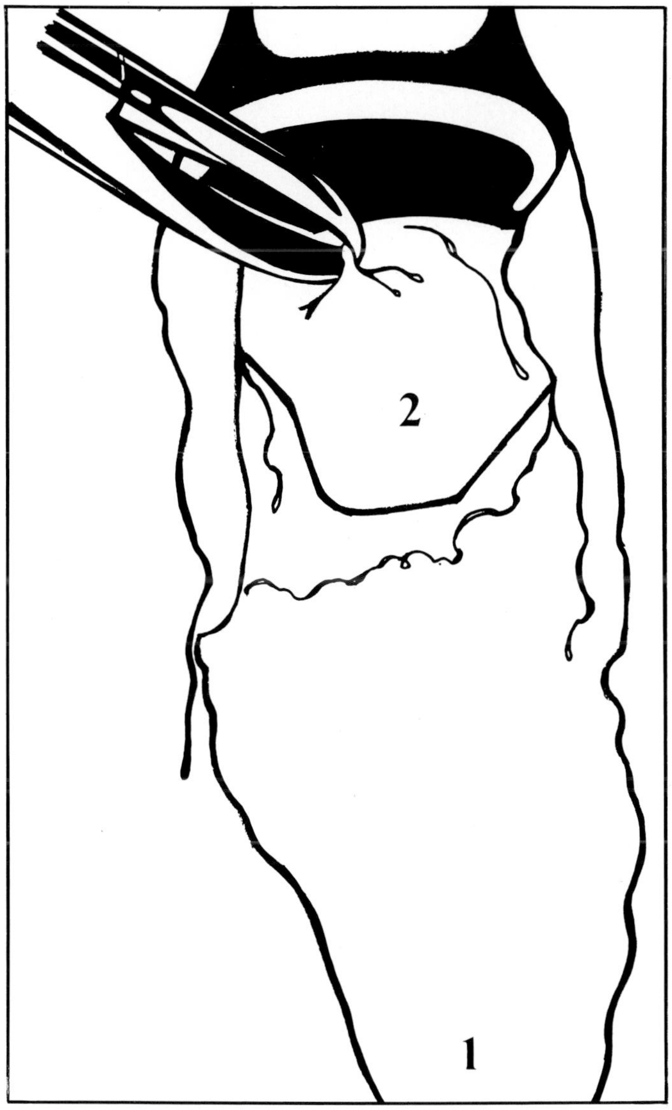

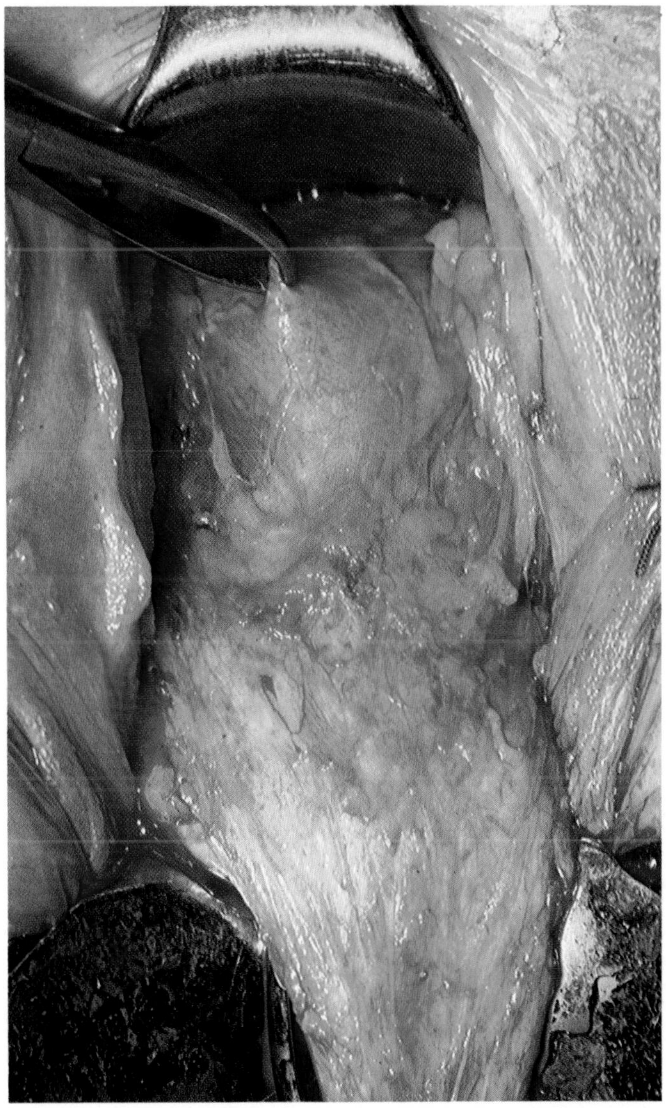

13

1 Triangle of vaginal skin
2 Utero-vesical pouch

13 Exposure of the anterior peritoneal (utero-vesical) pouch

The retractor is now used to gently pull back and protect the bladder, allowing the lower edge of the utero-vesical pouch to become obvious. This is recognised, as in this photograph, as a white or pale area owing to the double layer of peritoneum. Confirmation that this is the peritoneal sac can be obtained by picking up the anterior layer with forceps as shown. With previous inflammatory disease or endometriosis this pouch may be obliterated or difficult to define. In such circumstances it is wisest not to persevere because of the risk of opening the bladder and there are two safety measures that may be employed. Insertion of a bladder sound may show that it is safe to proceed but if in any real doubt it is better to wait till the pouch of Douglas is open and a finger can be passed over the broad ligament to define the anterior pouch.

14

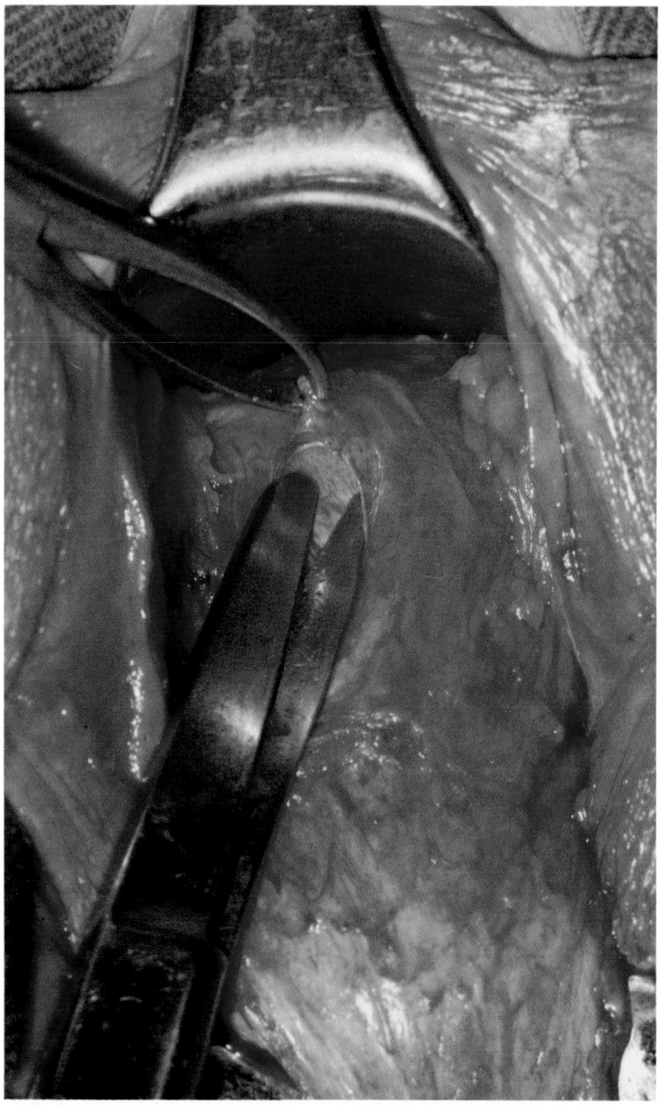

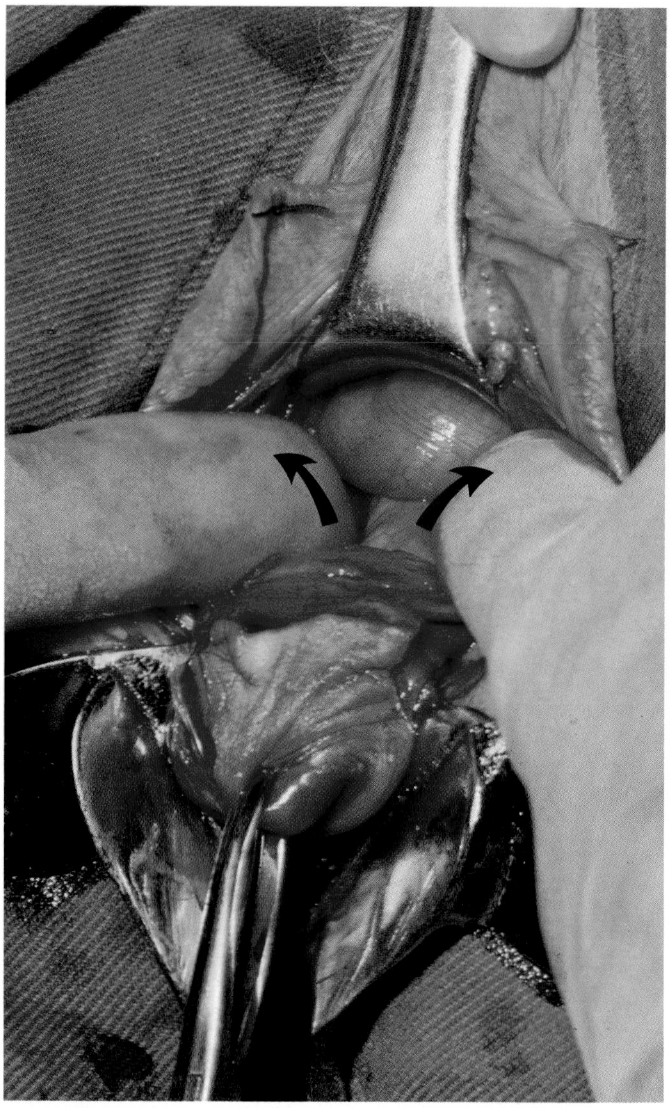

15

14 Opening the peritoneal cavity (anterior to the uterus)

The utero-vesical pouch has now been opened and the peritoneal cavity is exposed with the partially opened scissors. It is very unusual for there to be any collection of free fluid in the anterior pouch so that if fluid is encountered it is necessary to check that the bladder is intact.

15 Enlarging the peritoneal opening and displacing the bladder and ureters

The opening in the utero-vesical pouch is now enlarged. This is done by inserting the index finger of each hand and drawing the peritoneum laterally while keeping the fingers close to the uterus. This has the effect of displacing the bladder away from the uterus and at the same time the lower ureters are carried clear of the operation site in the direction arrowed.

As the pouch is enlarged a loop of small intestine or omentum is seen and confirms that the peritoneal cavity has indeed been opened.

Stage 3: Mobilization of uterine supporting and vascular ligaments

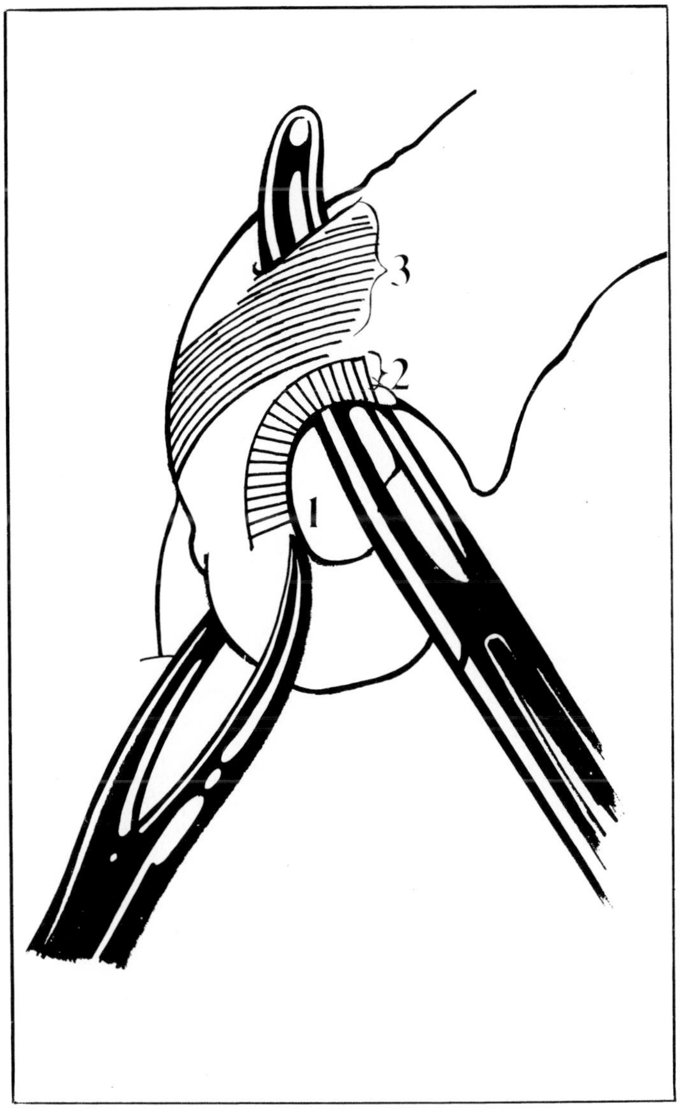

1 Area of pouch of Douglas
2 Utero-sacral ligaments (right)
3 Cardinal ligament (right)

19

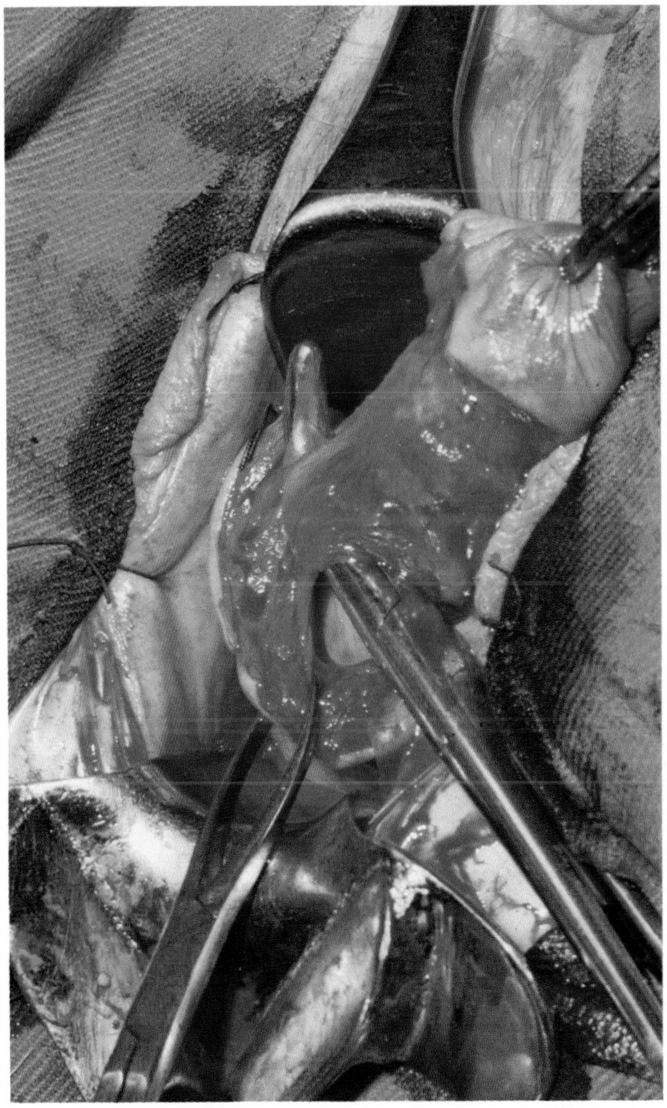

19 Definition of right utero-sacral and cardinal ligaments

The joint right utero-sacral and cardinal ligament is now defined, using cholecystectomy forceps. These ligaments merge as they join the cervix and make up the mass of tissue below the uterine vessels. The pedicle is fairly bulky (1 cm in diameter, approximately) and is fibromuscular. It contains no large arteries or veins. It is important at this stage to prepare and obtain a 'stalk' or length of free pedicle because that will subsequently be sutured to its fellow from the other side and they will form the main support of the vaginal vault. The uterine vessels lie just superior and are avoided in defining the ligamentous pedicle.

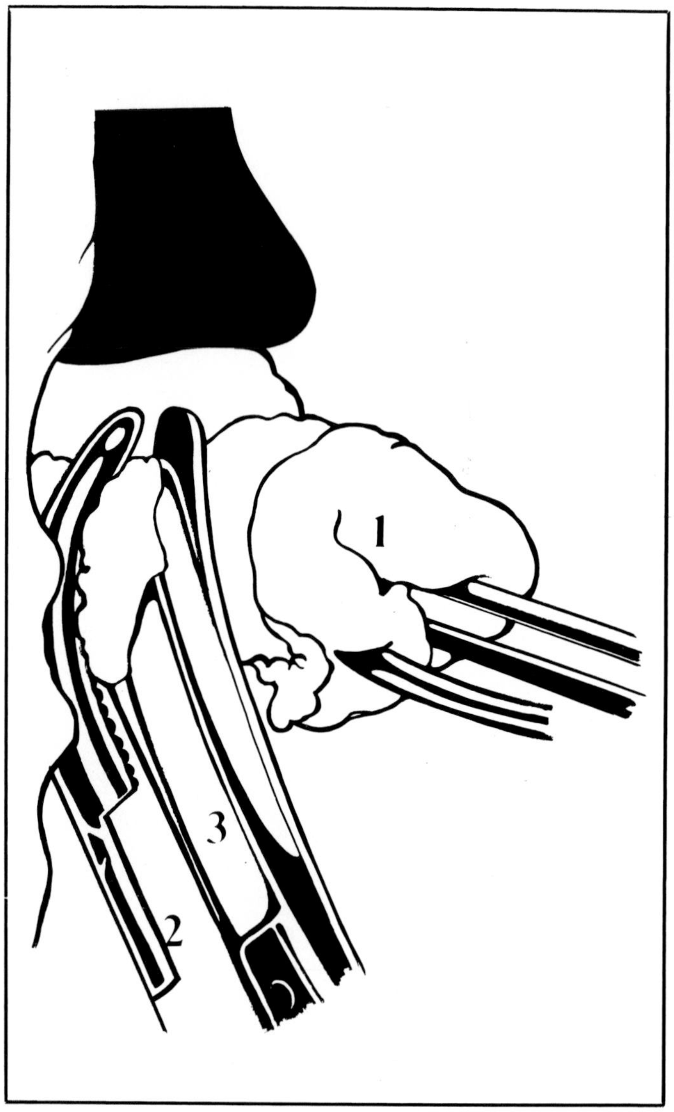

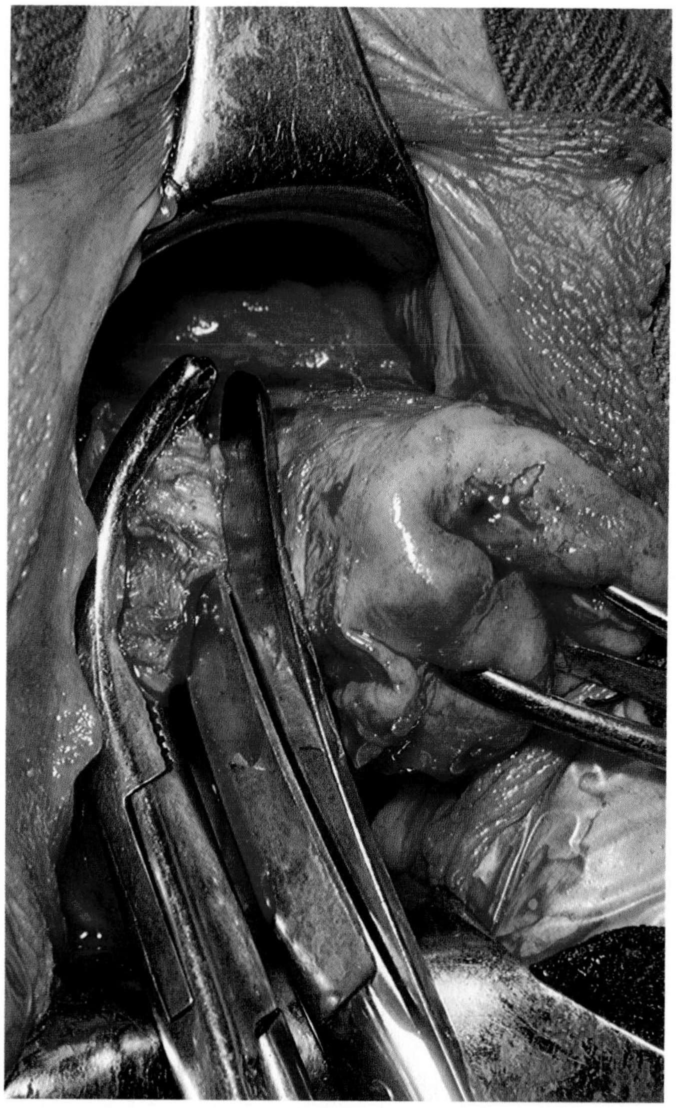

20

1 Cervix
2 Forceps clamping right utero-sacral and cardinal ligaments
3 Scissors dividing ligaments

20 Clamping and cutting right utero-sacral and cardinal ligaments

The right utero-sacral cardinal ligament has been clamped with cholecystectomy forceps. The forceps have been applied by inserting the tip of one blade through the defect made in the tissue and then closing the clamp. When cutting through the pedicle it is advisable to leave about 0.5 cm of uncrushed tissue distal to the forceps so that they do not slip off. Any vessels are thereby held taut and easily compressed. The advantage of leaving an adequate pedicle is seen at a later stage when double tying of these structures is described.

21

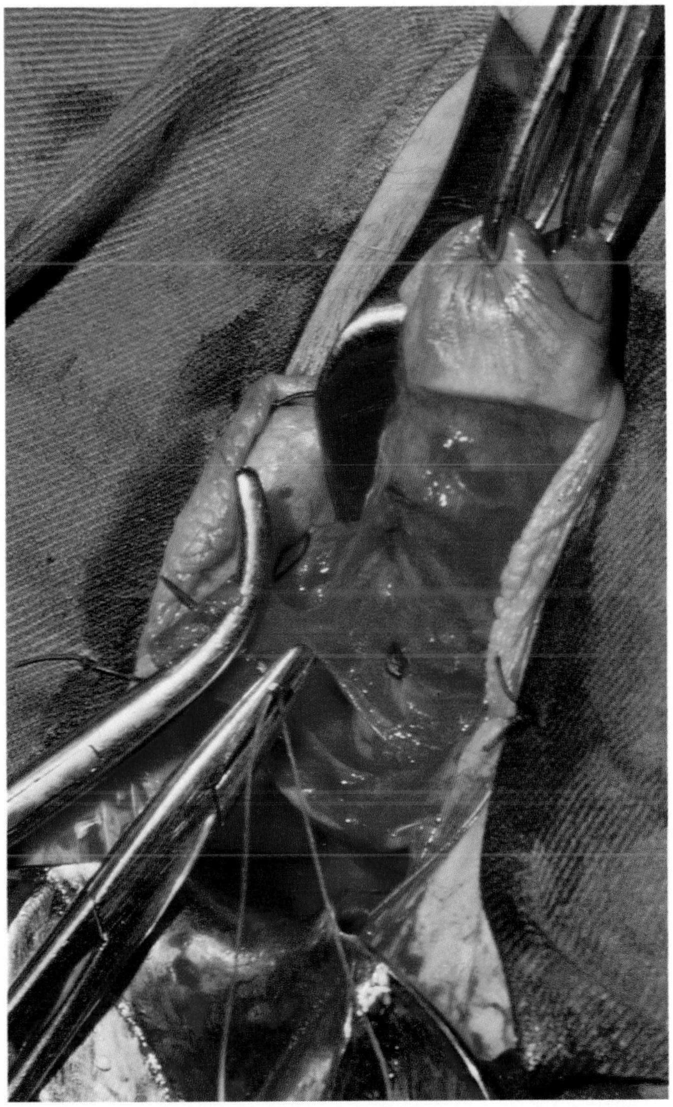

22

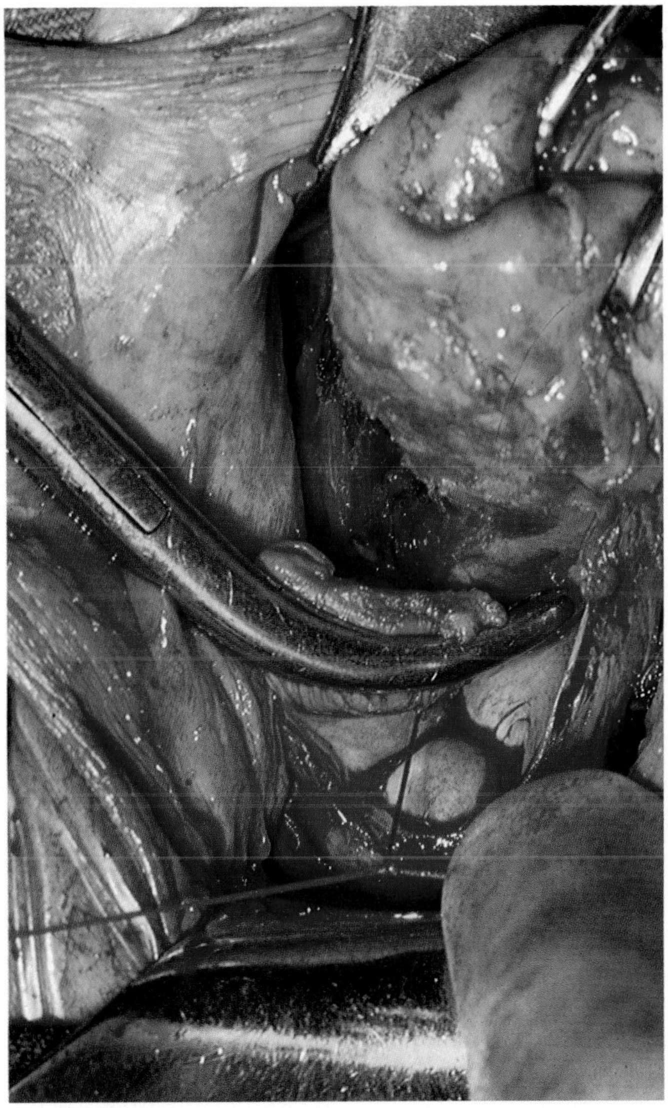

21 Transfixion of right utero-sacral and cardinal ligaments

The right utero-sacral ligament is now about to be ligated. A round-bodied Mayo needle carrying a PGA No. 0 suture transfixes the centre of the pedicle. The points of insertion should be approximately 1 cm from the actual forceps so that, when tying, the tissues can be safely gathered without slipping through. There is less likelihood of slipping and the ligature is more secure if the pedicle is transfixed centrally.

22 Ligation of right utero-sacral and cardinal ligaments

A single hitch is thrown under the point of the forceps as shown, then the two ends are brought back round the forceps to be tied in a surgical knot under the heel of the forceps. PGA suture is used and considerable power is required to obtain a firm knot. The suture is left long and is secured to the drapes. Double tying is not done at this stage and the reasons will be explained later. When actually tying the ligature it should be kept under direct vision continually and the assistant must release the clamping forceps very gradually. Immediately the suture is pulled up the assistant reaffixes the forceps to the end of the pedicle as a safety measure to keep the knot visible to the surgeon.

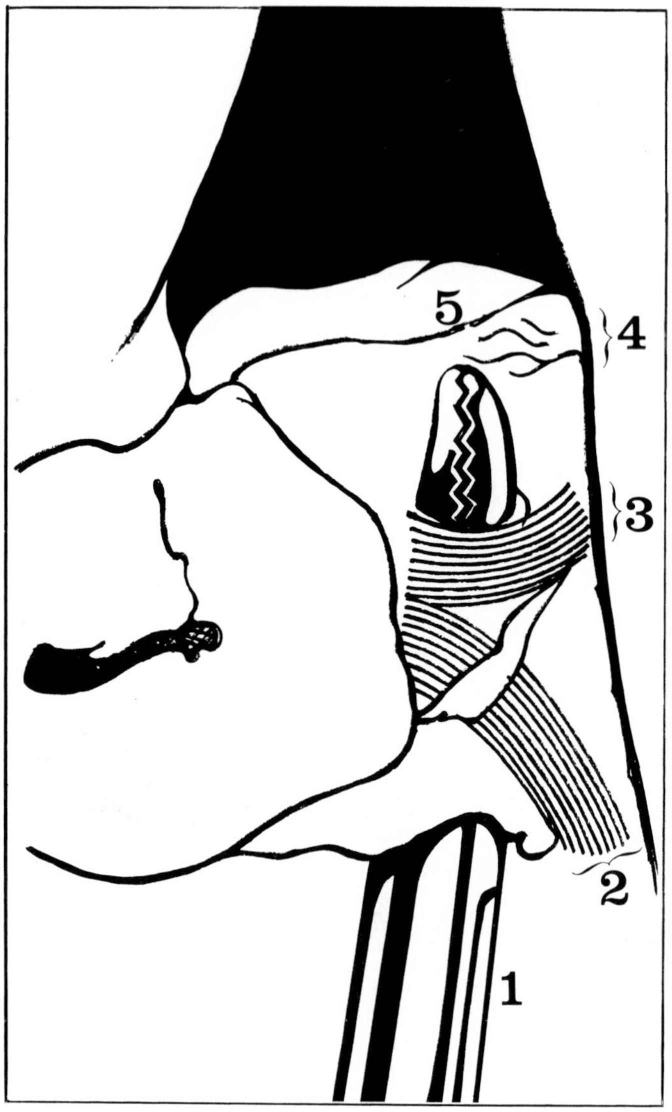

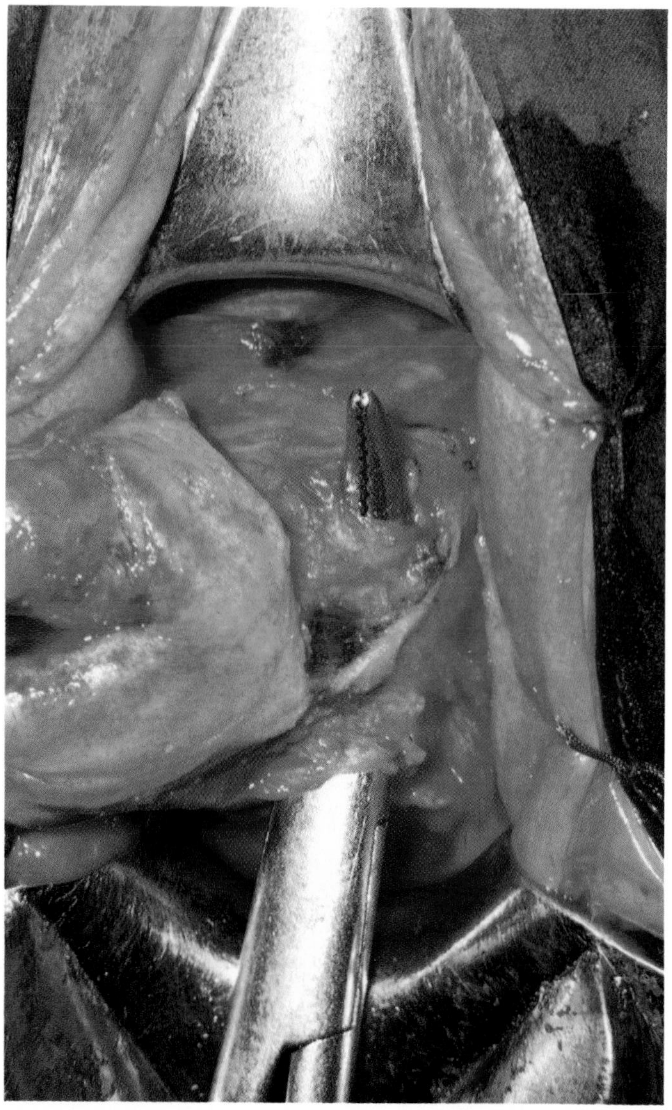

23

1 Forceps defining left utero-sacral and cardinal ligaments
2 Utero-sacral ligament
3 Cardinal ligament
4 Uterine vessels
5 Anterior aspect of broad ligament

23 Definition of left utero-sacral and cardinal ligaments

The left (joint) ligament is shown lying on the forceps which have been pushed through from the pouch of Douglas posteriorly. The utero-sacral and cardinal ligaments are seen to be largely fibrous. The vessels of the uterine plexus are just above.

24

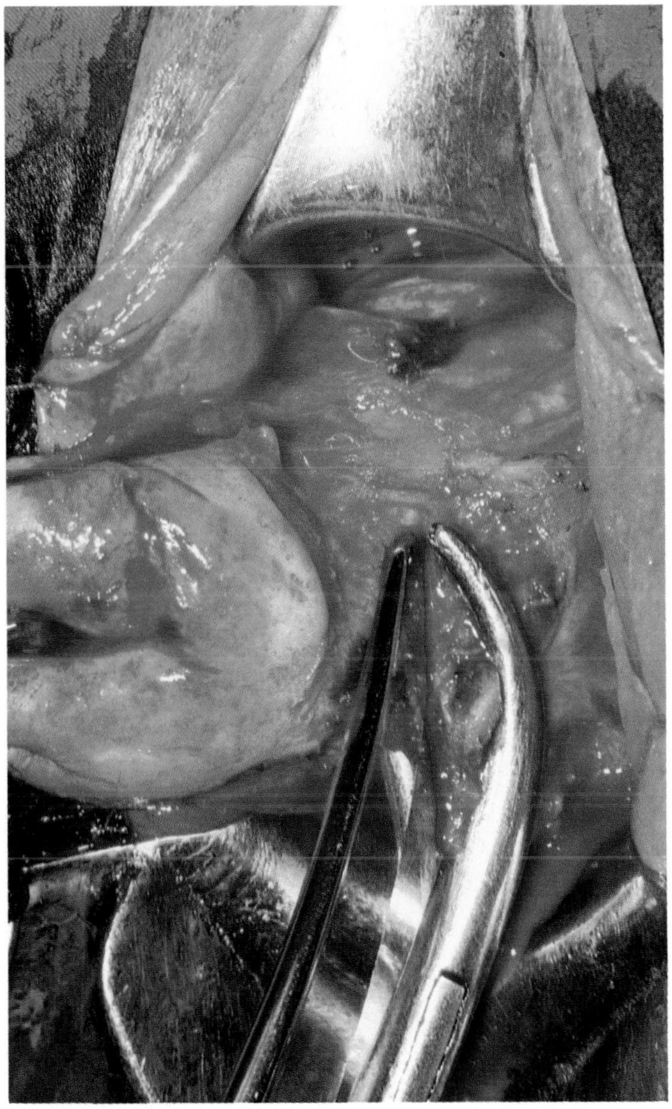

25

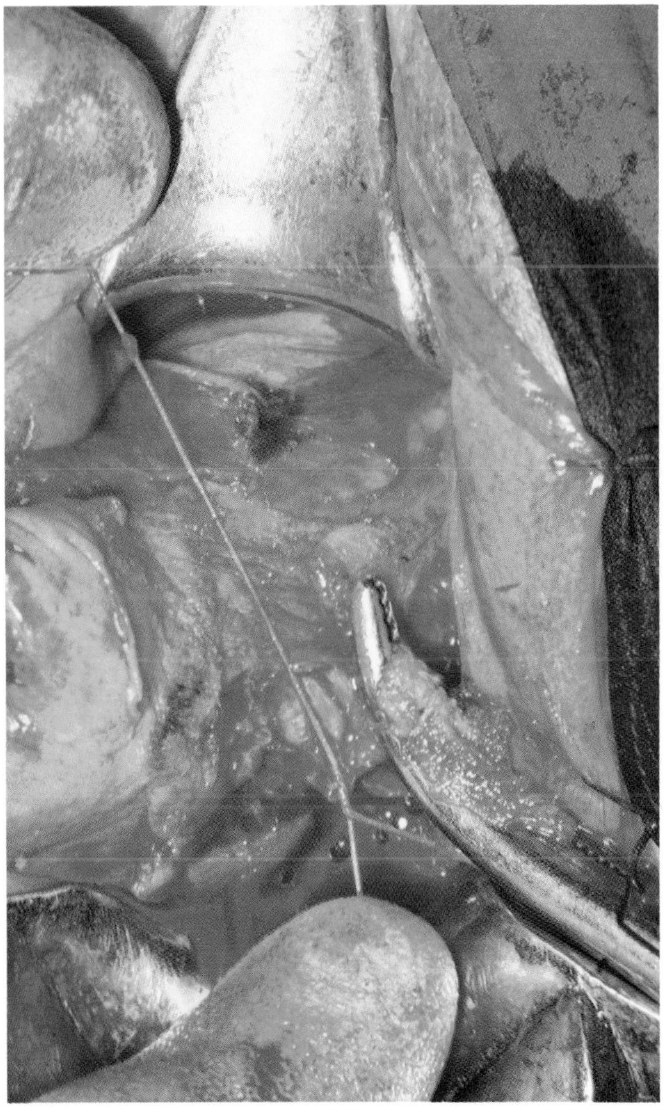

24 Clamping and detachment of left utero-sacral cardinal ligament

This is done as on the other side and it will be seen that an adequate cuff of tissue is left distal to the forceps.

25 Ligation of left utero-sacral cardinal ligament

The pedicle is secured by running up the suture as firmly as possible and the ends are kept long. With the completion of this step the uterus has lost its main support or anchor in the pelvis and becomes much more accessible.

26

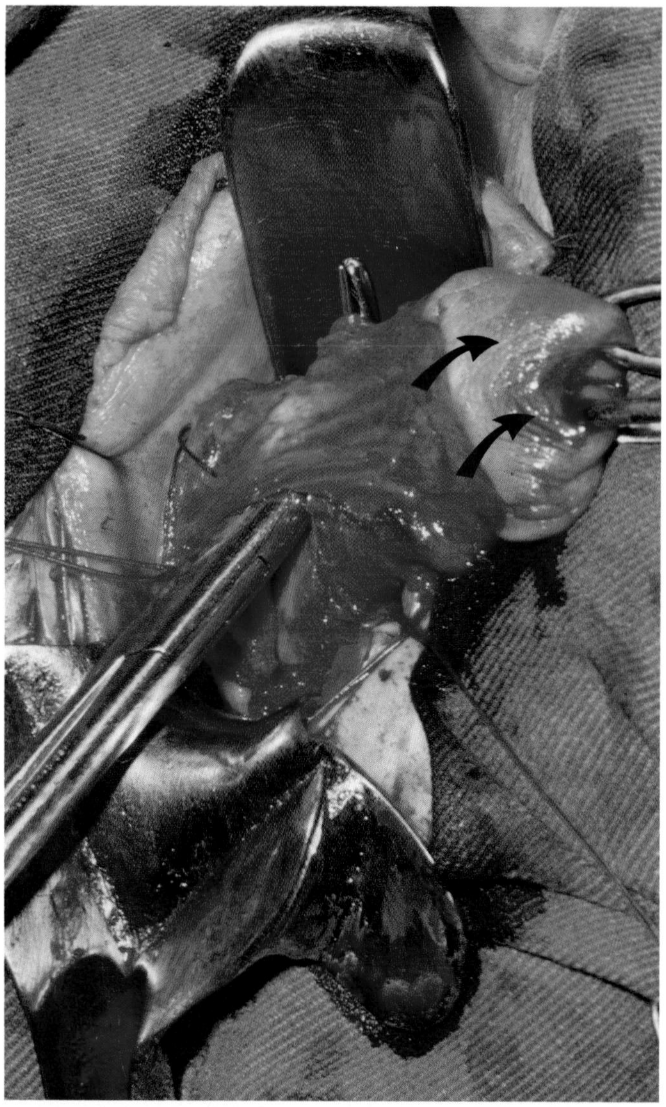

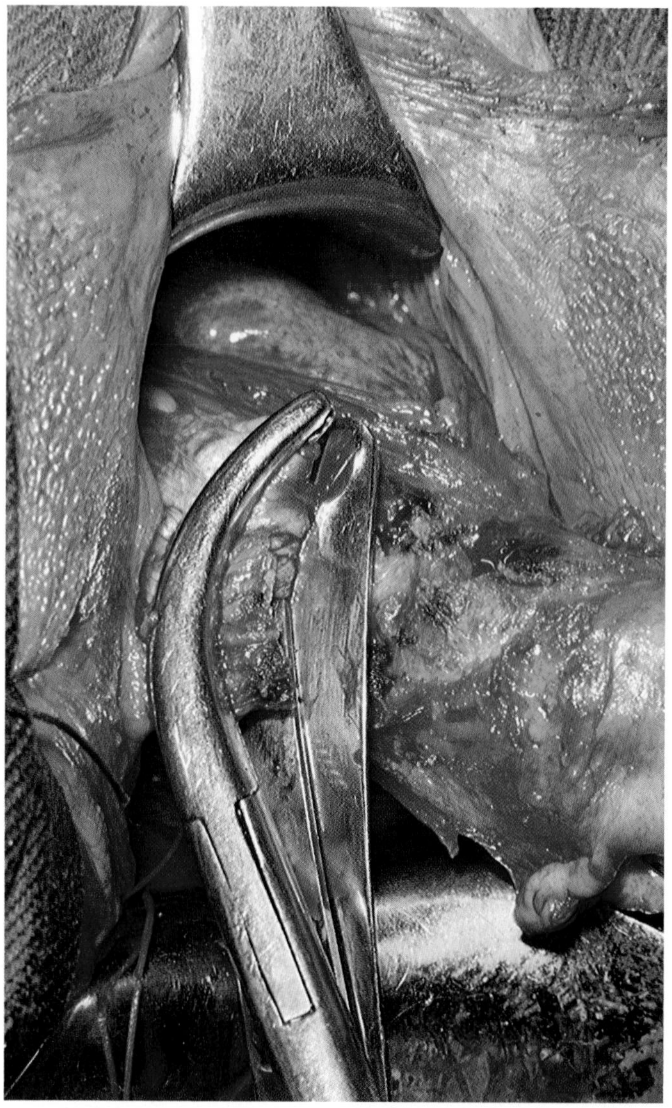

27

26 Definition of right uterine pedicle

The uterine pedicle refers to that containing the uterine arteries and veins, and is now defined on the right side. Since the operative approach is close to the uterus and since the pedicle is made up of branching and tributary vessels, it fans out into the lower broad ligament. Although it appears bulky it is largely vascular with very little fibromuscular content and is easily 'gathered' by the forceps and is not unduly bulky. The right pedicle lies on the forceps, the points of which have pierced the broad ligament at the level of the isthmus of the uterus.

27 Clamping and cutting right uterine pedicle

The forceps have been applied as described in stage 20. Note that an adequate cuff of non-crushed tissue has been retained distal to the clamping forceps. Division is by heavy scissors or scalpel. The uterine vascular pedicles must be clearly defined and clamped so that ligation is straightforward and safe.

28

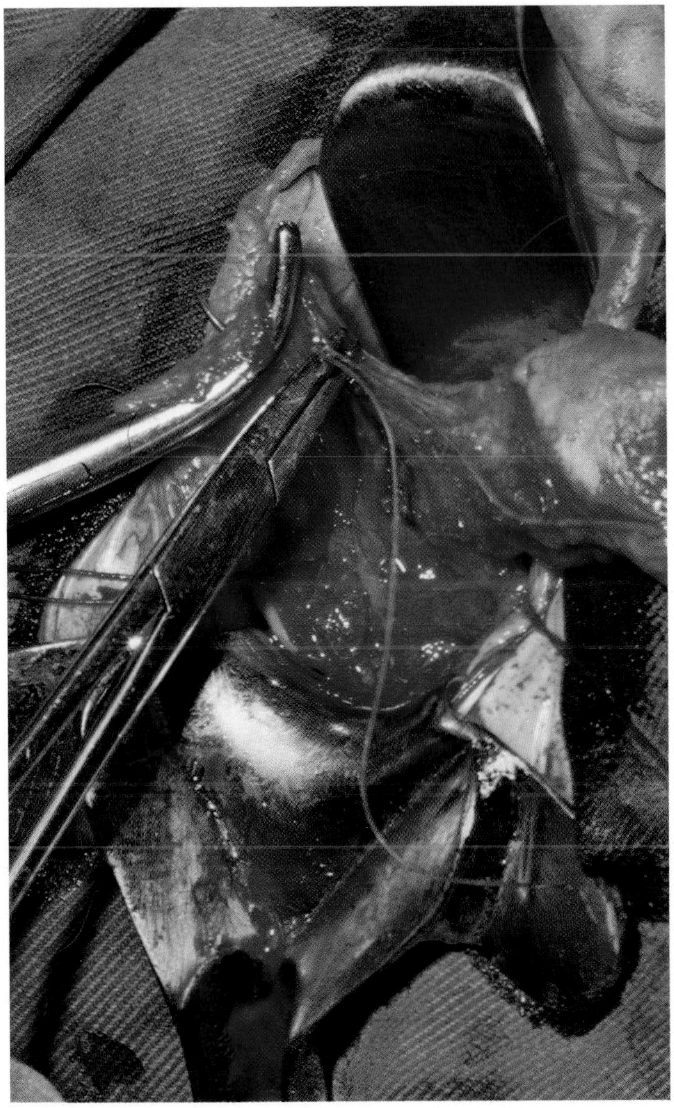

29

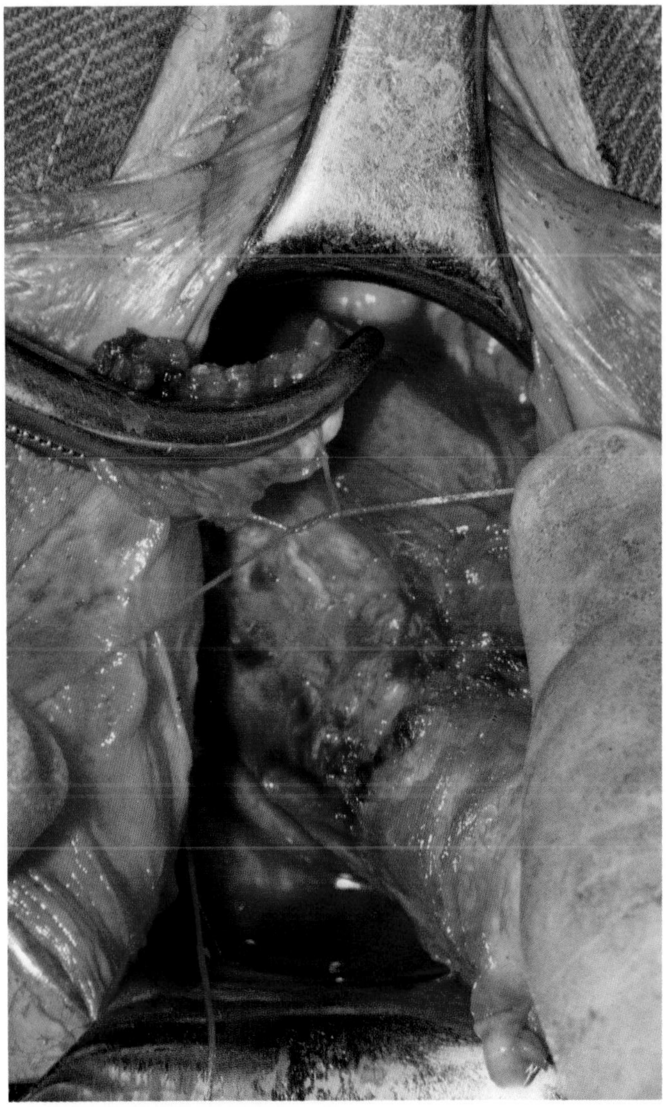

28 Transfixing the right uterine pedicle

The pedicle is cut 0.5 cm distal to the forceps as previously, and transfixed centrally. The uterine artery should be avoided while doing this and the needle should not be too close to the forceps, otherwise the first hitch under the tip of the forceps, which is tightened before their removal, will not be firm.

29 Tying the right uterine pedicle

The right uterine pedicle is single tied as previously and the ends of the suture left long and fixed to the drapes. The assistant keeps control of the pedicle until ligation is complete. Although the forceps have to be released while the suture is being run up, they are immediately re-tightened and are not removed from the pedicle till the surgeon has completed ligation.

30

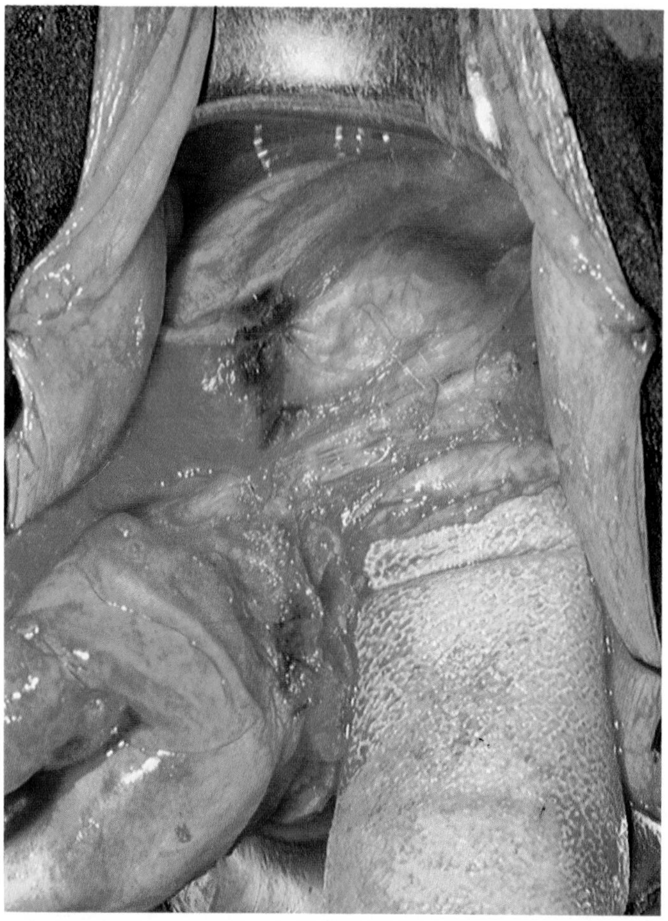

31

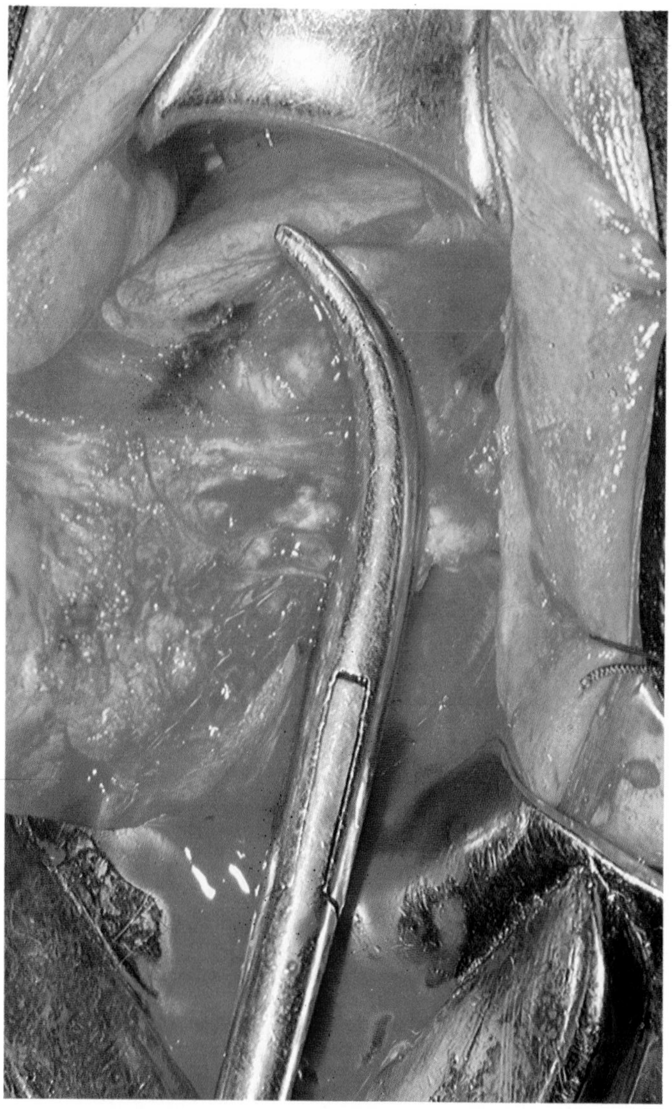

32

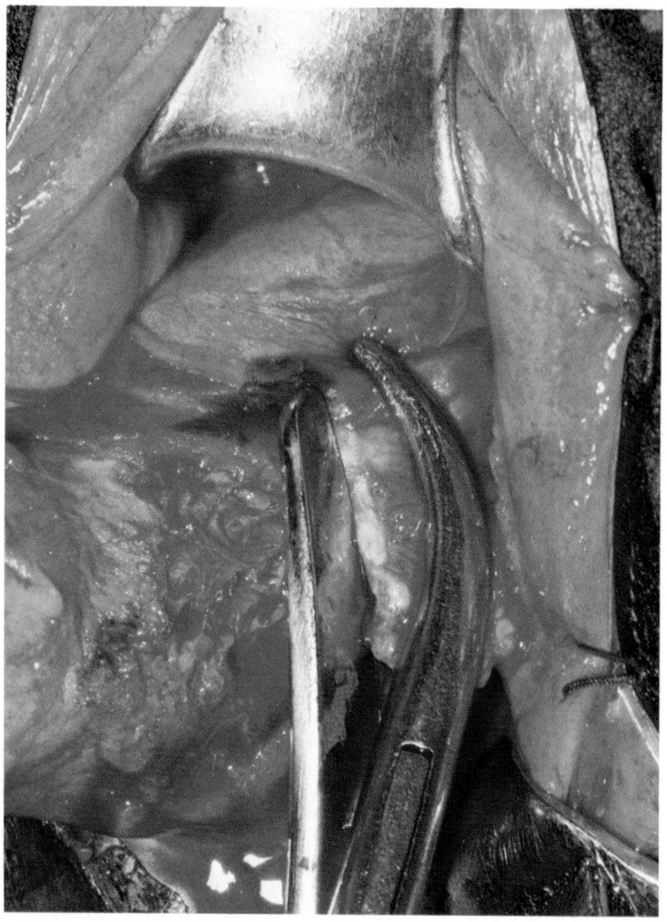

30–32 Definition, clamping and detachment of left uterine pedicle

The left uterine vascular pedicle is easily defined by a finger inserted into the pouch of Douglas. The uterine artery is seen at its centre with the peritoneal edge of the anterior pouch just above. The subsequent steps are carried out exactly as on the other side.

33

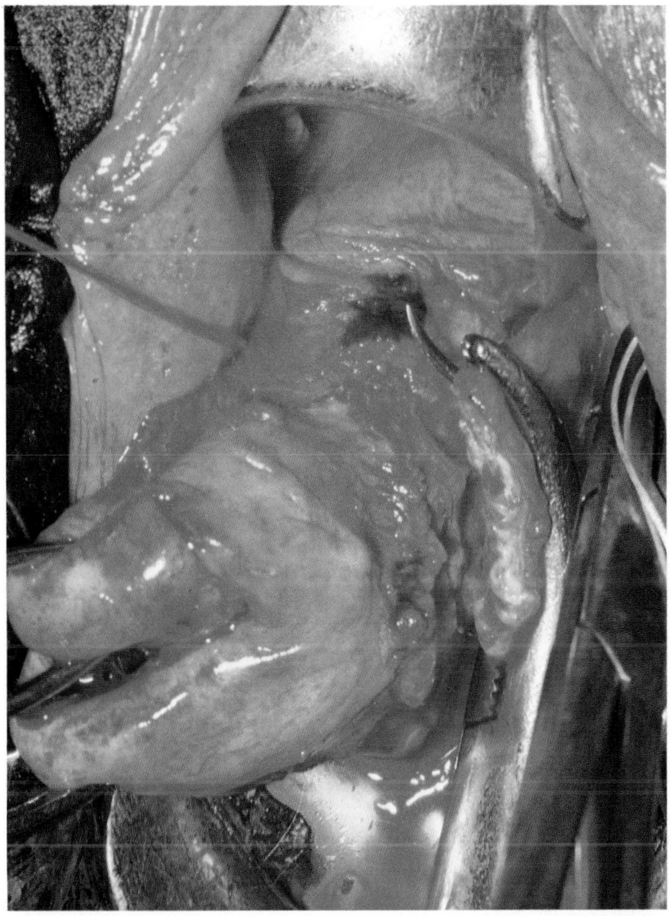

34

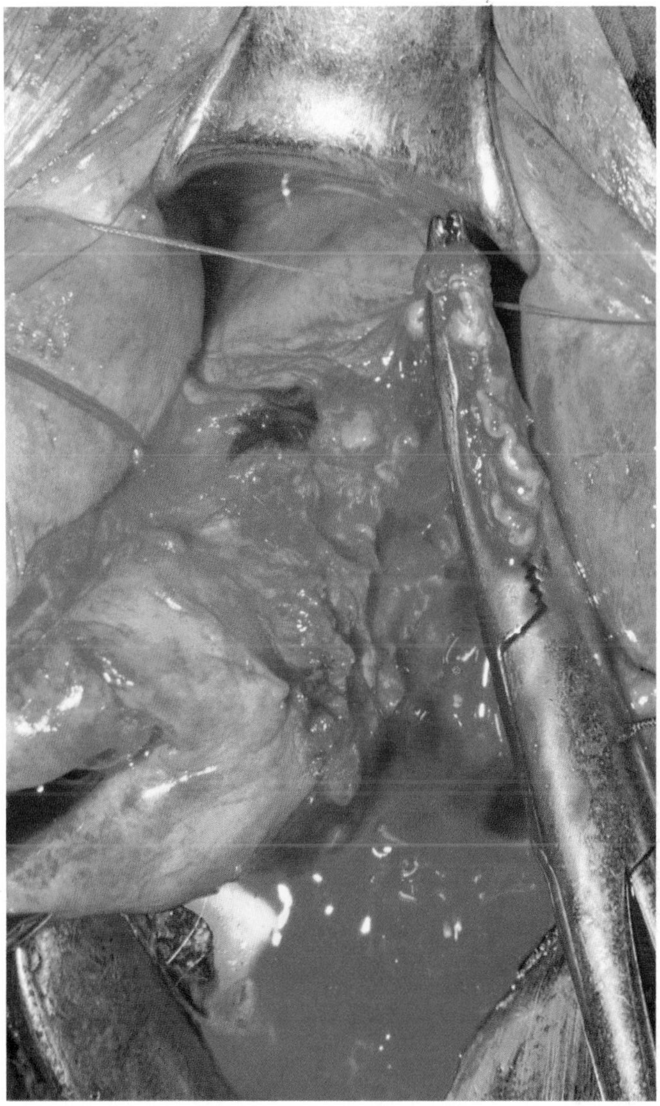

35

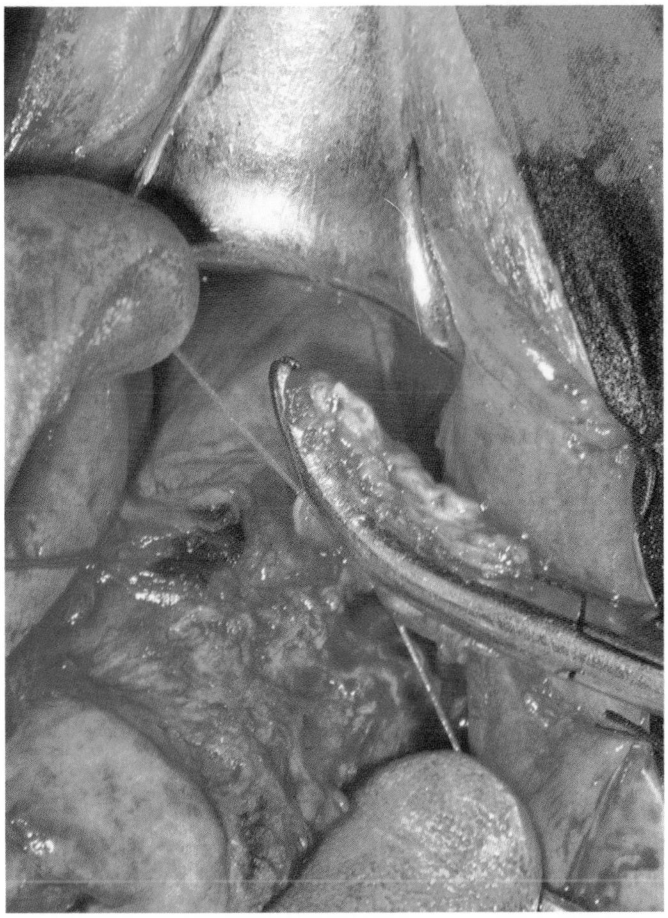

33–35 Securing the left uterine pedicle

The operation proceeds as on the opposite side with transfixion and ligation of the pedicle in standard fashion.

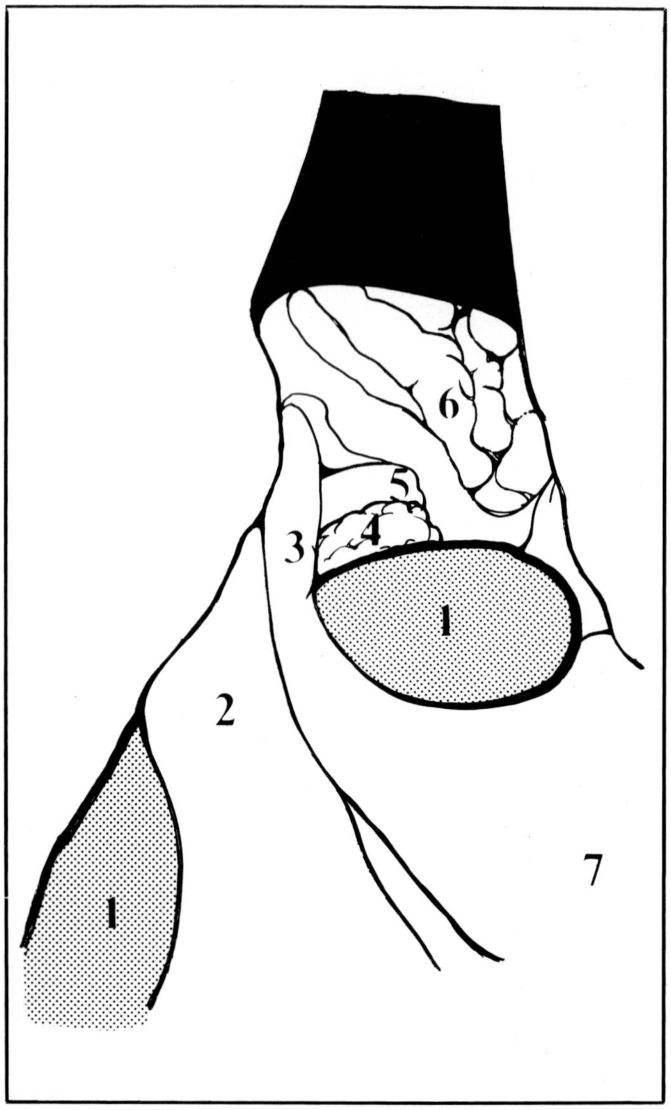

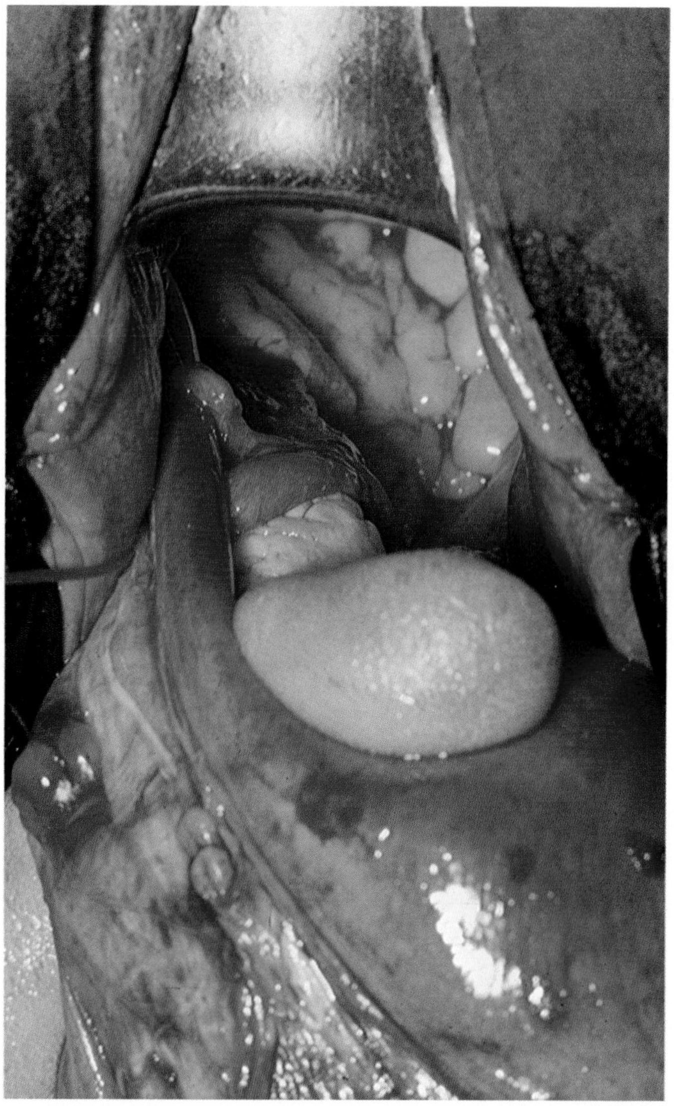

36

1 Left forefinger inserted behind right broad ligament pedicle
2 Right broad ligament
3 Right round ligament
4 Right ovary
5 Right fallopian tube
6 Small intestine and omentum
7 Uterus

36 Definition of right broad ligament pedicle

The uterus is delivered into the wound allowing definition of the right broad ligament pedicle which lies on the surgeon's left forefinger. The round ligament is in the centre of the picture as it joins the uterus and the fallopian tube and the ovary lie posterior and medial to it. Omentum and small intestine are seen intra-peritoneally just below the retractor.

37

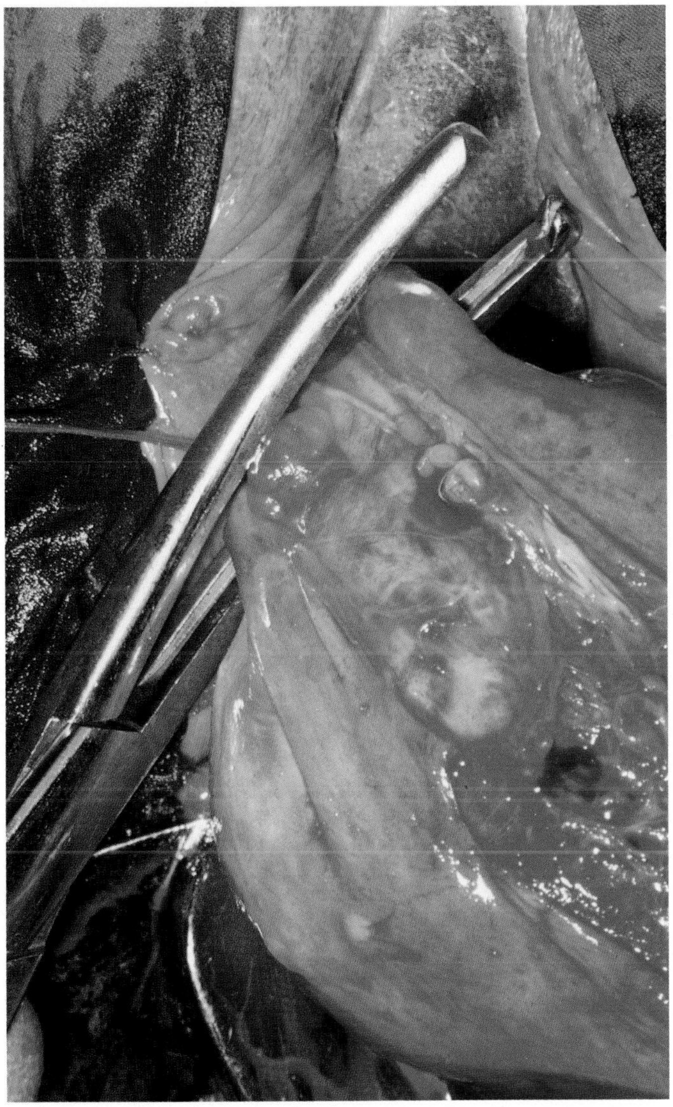

38

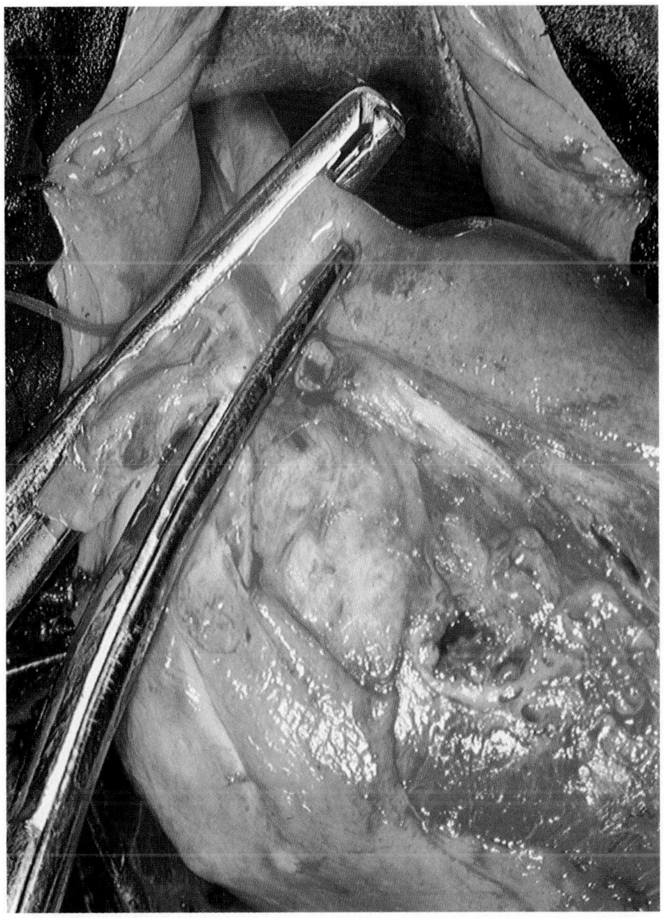

39

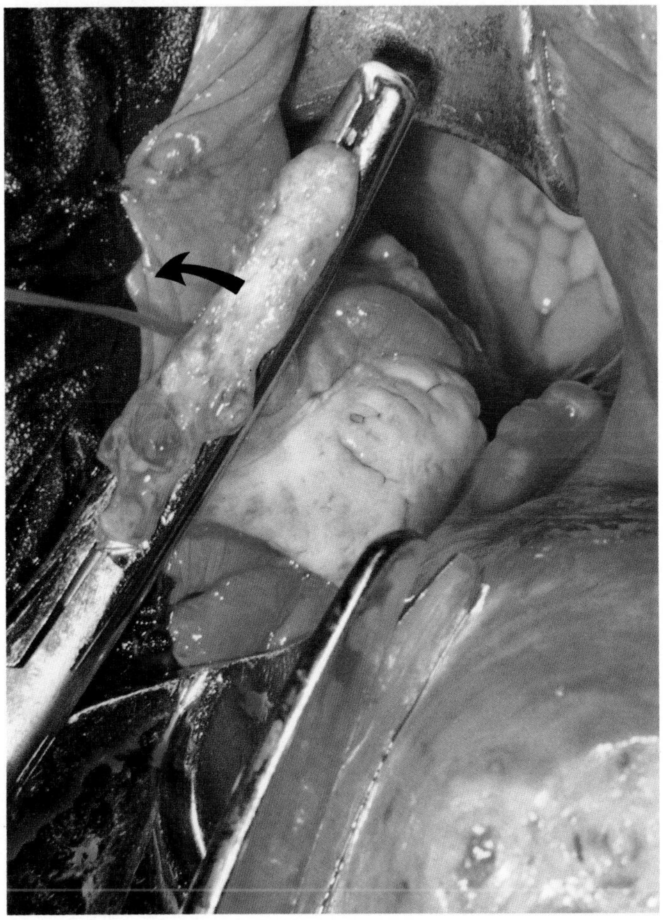

37–39 Clamping and detaching of right broad ligament pedicle
The bulky pedicle is clamped in **37** by heavy Maingot's forceps. This instrument is ideal for the purpose because of its long strong blades and the longitudinal ridging obviates any slipping. The tube and round ligament are clearly visible. The pedicle is cut with strong scissors in **38** and in **39** the detached pedicle falls away as arrowed to reveal the ovary and the ovarian ligament posteriorly.

40

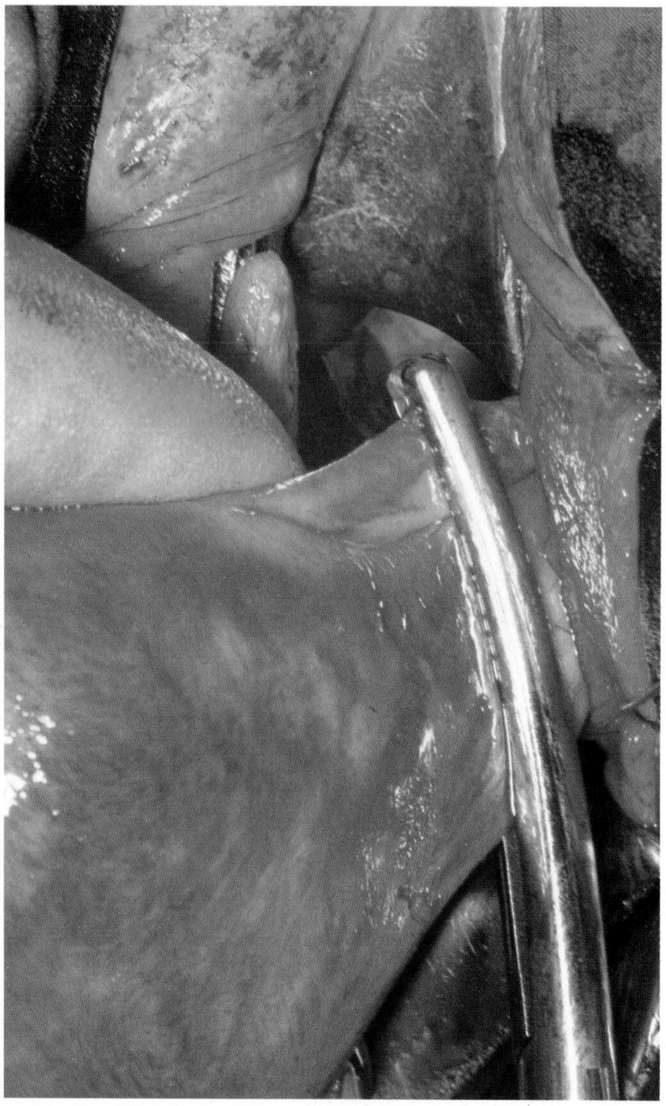

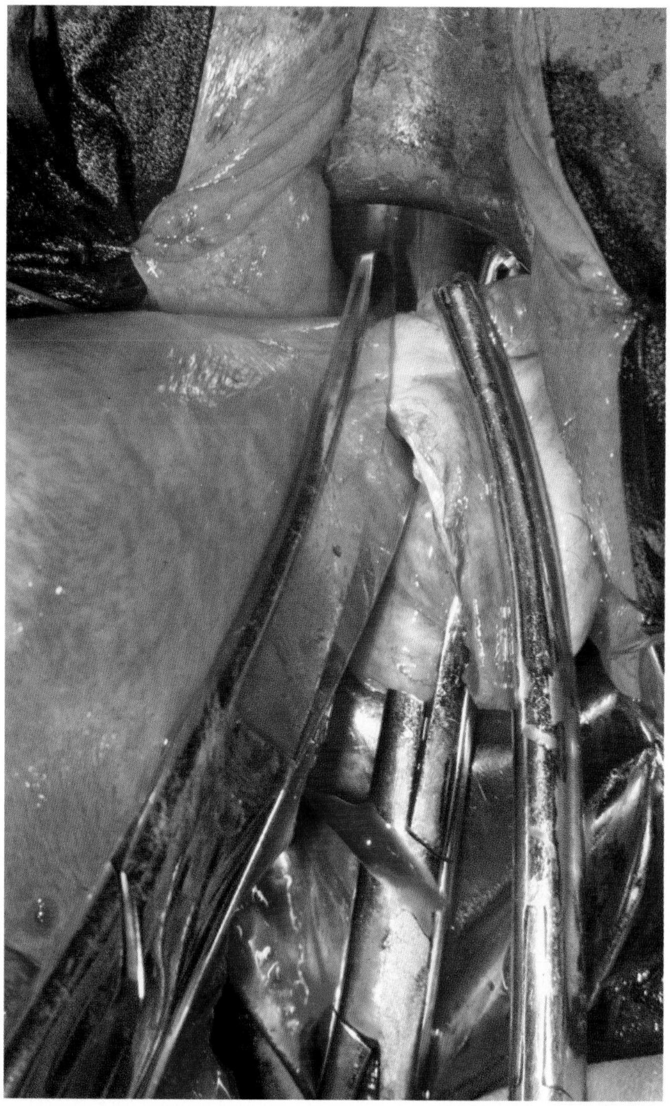

41

40 Definition and clamping of left broad ligament pedicle

The uterus is now attached only by the left broad ligament. Traction on the right cornu of the uterus is used to put the ligament on the stretch and it is clamped as shown. The right broad ligament clamp is seen in the background.

41 Division of left broad ligament pedicle

It is detached exactly as on the other side and as shown.

42 View following removal of uterus

Both ovaries are now clearly seen and it is at this stage that a routine examination is made during vaginal hysterectomy. If any pathology such as cyst on the ovary is encountered it is dealt with before proceeding further. In such circumstances salpingo-oophorectomy is feasible and comparatively safe but operations on the ovary tend to be followed by bleeding with possible vault infection. This emphasises the importance of not embarking on vaginal hysterectomy if there is pre-operative clinical evidence of significant adnexal pathology (e.g. endometriosis).

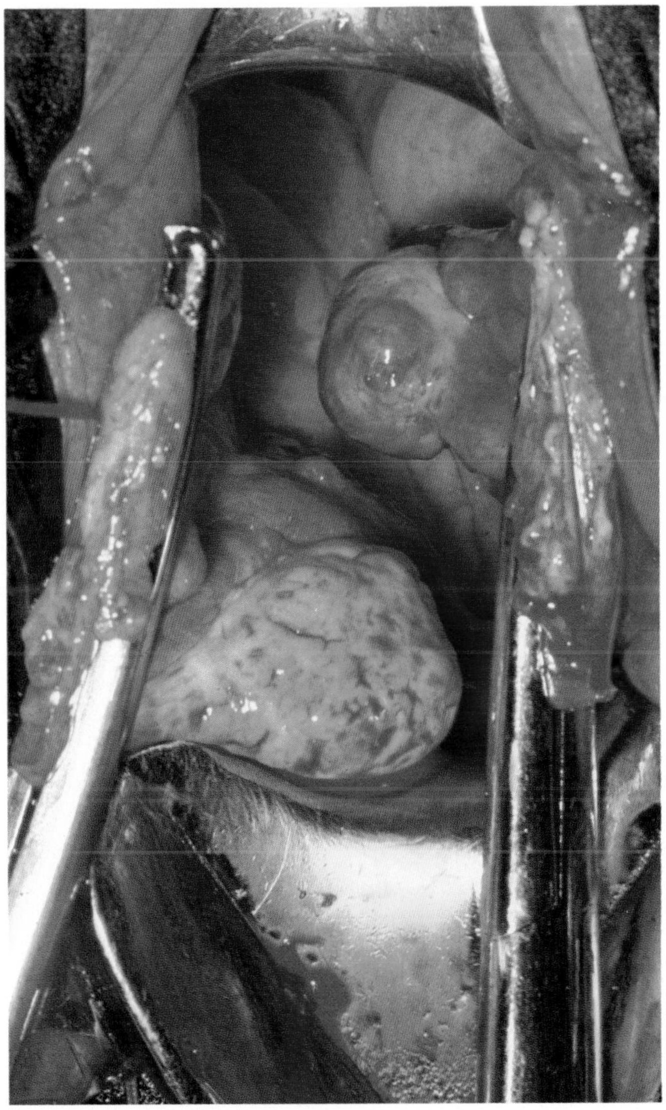

42

43

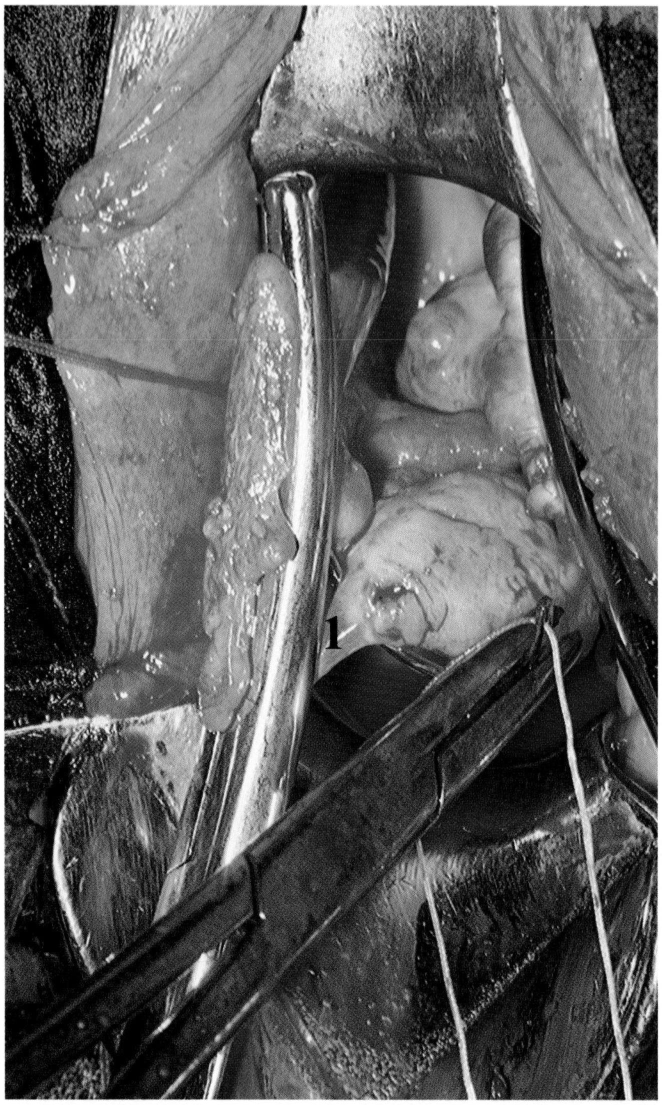

44

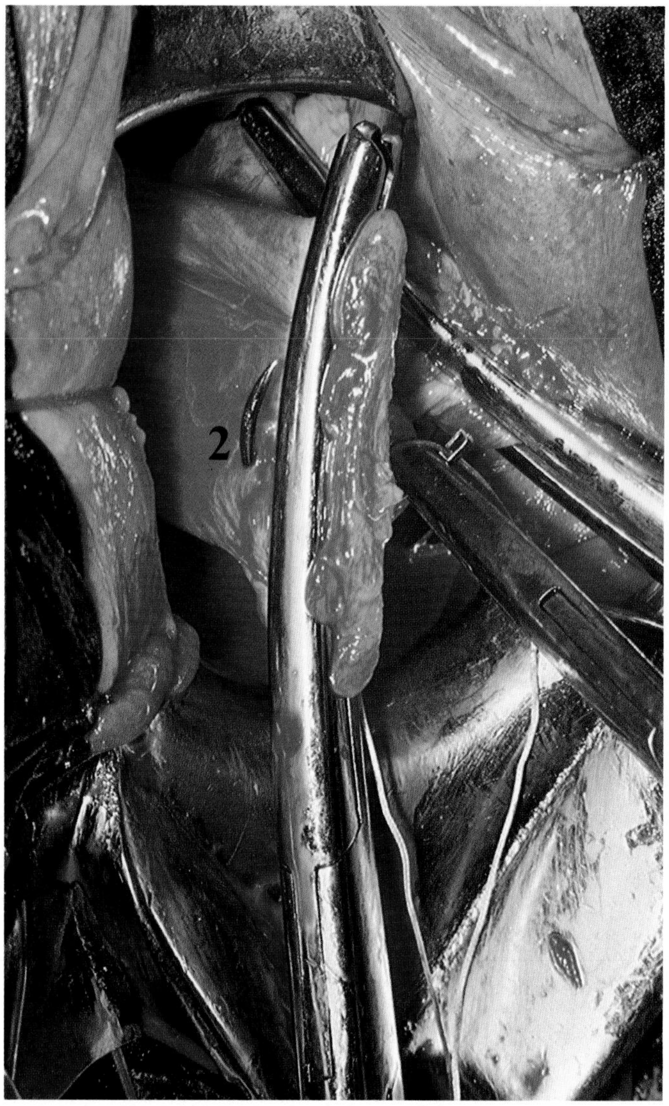

43 Transfixing right broad ligament pedicle (i)

In ligation of the broad ligament pedicles the fibromuscular round ligament should be used as an anchor for the suture and it is wise to include the ovarian ligament also. The pedicle is necessarily bulky so that it is difficult to compress adequately and there is the risk of structures escaping from the ligature. The needle is seen to have transfixed the right ovarian ligament as marked (1) before piercing the pedicle at its mid-point.

44 Transfixing right broad ligament pedicle (ii)

As the pedicle is rolled medially the needle is brought through the centre of the round ligament as shown (2).

45

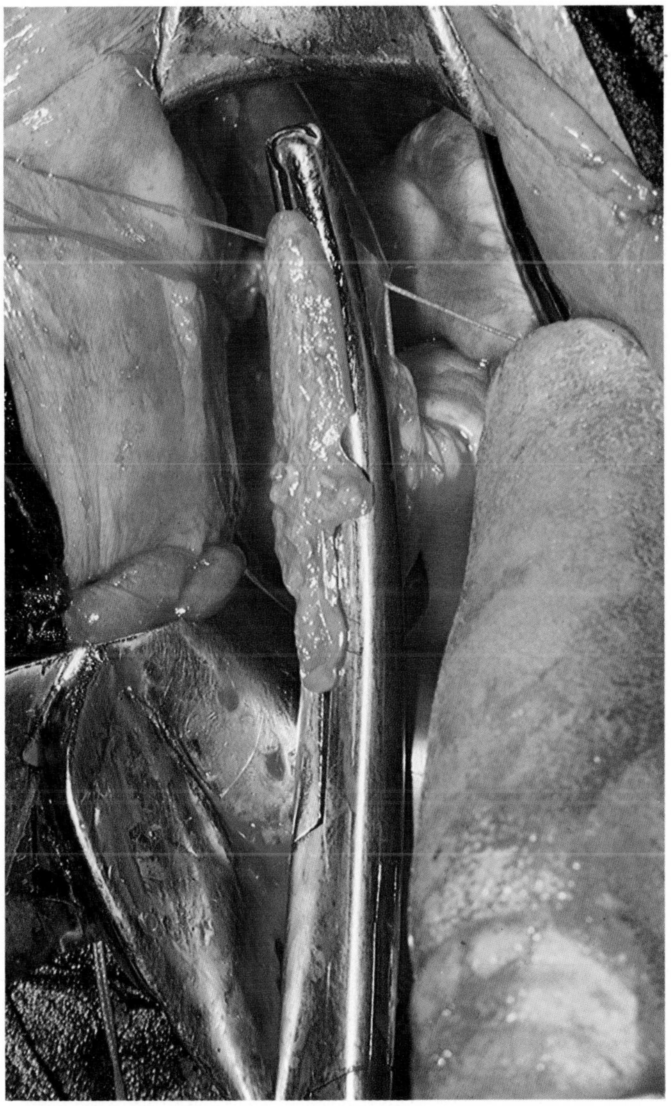

46

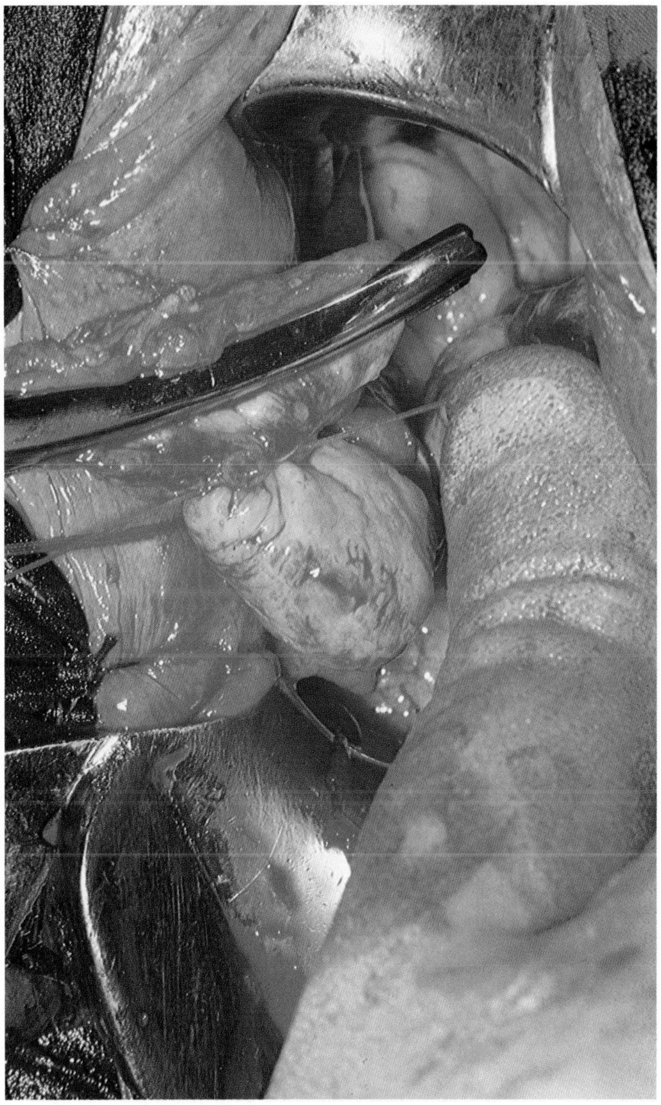

45 Tying right broad ligament pedicle (i)

The ligature is shown being single tied in the usual fashion. Considerable force is needed if PGA sutures are used. The ends are left long and fixed to the drapes.

46 Tying right broad ligament pedicle (ii)

47
 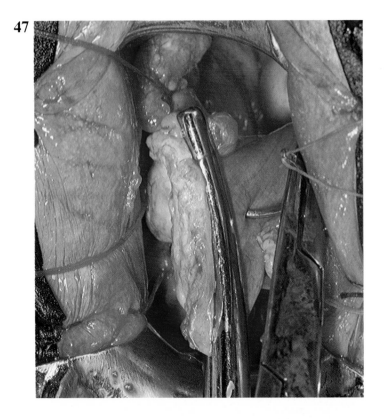

48
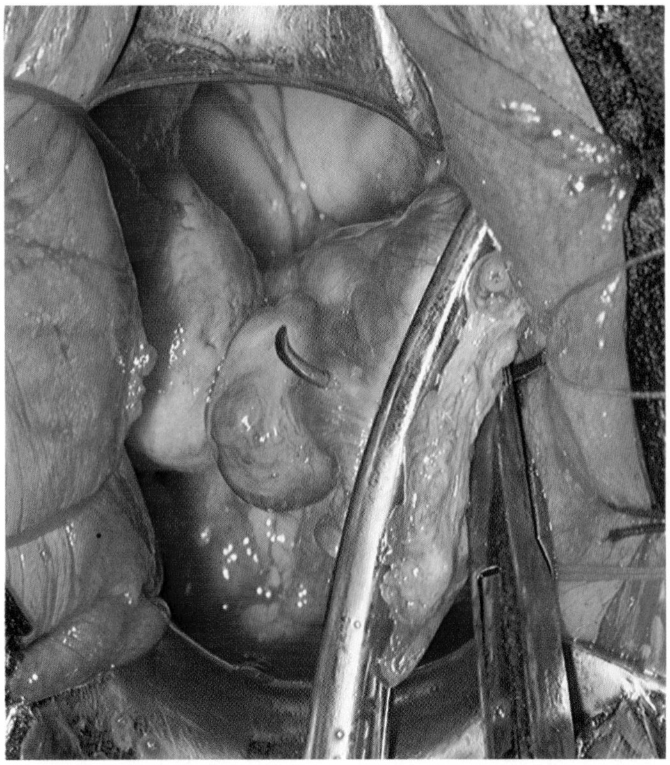

49
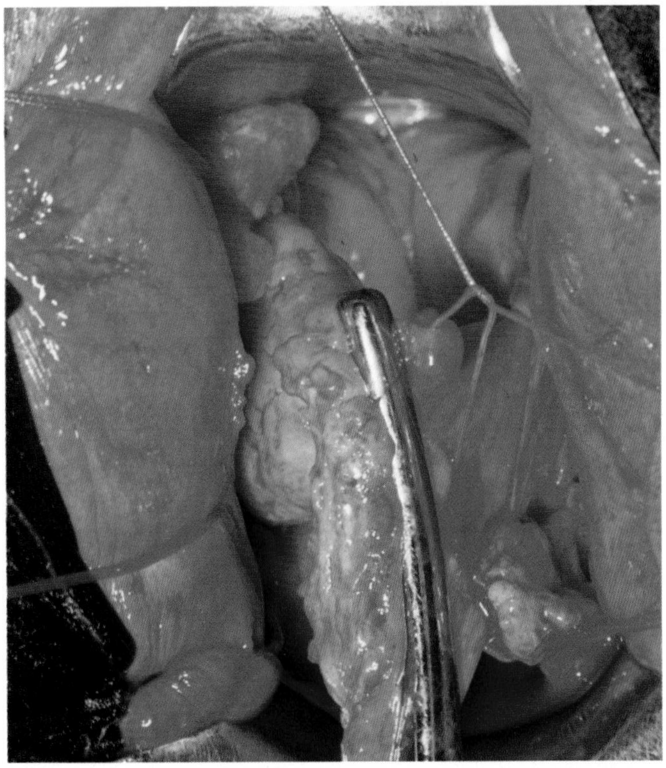

50
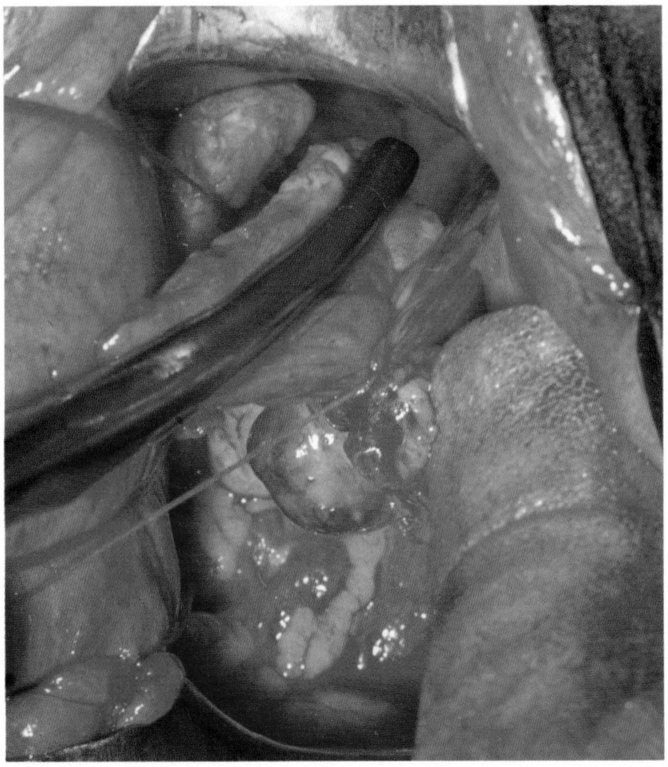

47–50 Transfixion and tying left broad ligament pedicle

The left broad ligament pedicle is shown being secured in the same way as the right. In this instance the needle pierces the round ligament first, then the centre of the pedicle and finally the ovarian ligament.

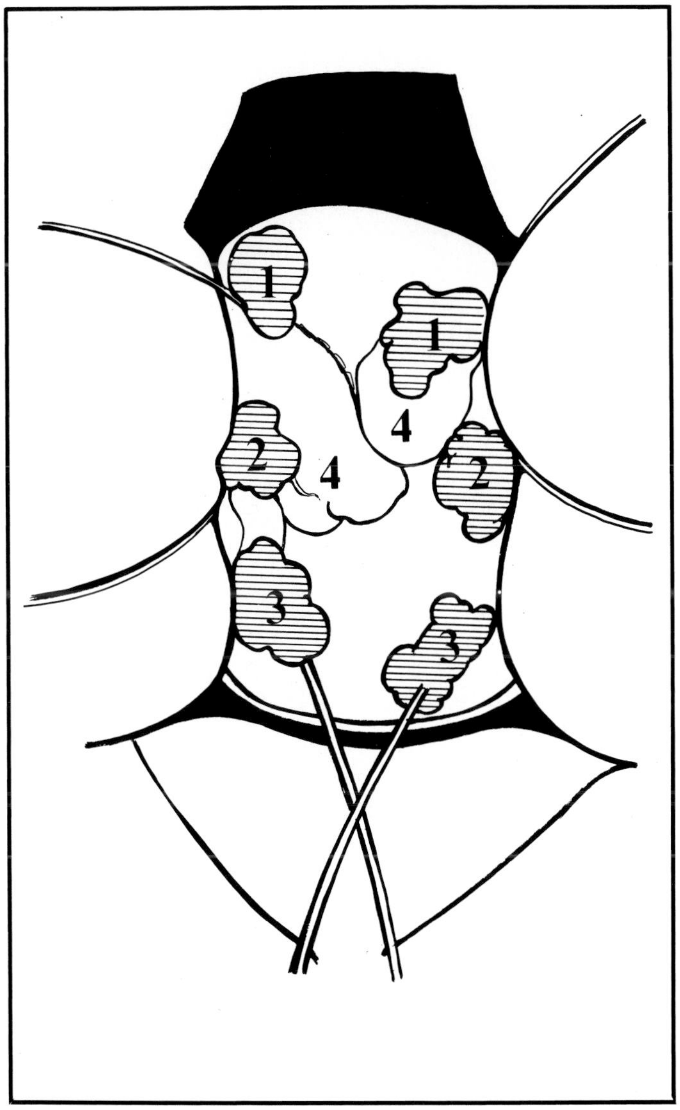

Shaded areas indicate the ligated pedicles
1 Broad ligament pedicle
2 Uterine pedicle
3 Utero-sacral and cardinal pedicle
4 Ovaries

51

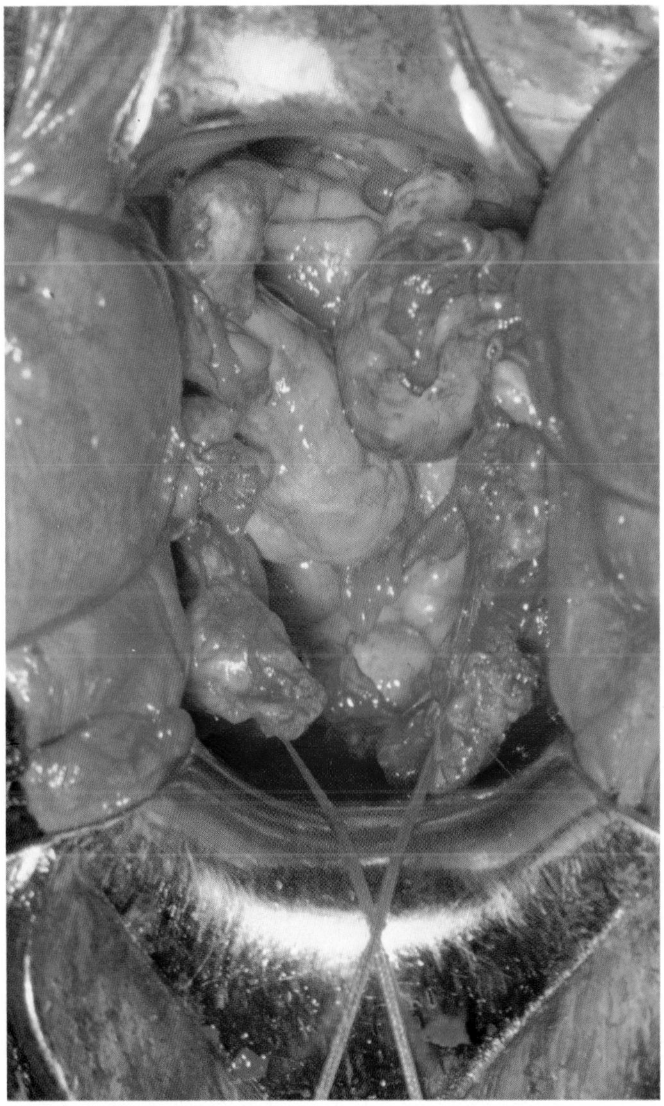

51 Appearance following removal of uterus

The three pedicles on each side have now been secured and the peritoneal cavity awaits closure. Gentle traction on the uncut sutures displays the pedicles – the broad ligaments near the top of the picture, the uterine pedicles half way down and the utero-sacrals just above the Auvard speculum with their sutures crossing over each other.

52

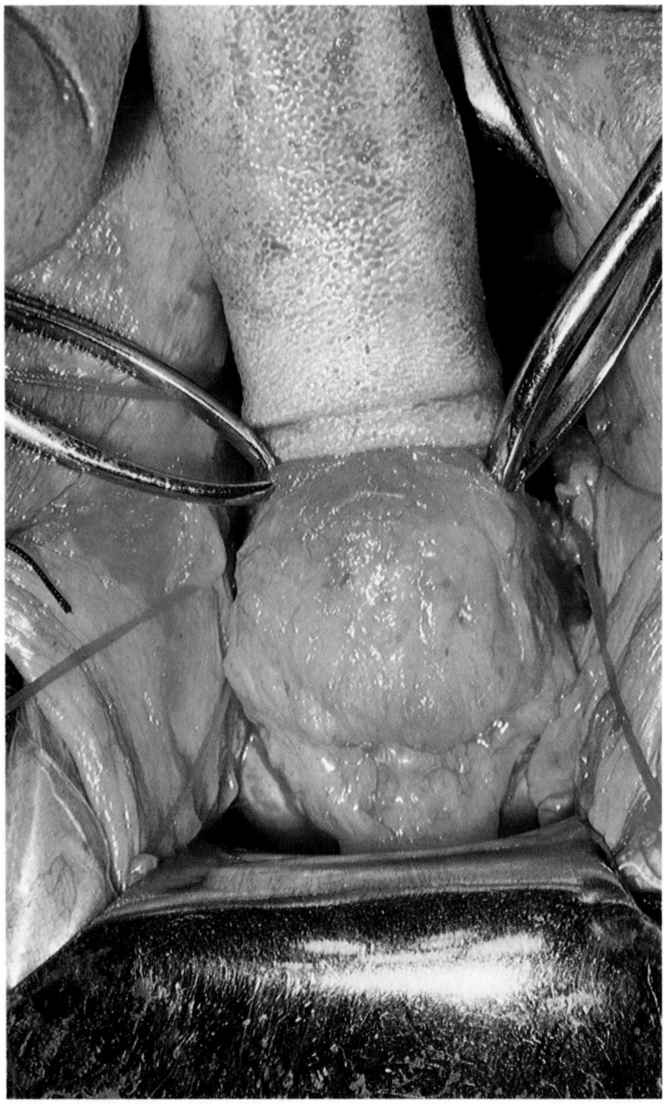

53

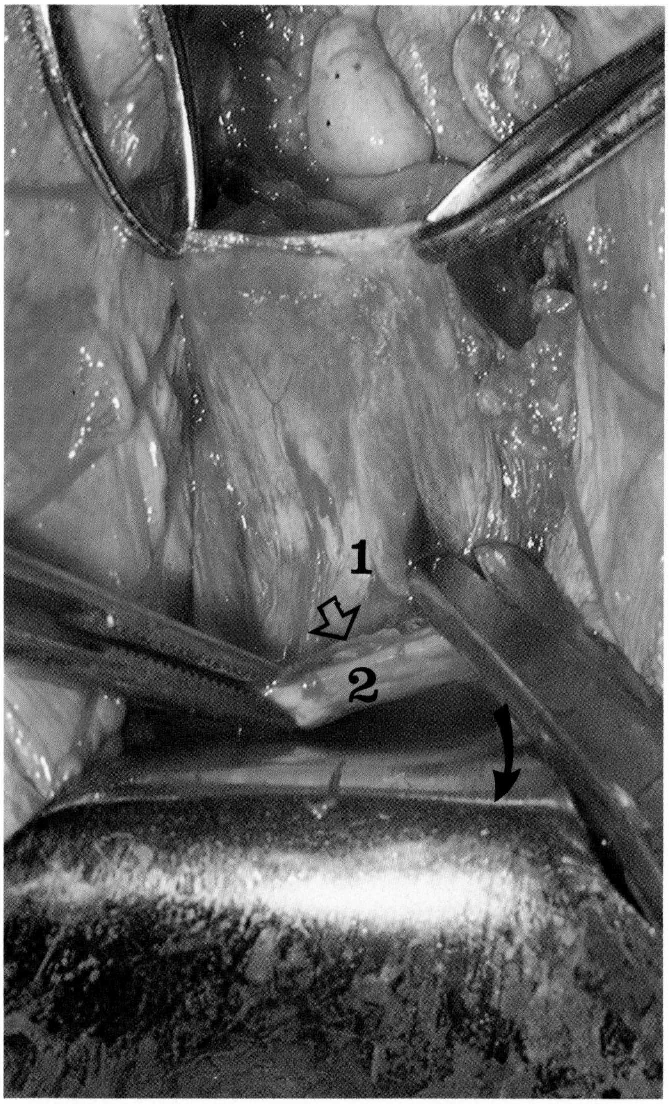

52 Elimination of posterior pouch (i)

This entails dissection of the peritoneum of the pouch of Douglas to eliminate any sacculation in that area. This is a very important part of the operation because it is by herniation of the peritoneal sac between the utero-sacral ligaments that recurrence takes place. The peritoneum with its covering of extra peritoneal fat is raised on the finger while the edge is held with two pairs of Littlewood's forceps.

53 Elimination of posterior pouch (ii)

The peritoneum is dissected off the utero-sacral ligaments with scissors and separation is easy once the plane of cleavage has been found. This always lies very close to the peritoneum which comes up as a thin layer. The anterior leaf of the peritoneum is held upwards and forwards by two pairs of Littlewood's forceps, and it has all the features of a hernial sac. Any excess tissue is trimmed off. The dark arrow shows the direction of pressure: the outline arrow indicates the plane of cleavage between the enterocele sac (1) and the vaginal edge (2).

Stage 4: Closure of peritoneal cavity

The aim is to close the cavity while leaving all the six pedicles extraperitoneally. A purse-string suture is not very satisfactory because it is difficult to place and difficult to run up tight. Too many important structures in any case become dependent on a single suture strand. We prefer to close the cavity with interrupted sutures as will be demonstrated. The two lateral stitches close the angles of the peritoneal opening while keeping the ligated pedicles extraperitoneal and then the centre part is closed with three single stitches. An atraumatic needle carrying a PGA No. 0 suture picks up the following structures on each side:

1 The lateral aspect of the anterior peritoneal leaf
2 A portion of the round ligament
3 The ovarian ligament
4 A portion on the utero-sacral ligament
5 The lateral aspect of the posterior leaf of peritoneum

The line of this suture is above and medial to the three pedicles which are gently pulled down by the assistant while it is being placed.

54
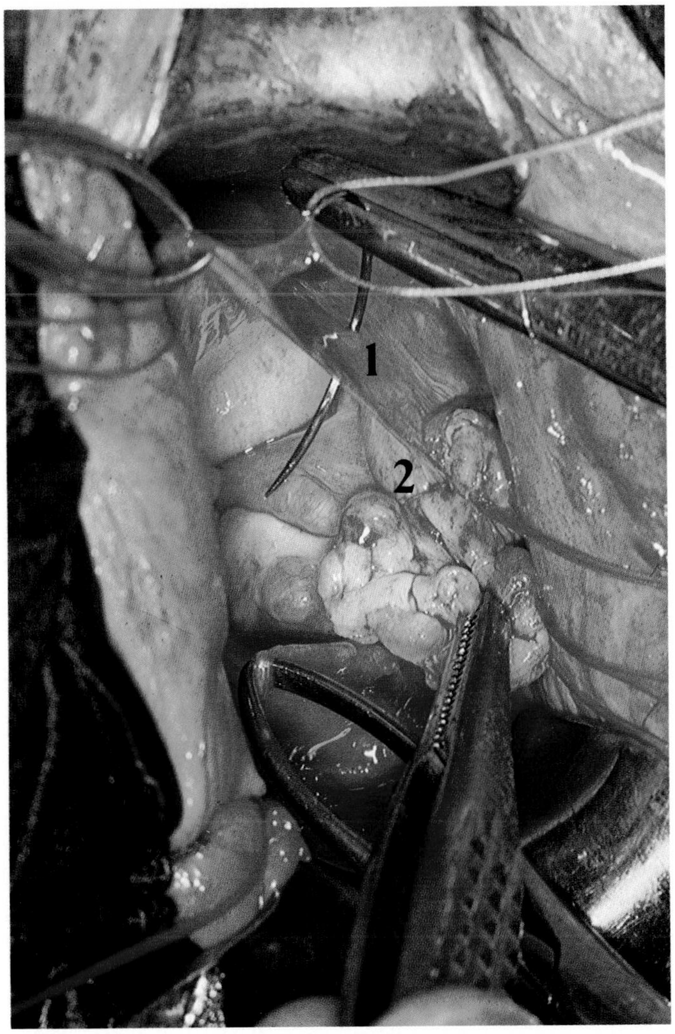

54 Closure of peritoneal cavity – left side (i)
The needle has picked up the lateral peritoneal leaf (1) and the round ligament (2) is thrown into relief by traction on the broad ligament pedicle.

55
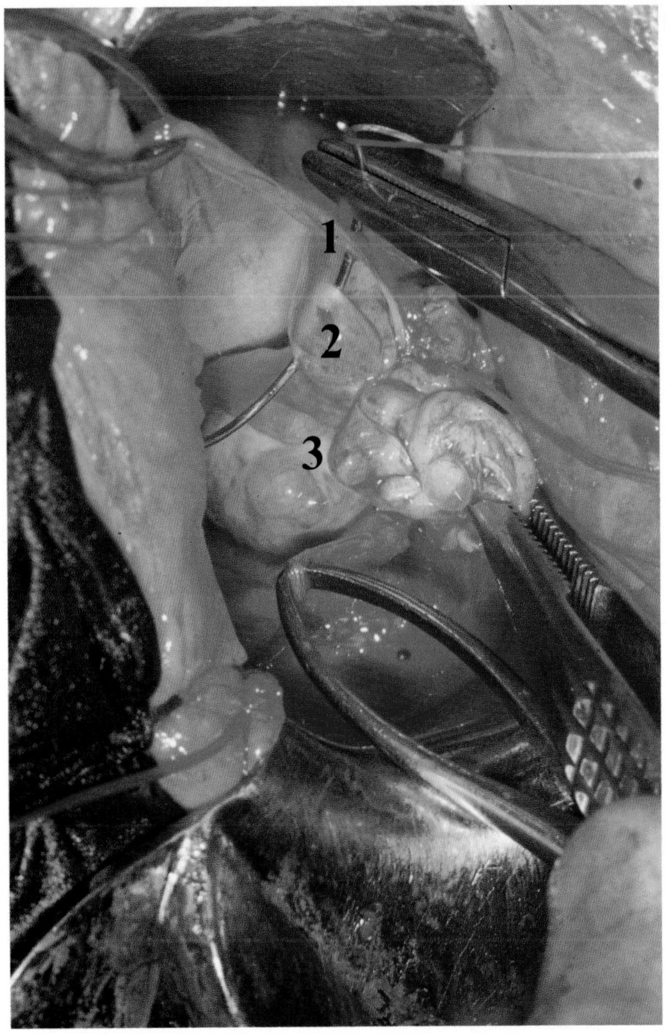

55 Closure of peritoneal cavity – left side (ii)
The round ligament has been transfixed and the dissecting forceps retract the broad ligament pedicle laterally to show the ovarian ligament (3).

56

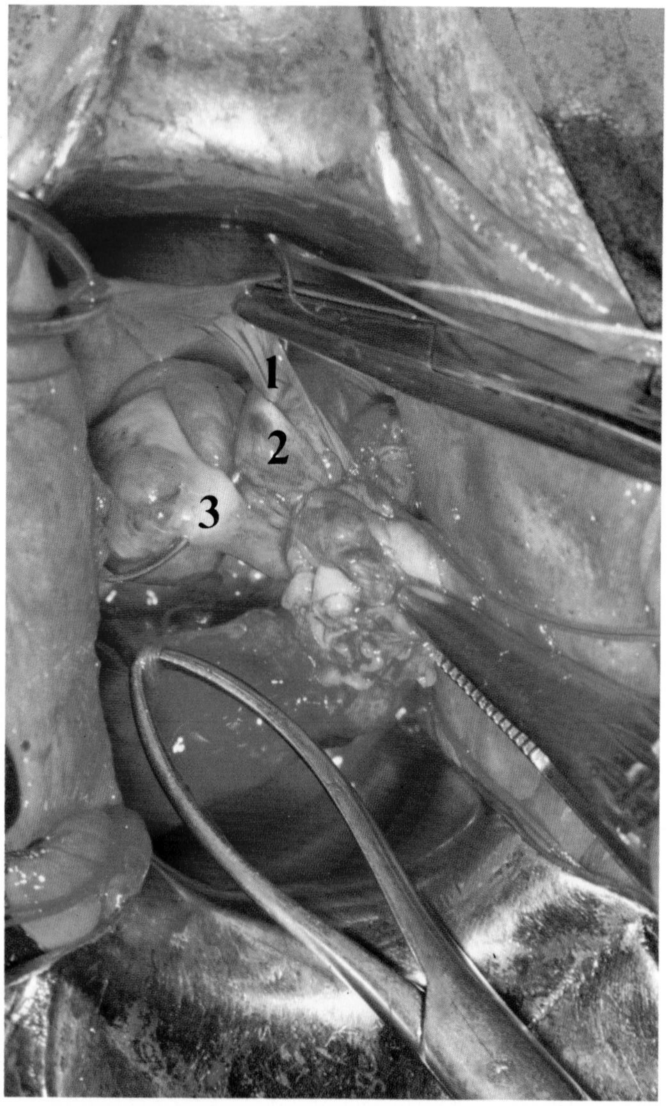

57

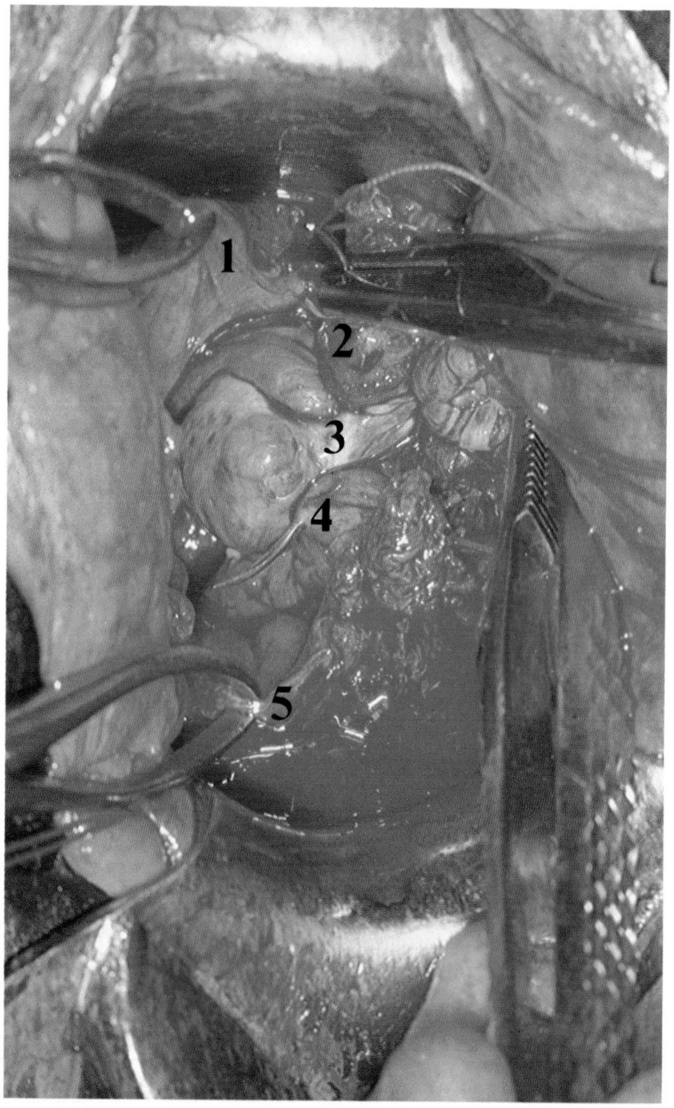

56 Closure of peritoneal cavity – left side (iii)

The ovarian ligament (3) has been transfixed by the needle while the dissecting forceps keep the pedicle taut.

57 Closure of peritoneal cavity – left side (iv)

The utero-sacral ligament (4) is displayed by traction on the suture and has been picked up by the needle. Only the posterior peritoneal leaf (5) remains to be included.

58

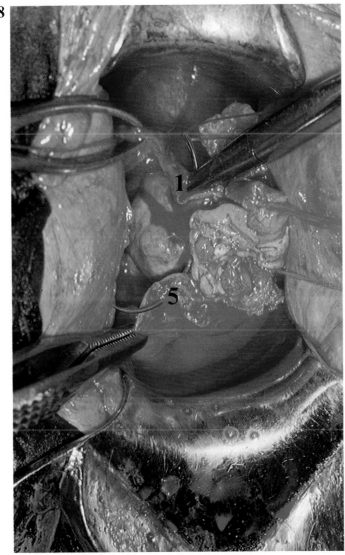

59

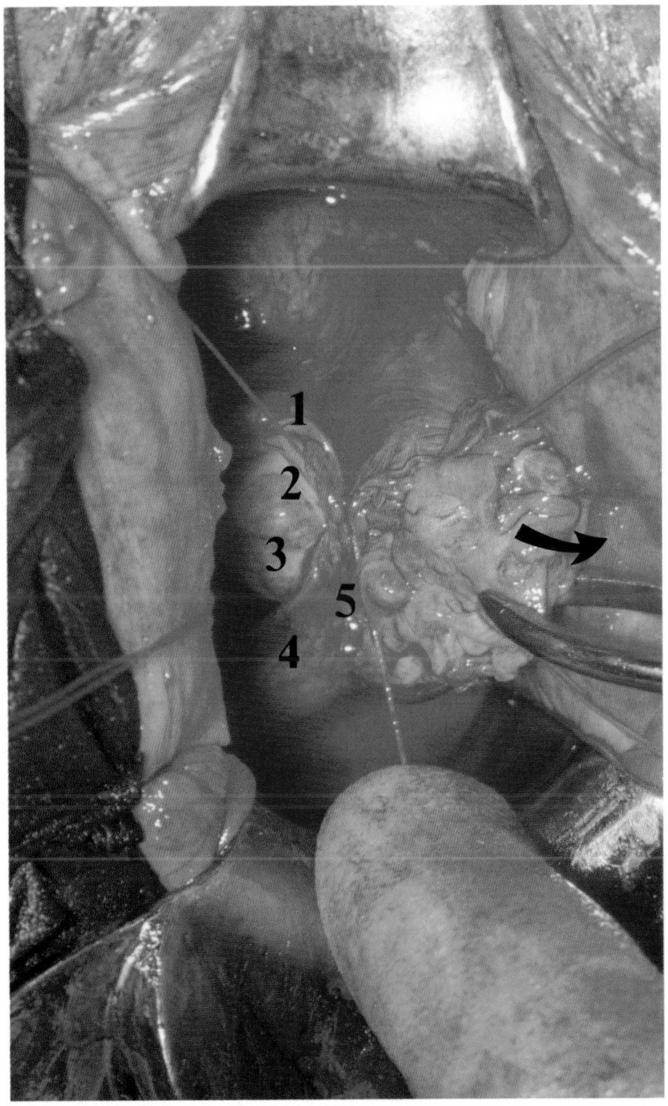

58 Closure of peritoneal cavity – left side (v)

The needle finally picks up the lateral aspect of the posterior peritoneal leaf (5). As the two layers of peritoneum come together the intervening course of the stitch is occluded but the long sutures show the position of the three pedicles.

59 Closure of peritoneal cavity – left side (vi)

The left side of the peritoneal opening is closed as the stitch is tied and the various pedicles again come into view as the three long sutures and Littlewood's forceps pull laterally (arrowed). The pedicles themselves are identifiable by their sutures and are all extraperitoneal.

60

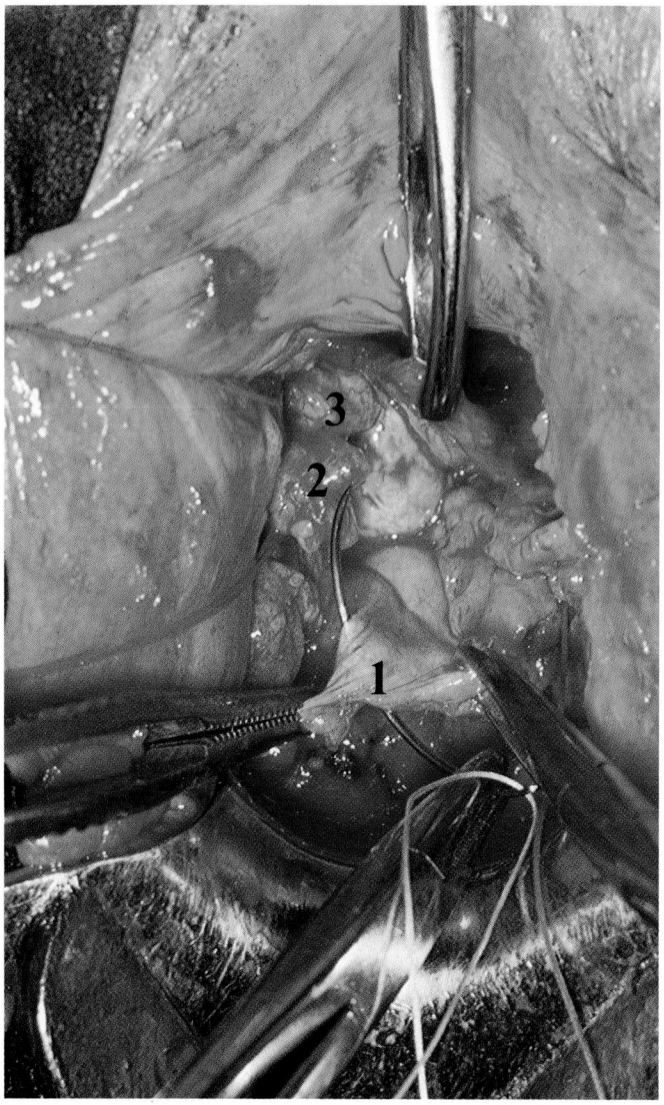

61

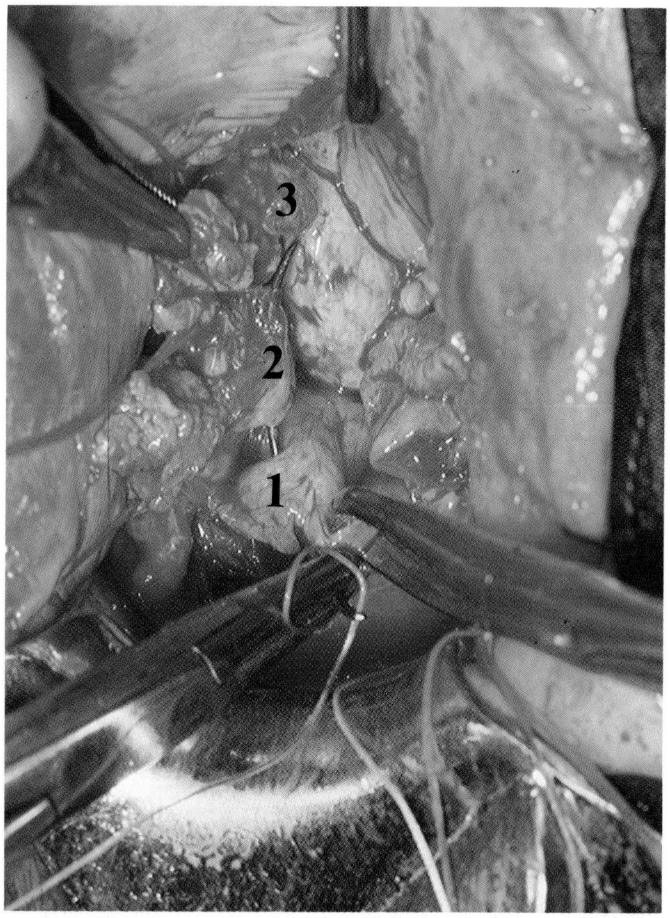

62

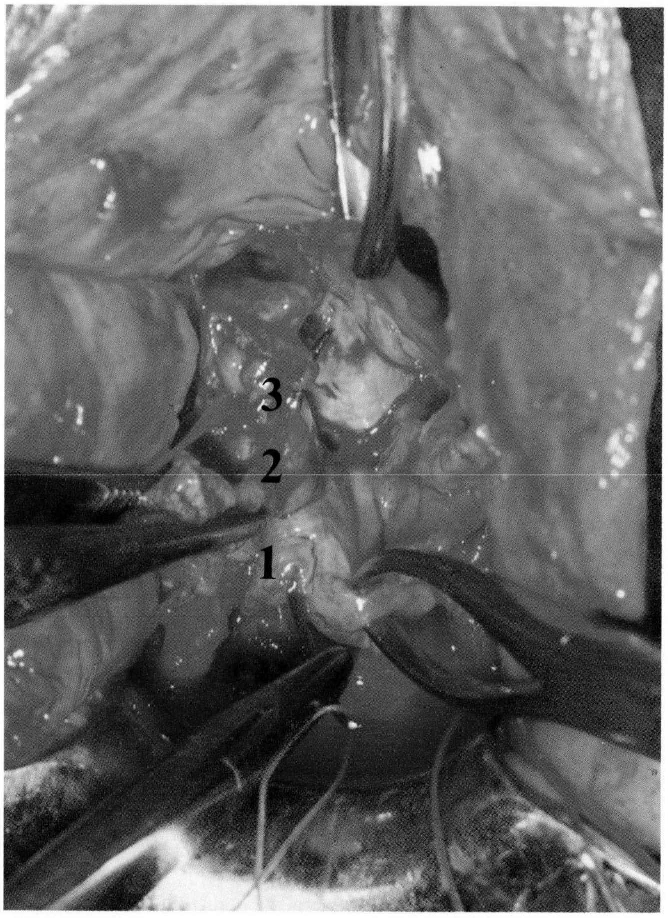

60–62 Closure of peritoneal cavity – right side (i) (ii) (iii)

The same procedure is followed on the right side in the reverse direction to suit the surgeon's hand. The needle traverses the right side of the posterior peritoneal leaf (1), catches the right utero-sacral ligament (2) and transfixes the right ovarian ligament (3).

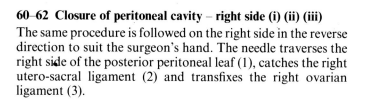

63
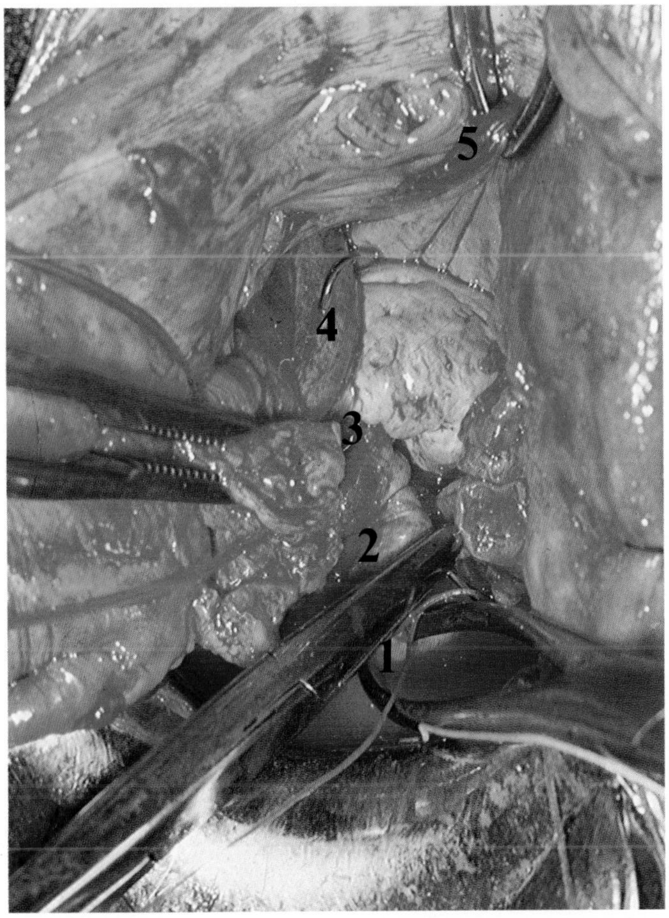

64
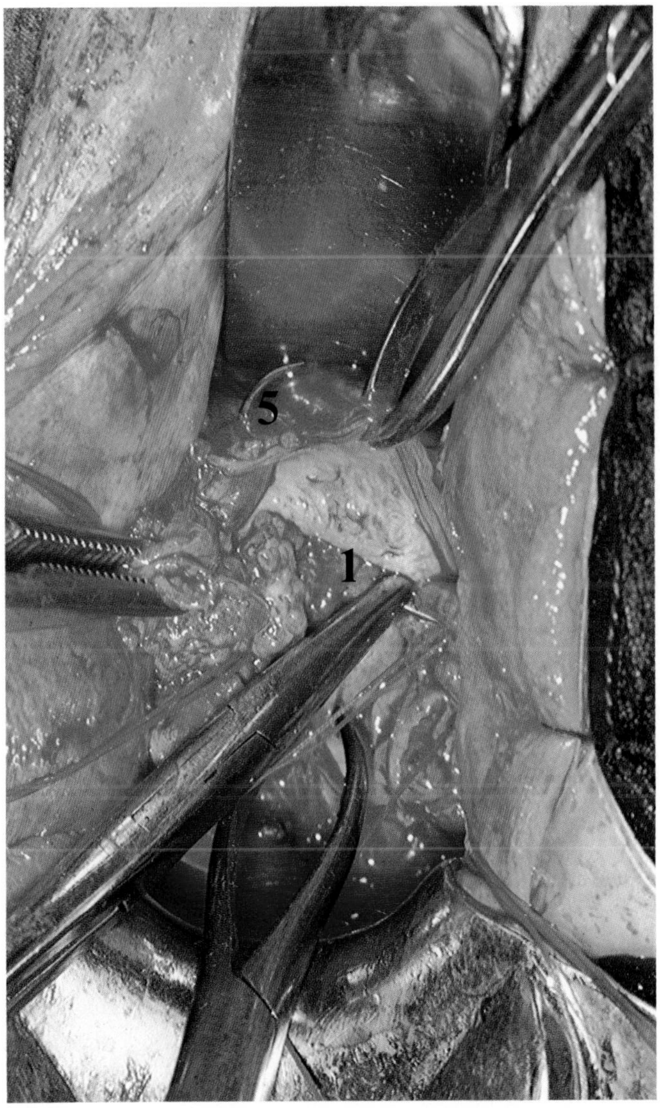

65
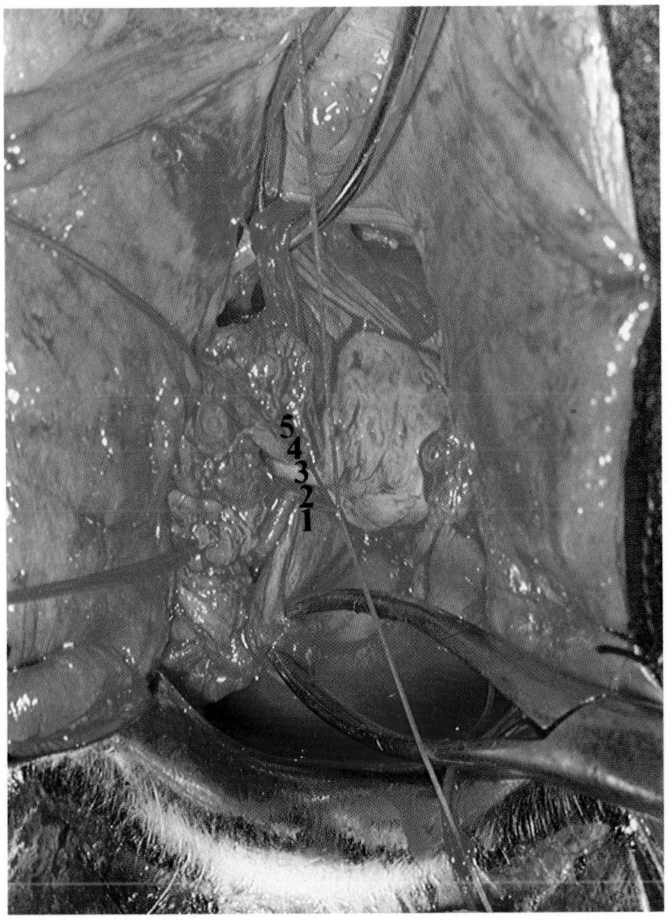

63–65 Closure of peritoneal cavity – right side (iv) (v) (vi)

The round ligament (4) and the lateral aspect of the anterior peritoneal leaf (5) are picked up in turn and the stitch is tied with the three pedicles indicated by their attached sutures lying extraperitoneally. The right ovary is clearly seen in the remaining central peritoneal opening.

66

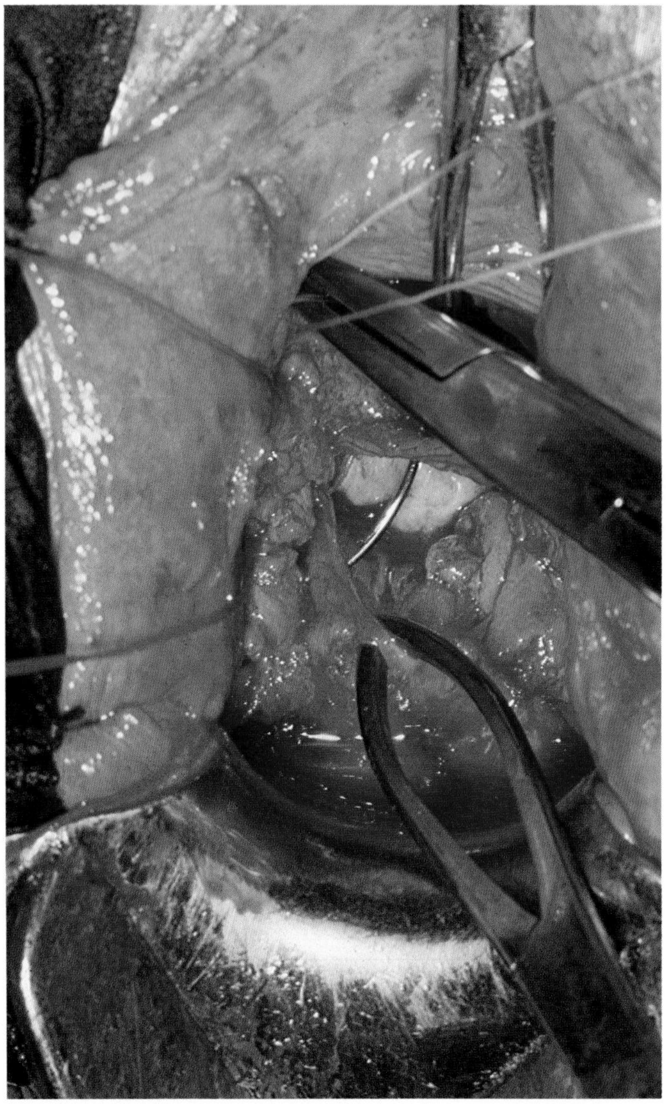

67

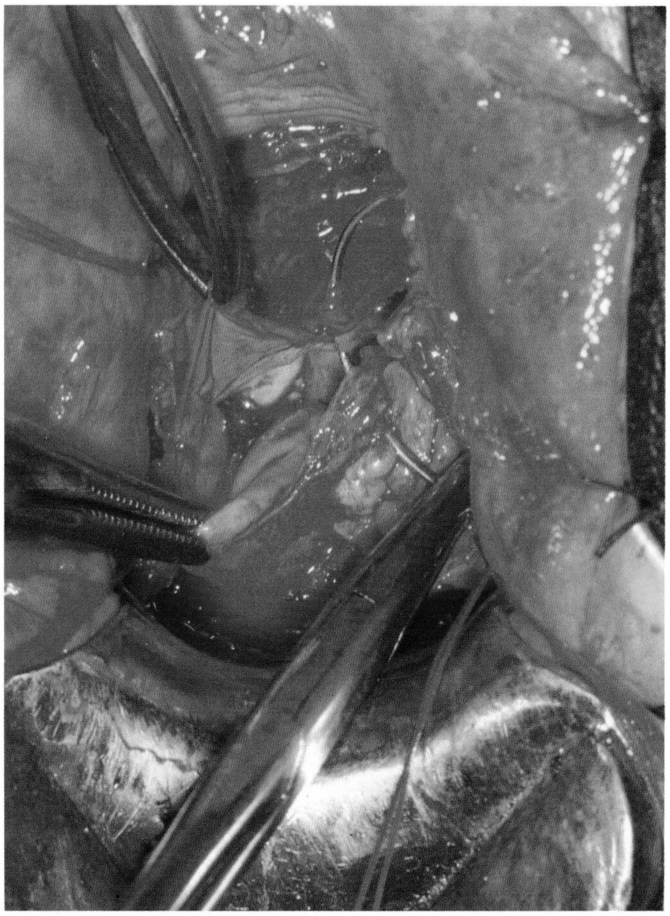

68

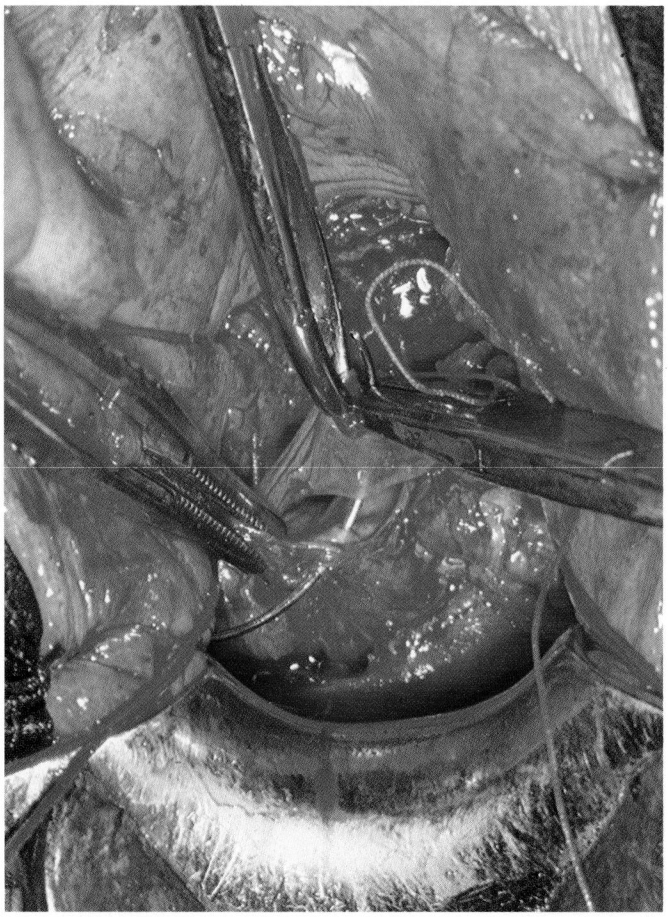

66–68 Closure of peritoneal cavity completed (i) (ii) (iii)

In the first illustration an interrupted stitch closes the right side of the central opening, in the second the left side and in the third a final stitch completes the closure. A continuous stitch would serve equally well.

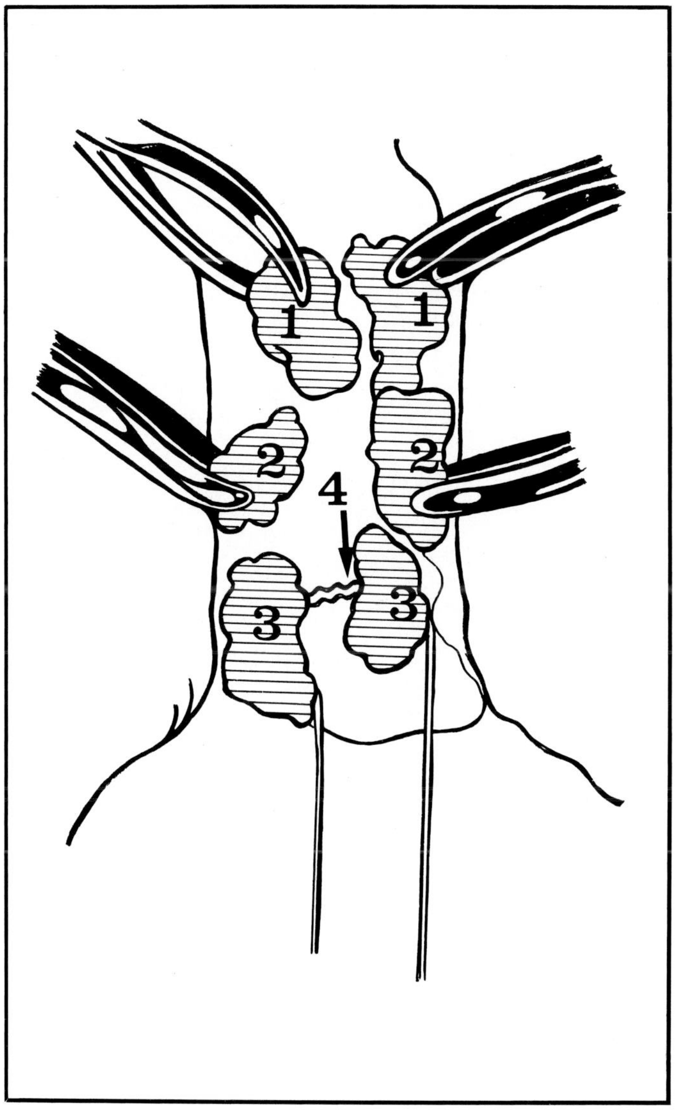

69

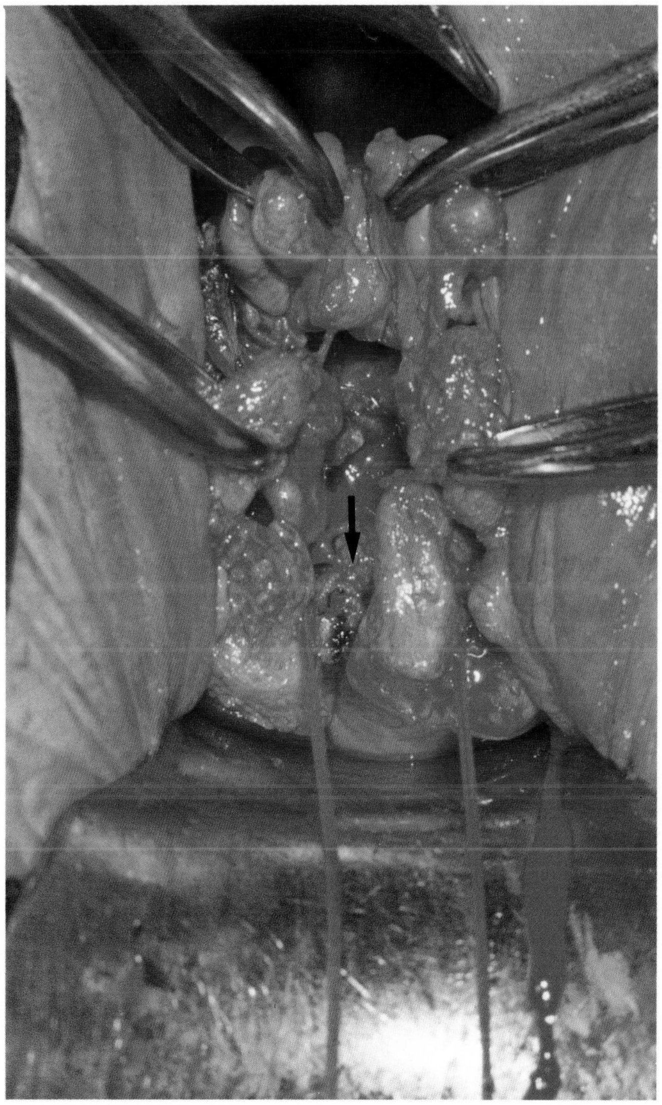

Shaded areas indicate the ligated pedicles
1 Broad ligament pedicle
2 Uterine pedicle
3 Utero-sacral and cardinal pedicle
4 Closed peritoneal suture line

69 Closure of peritoneal cavity completed (iv)

The peritoneum is now closed. Note that the three pedicles on each side are lying extraperitoneally. The closed peritoneal suture line (arrowed) lies directly between the utero-sacral pedicles and is well away from the broad ligament pedicles. This is a constant finding at this stage and seems to indicate that the broad ligaments have no direct relationship to the vaginal vault and its support. These pedicles are not therefore used for that purpose.

Stage 5: Double tying of pedicles in vaginal hysterectomy

The commonest cause of morbidity in vaginal hysterectomy is directly related to incomplete haemostasis and the main source of the bleeding or oozing is from the pedicles. These are inclined to be bulky and difficult to ligate sufficiently tightly especially when using PGA suture material. We repeatedly find that after a lapse of 10 to 15 minutes a securely tied pedicle starts to ooze because of a shrinkage in the pedicle volume and consequent slackening of the ligature. This is less likely to happen with catgut with its inherent elasticity, but it is a problem with PGA. Because of this problem and because we consider that PGA has considerable advantages for vaginal surgery (as explained earlier) we prefer to ligate singly in the first place and return to repeat ligation definitively in each of the six pedicles after the peritoneum has been closed.

70

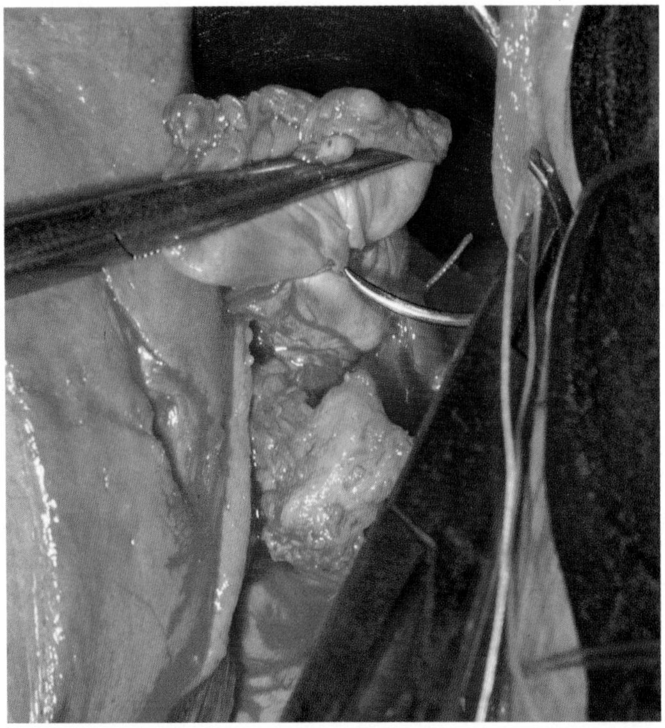

71

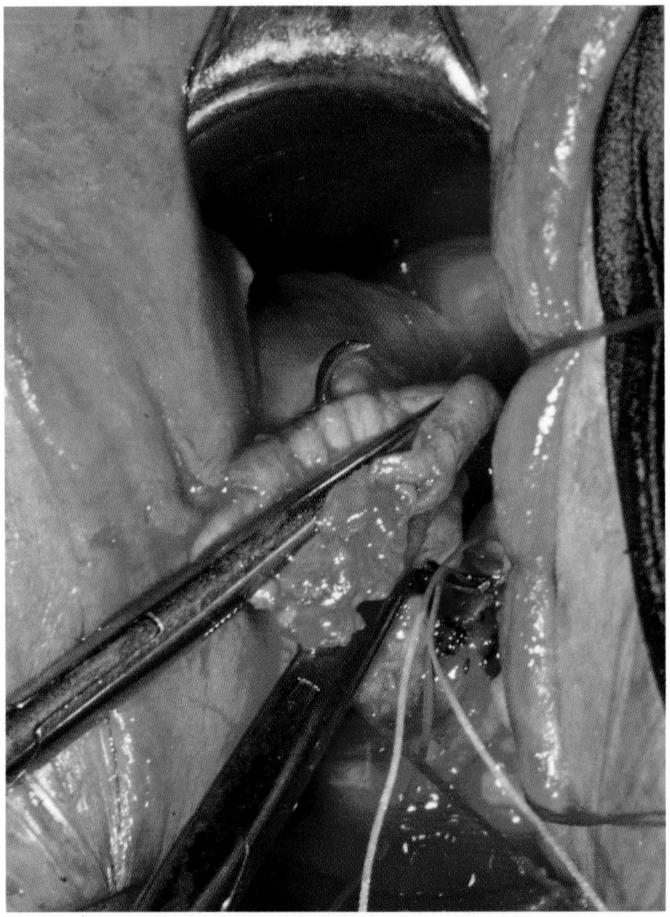

72

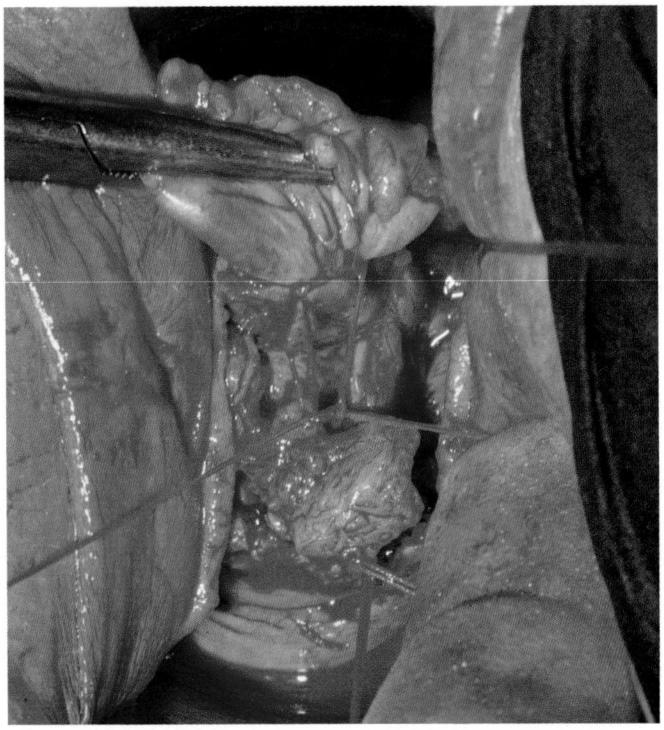

70–72 Religation of right broad ligament pedicle

The pedicle is held with fine forceps and transfixed immediately proximal to the previous ligature (**70**). The needle point emerges proximal to the ligature (**71**). The suture is tied (**72**). The suture ends are subsequently cut short.

73

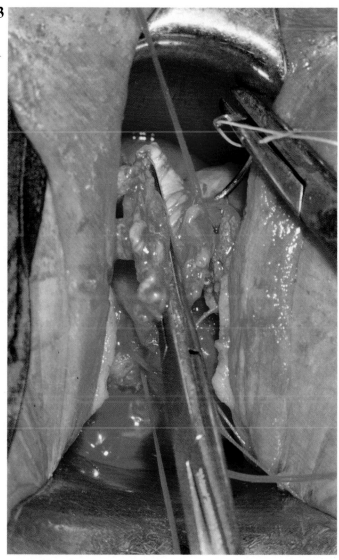

74

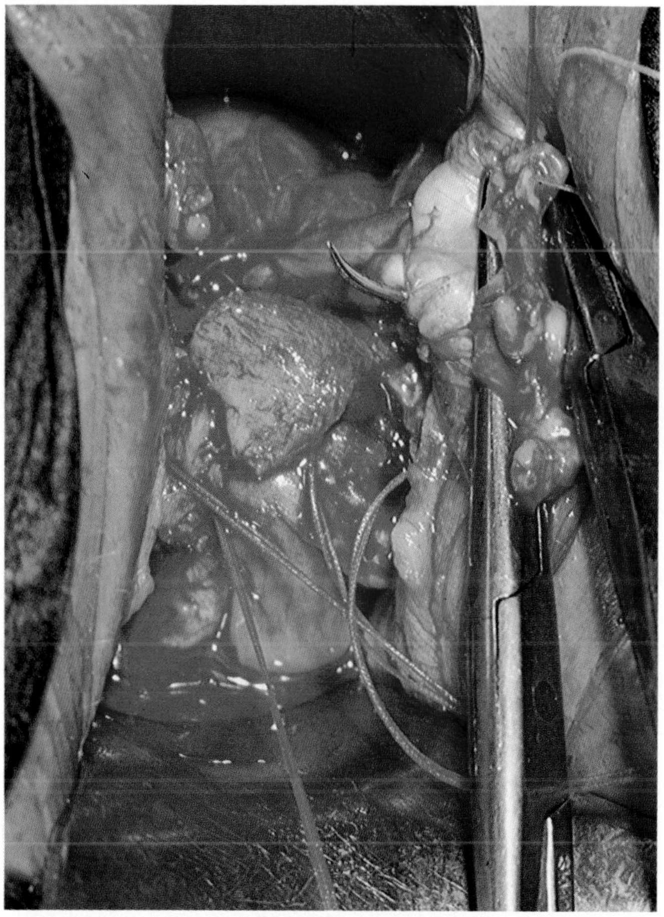

75

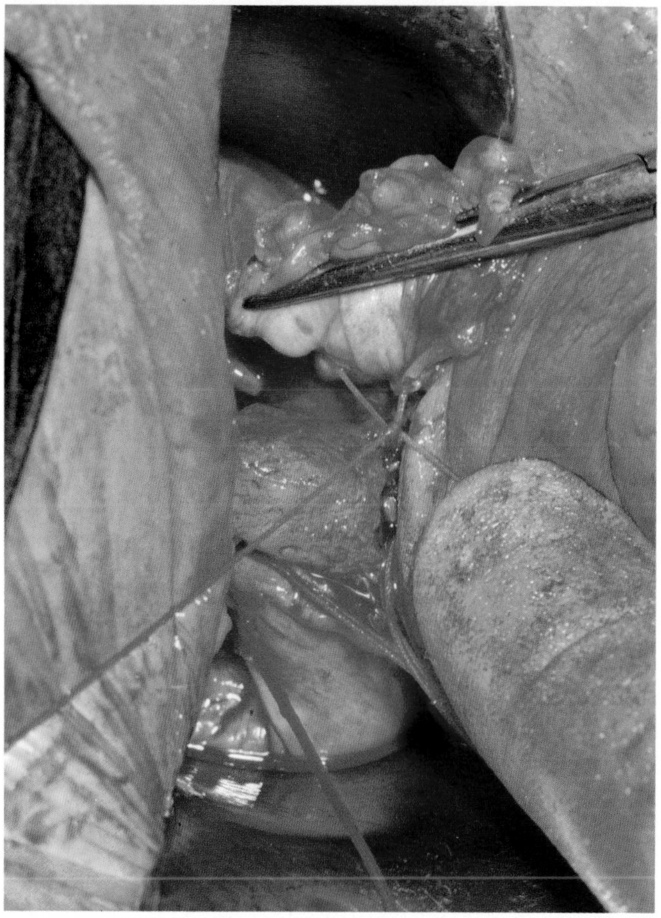

73–75 Religation of left broad ligament pedicle

The same sequence is shown in relation to the left pedicle and again the sutures will be cut short. Note how the ovarian ligament shows up in this illustration.

76

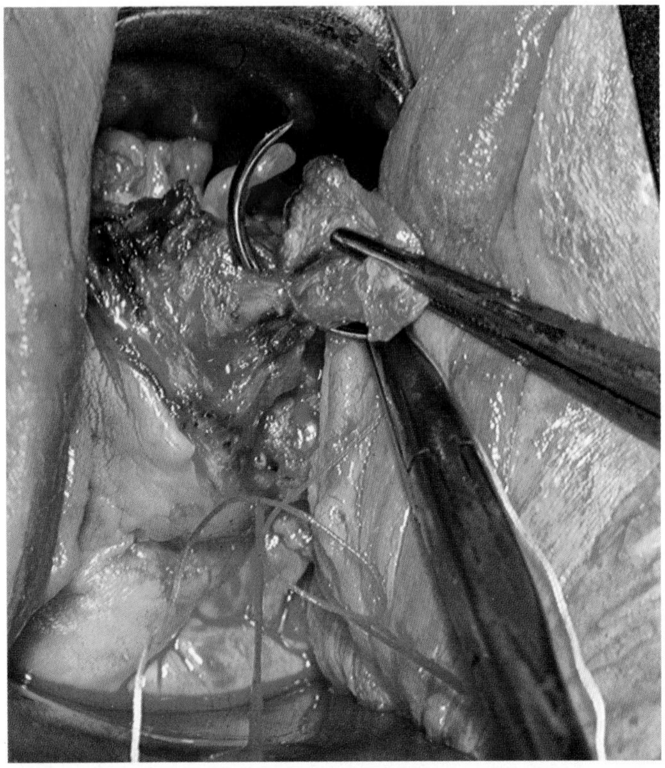

77

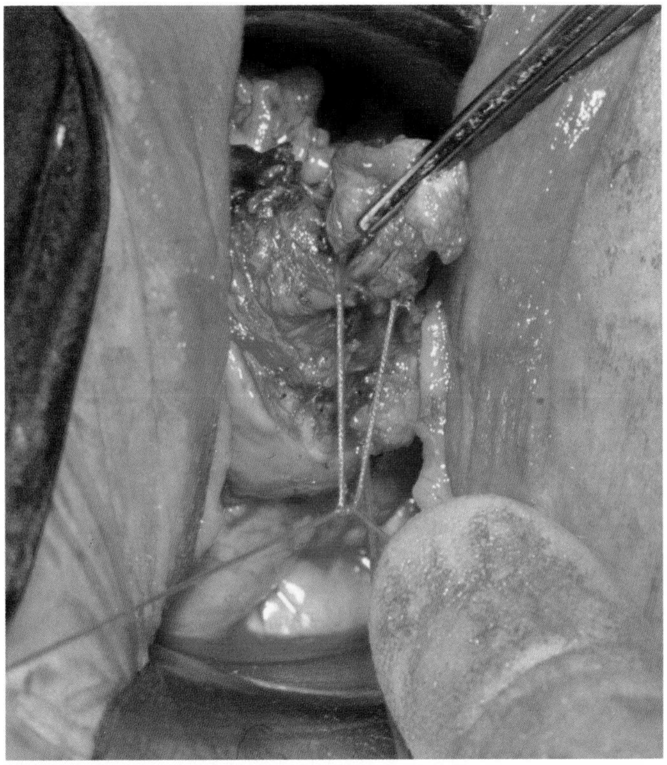

78

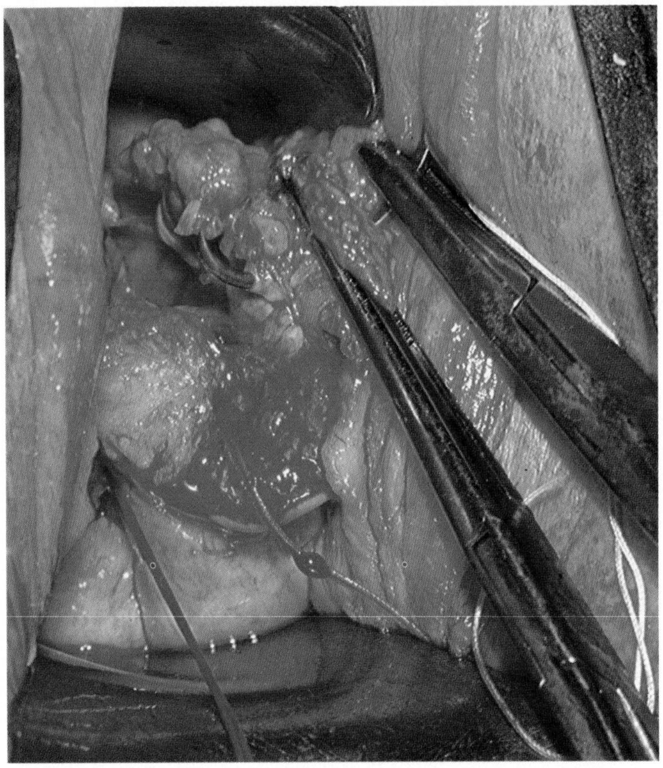

79

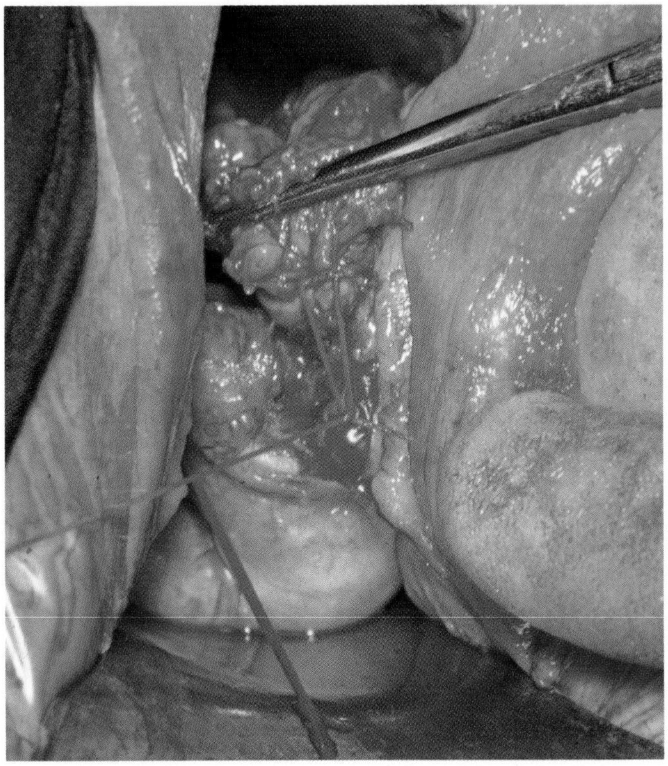

76–79 Religation of right and left uterine pedicle

Transfixion is just proximal to the previous ligature with subsequent tying of the suture. The uterine artery or any large vessel is of course avoided by the needle as far as possible. The ligature will be cut short. The right pedicles are in **76** and **77**; the left pedicles in **78** and **79**.

80

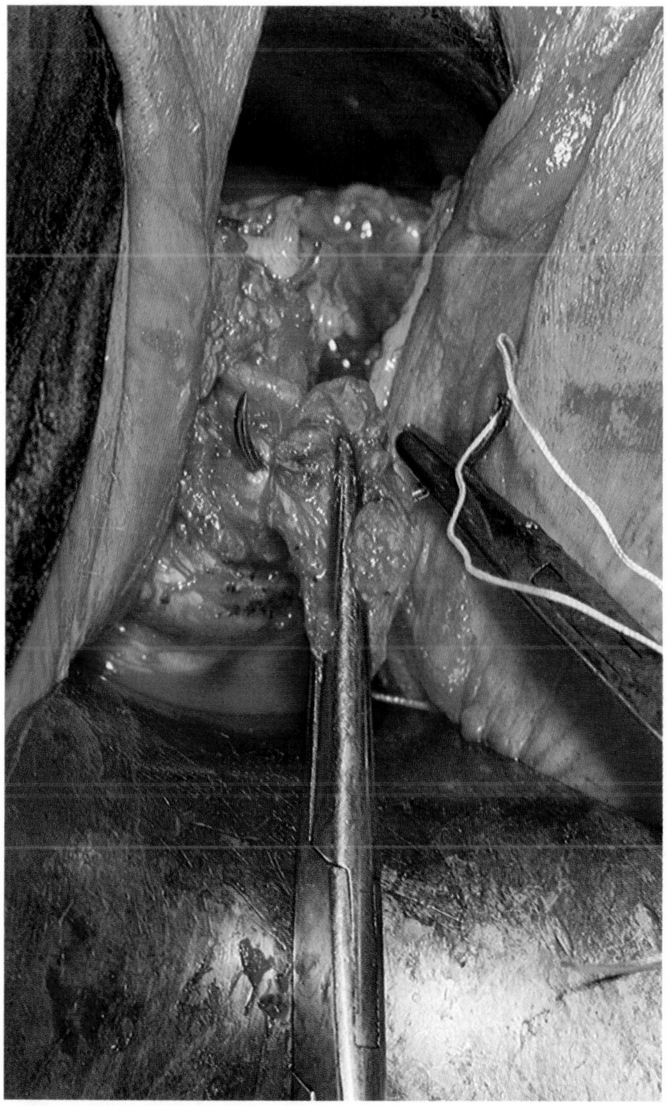

81

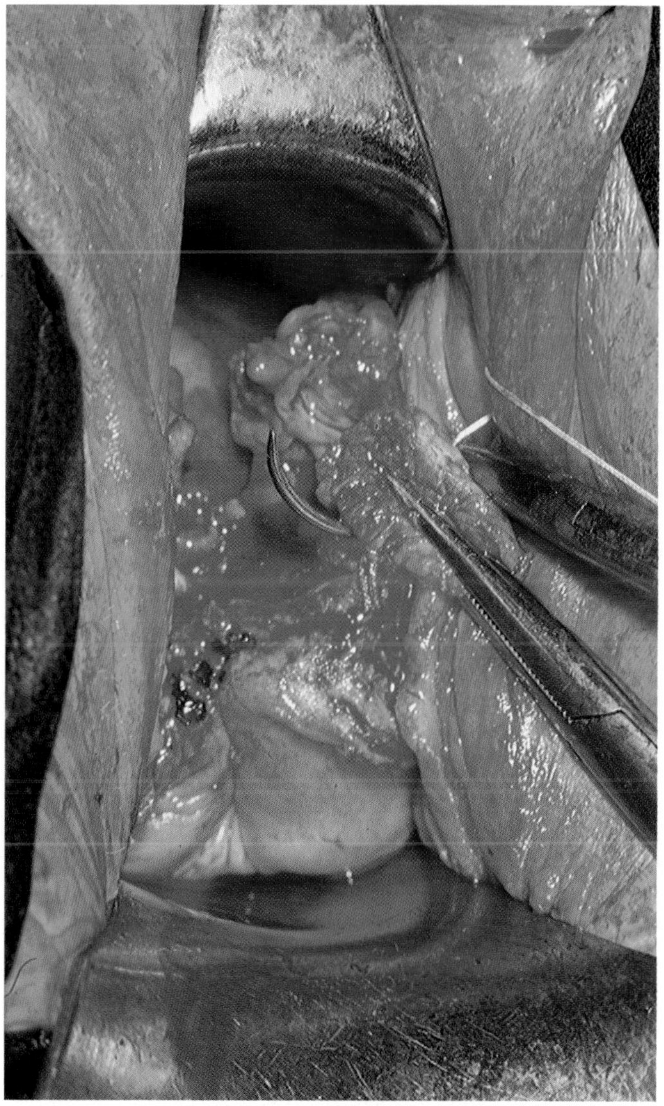

80 and 81 Religation of utero-sacral cardinal ligaments

These pedicles are religated in the same way as the others. **80** and **81** show the right and left pedicles respectively being transfixed in the usual way. They are tied as previously, but the ends of the suture are kept long in this instance.

Stage 6: Reconstruction of the vault of the vagina

The main agents in forming the new vault of the vagina are the combined utero-sacral and cardinal ligaments from each side. They are sutured together in the mid-line to form an apex or centrepoint of the vault. Joining the medial borders of the utero-sacral component eliminates the pouch of Douglas and closes all potential hernial space posteriorly. The uterine pedicles have no part in giving mechanical support since they are almost entirely vascular and in the interests of haemostasis they should not have excessive tension applied to them. The broad ligament pedicles are not stitched together to reinforce the vault because this will subject them to undue and excessive tension. The anterior part of the vault will derive any additional support required from the reconstituted pubo-cervical fascia.

82

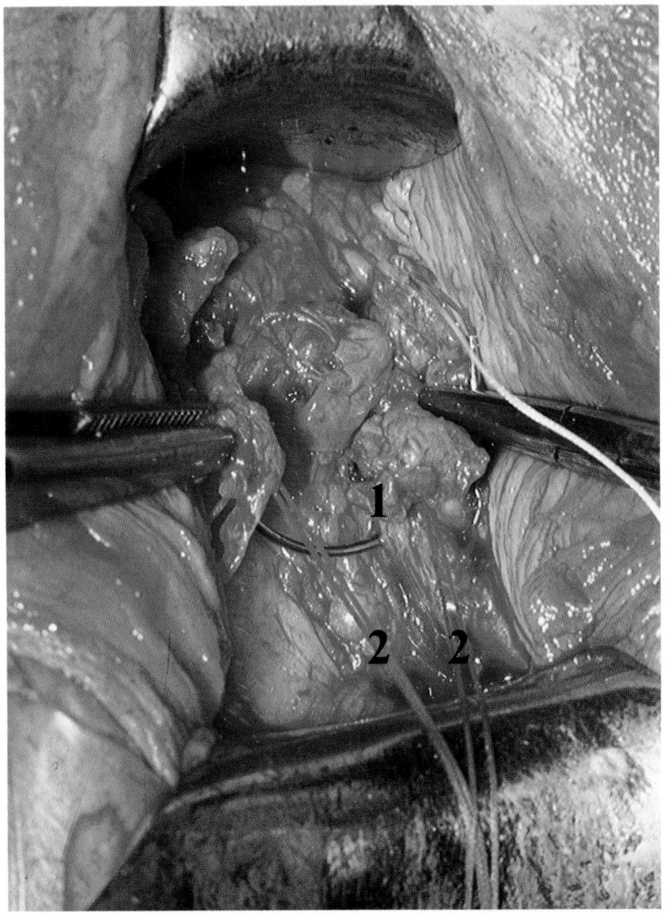

83

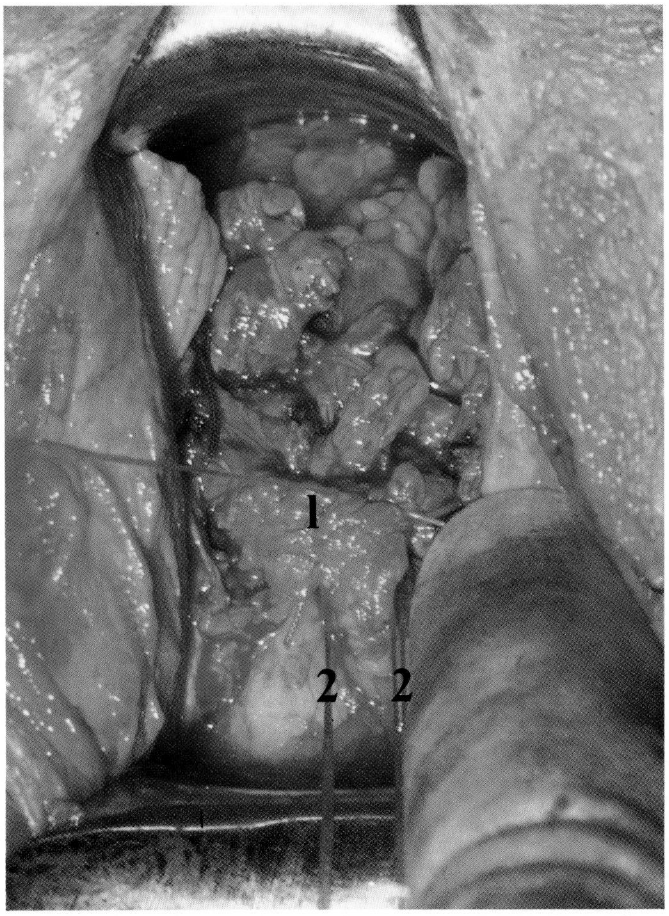

82 Approximation of utero-sacral cardinal ligaments (i)

The utero-sacral cardinal ligaments are approximated in the mid-line by a PGA No. 0 suture which encircles the medial two-thirds of each pedicle on the superior surface 1 cm proximal to the double ligatures. The assistant holds the pedicles in proximity by the long sutures while this stitch is inserted. This stitch is numbered 1 and is the only one on the anterior or upper aspect. The utero-sacral long sutures are indicated as 2 on the illustrations.

83 Approximation of utero-sacral cardinal ligaments (ii)

This shows the suture tied and the ligaments approximated on the upper or anterior surface.

84

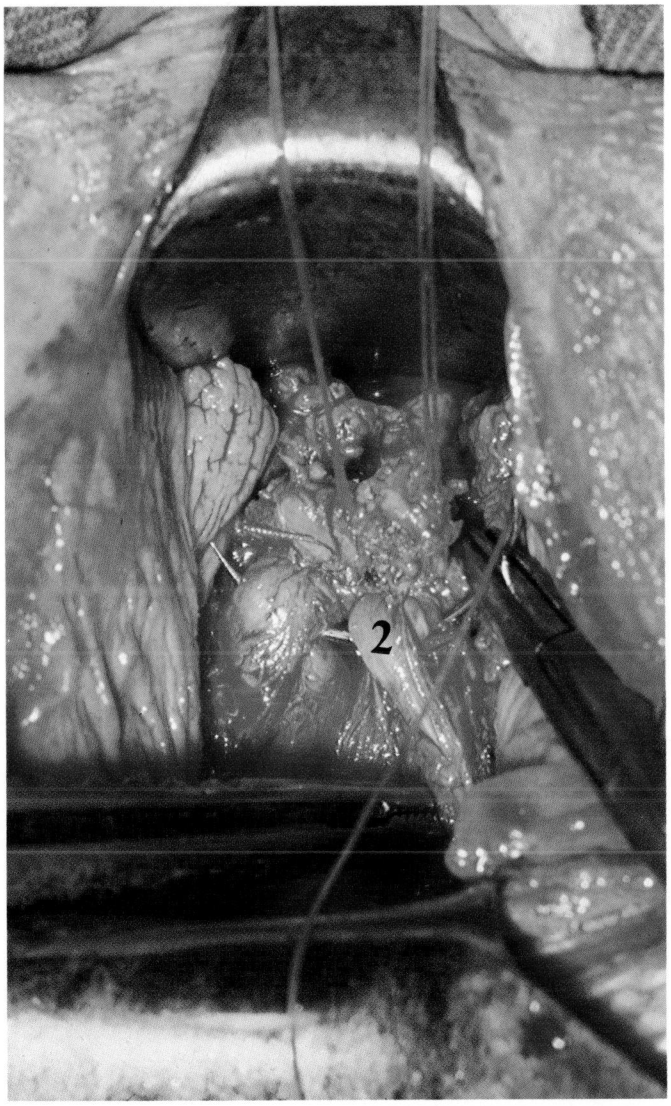

85

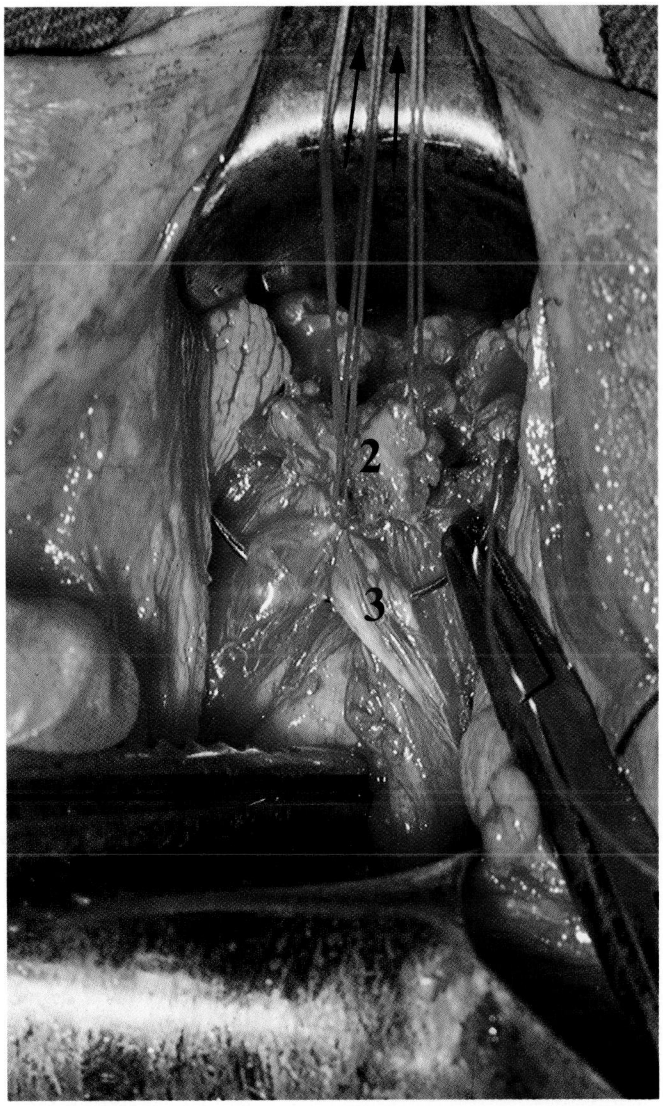

84 Approximation of utero-sacral ligaments posteriorly (i)

The utero-sacral cardinal ligaments are lifted upwards to give access to the utero-sacral ligaments proper. Their medial surfaces will be stitched together to obliterate the pouch of Douglas and two sutures usually suffice. The needle has transfixed the medial border of the ligaments 1 cm proximal to the double ligature ready to approximate them in the mid-line (2).

85 Approximation of utero-sacral ligaments posteriorly (ii)

The first suture has been tied and cut (2) and the placement of a second similar suture is shown (3). When this has been tied the posterior aspect of the vault is firmly supported. In the placement of these last two stitches the long sutures holding the utero-sacral ligaments have been elevated as arrowed.

86

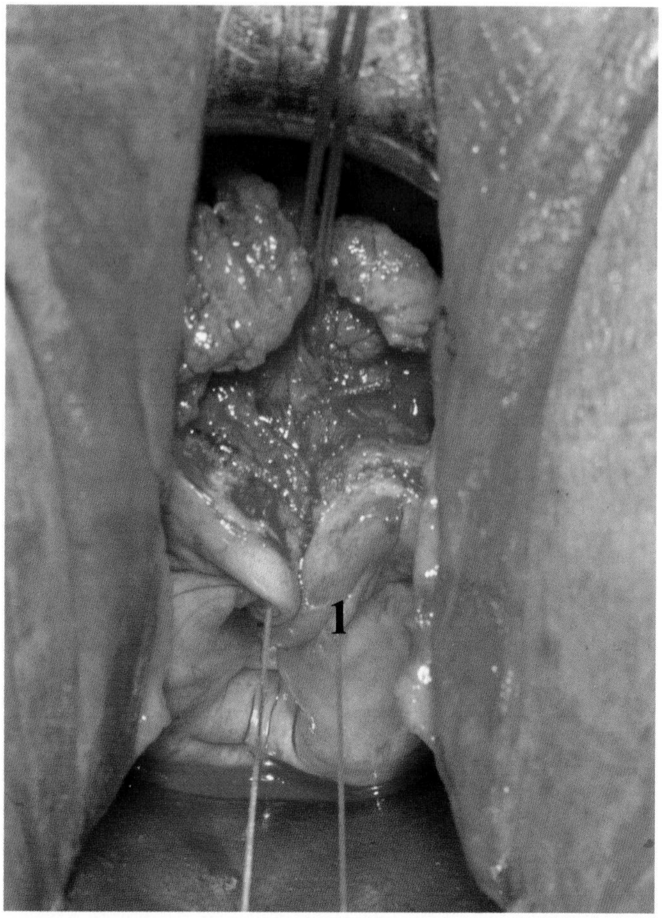

87

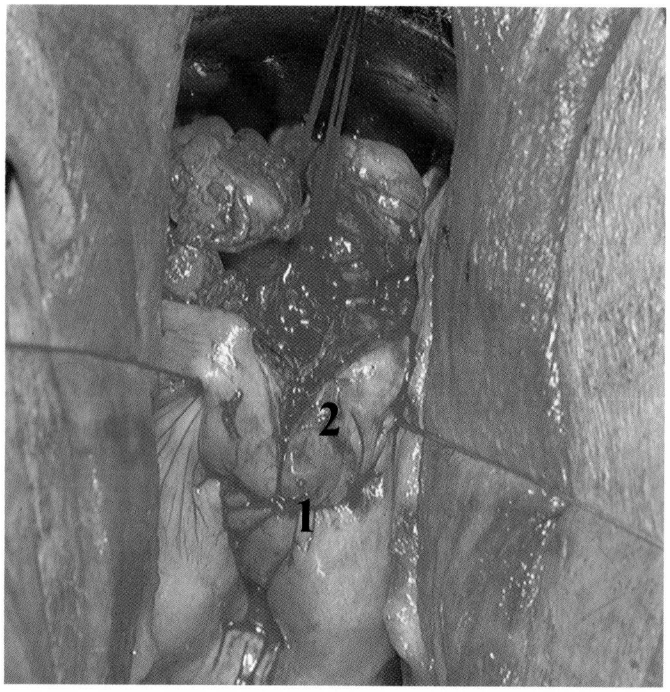

88

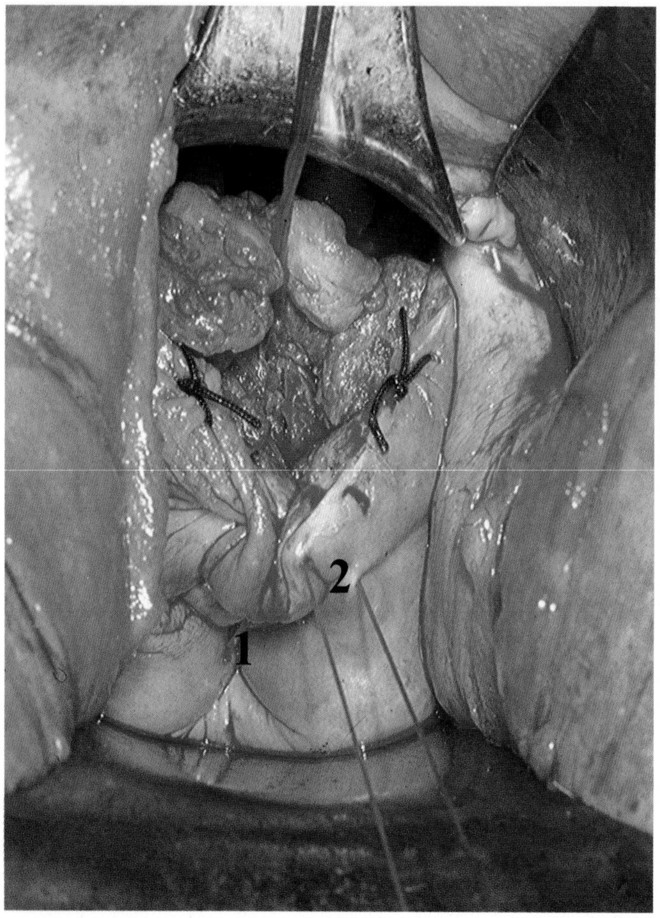

89

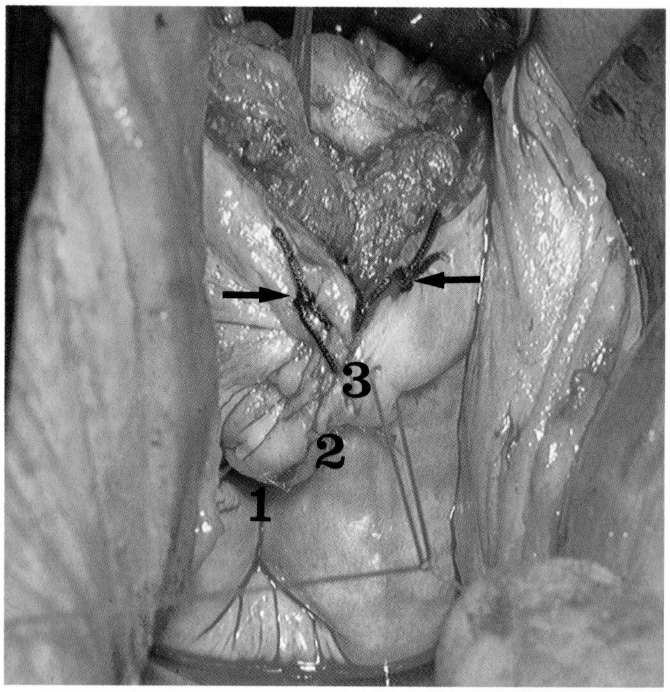

86–89 Resuture of vaginal vault

The vaginal skin at the vault is closed by a series of interrupted sutures from above downwards and the guidance given by the marking sutures aids symmetrical closure. The skin sutures should not be so tight as to cut into the tissues during the phase of post-operative oedema. They should be fairly widely spaced to allow drainage of minor bleeding or oozing from small vessels and thereby avoid haematomata. The sutures are numbered in progression of placement. Arrows indicate the original marking sutures.

Stage 7: Anterior vaginal wall repair

Some degree of anterior wall support is required in every case of vaginal hysterectomy and is carried out as described in the section dealing with 'anterior colporrhaphy and posterior colpoperineorrhaphy' (page 71). The pubocervical fascia is separated from the overlying skin layer on each side and the two edges are brought together in the mid-line by a continuous PGA No. 00 suture extending from below the external urethral meatus to the vault located at the junction of the utero-sacral cardinal pedicles.

90

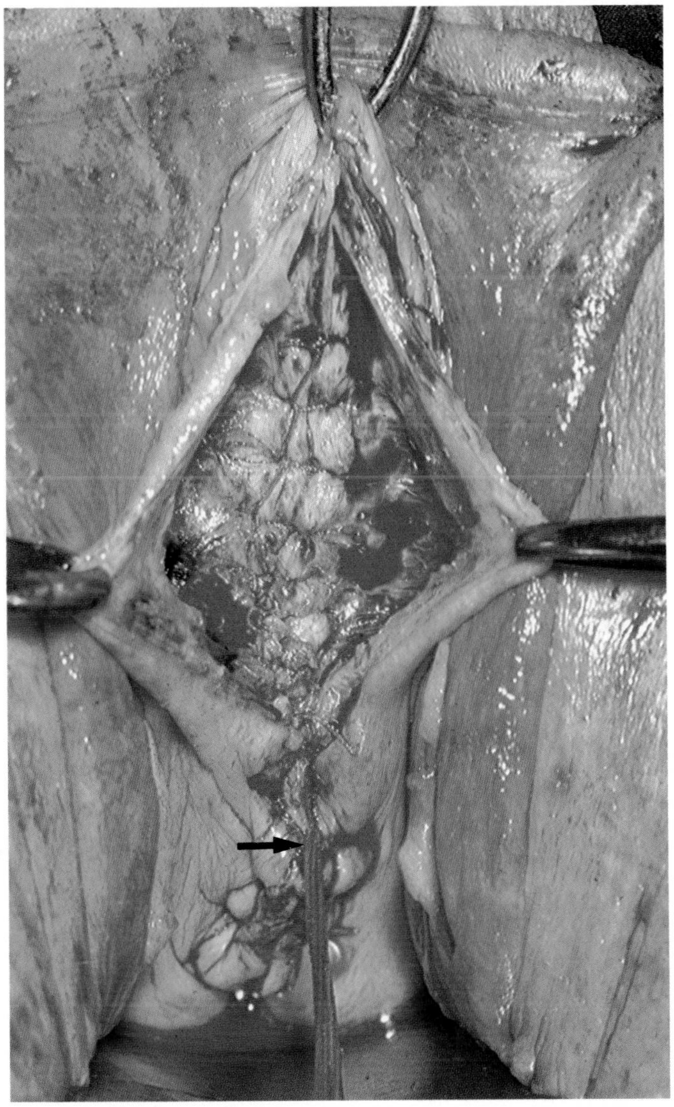

91

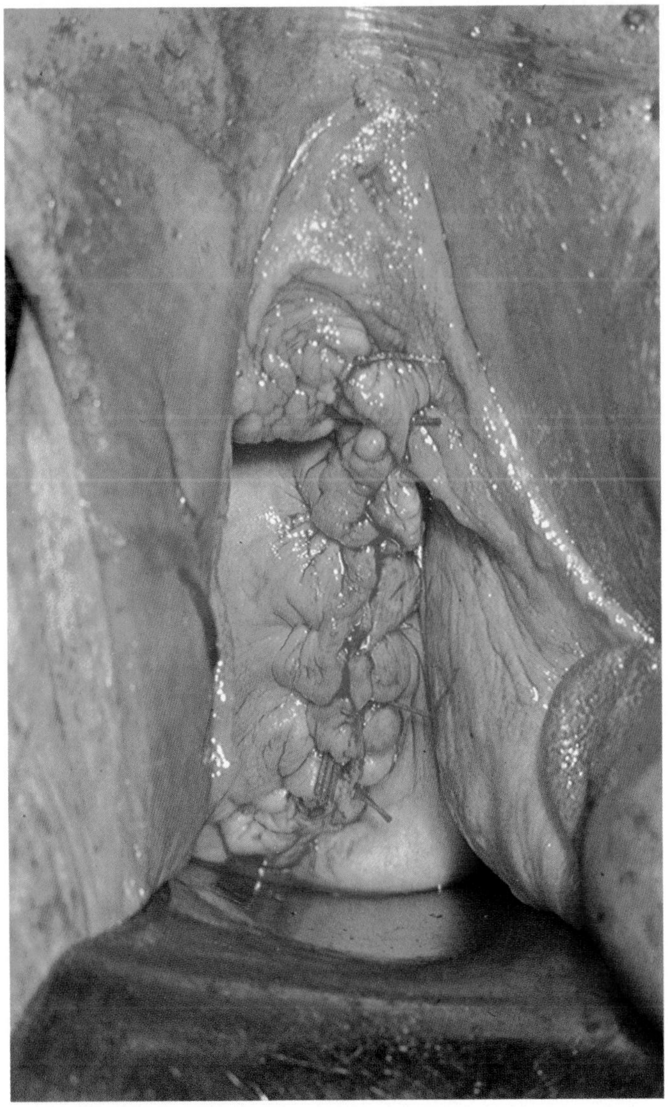

90 Reconstitution of anterior vaginal wall (i)
The pubocervical fascia from each side is shown sutured in the mid-line to support the bladder base and the anterior vault of the vagina. The utero-sacral holding sutures (arrowed) are about to be cut short. Some surgeons leave the cut ends long to act as a wick drain at the vault. This is unnecessary with PGA suture material but may have some advantage with catgut.

91 Reconstitution of anterior vaginal wall (ii)
The skin closure has been completed.

Stage 8: Posterior vaginal wall repair

Routine posterior repair in prolapse operations has on occasion been followed by coital problems and there is a tendency to question the need for this step unless obviously required. It seems that the pendulum has swung too far the other way, for we repeatedly see cases where a necessary posterior repair was omitted and the patient needs further surgery. In fact most women requiring a vaginal hysterectomy and anterior repair need some reinforcement of the lower posterior wall and perineum.

92

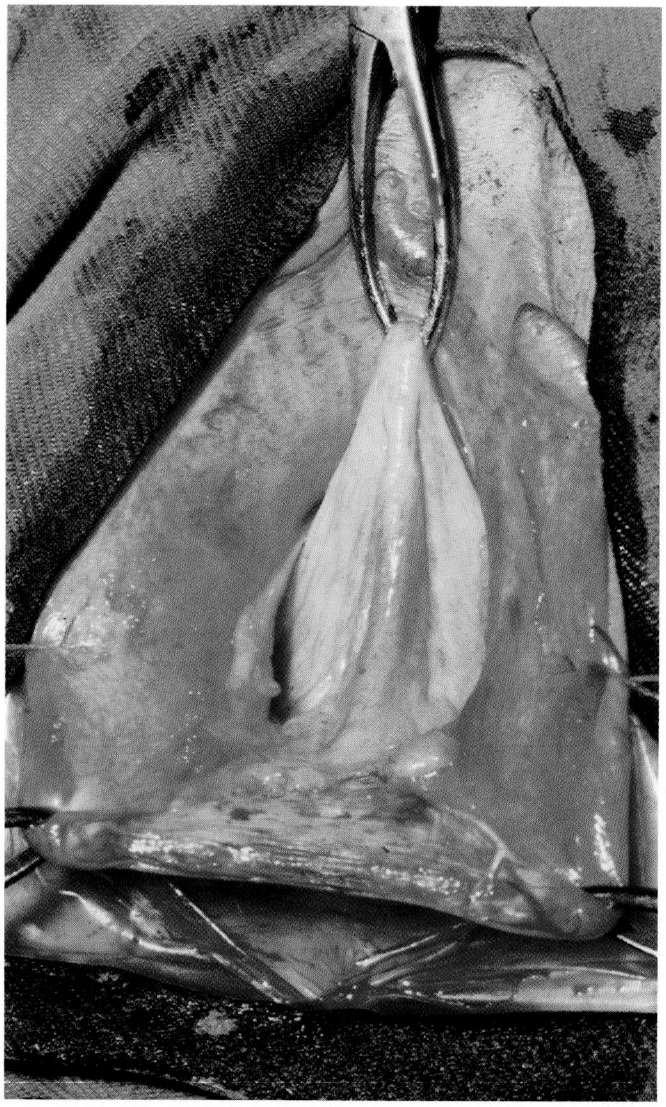

93

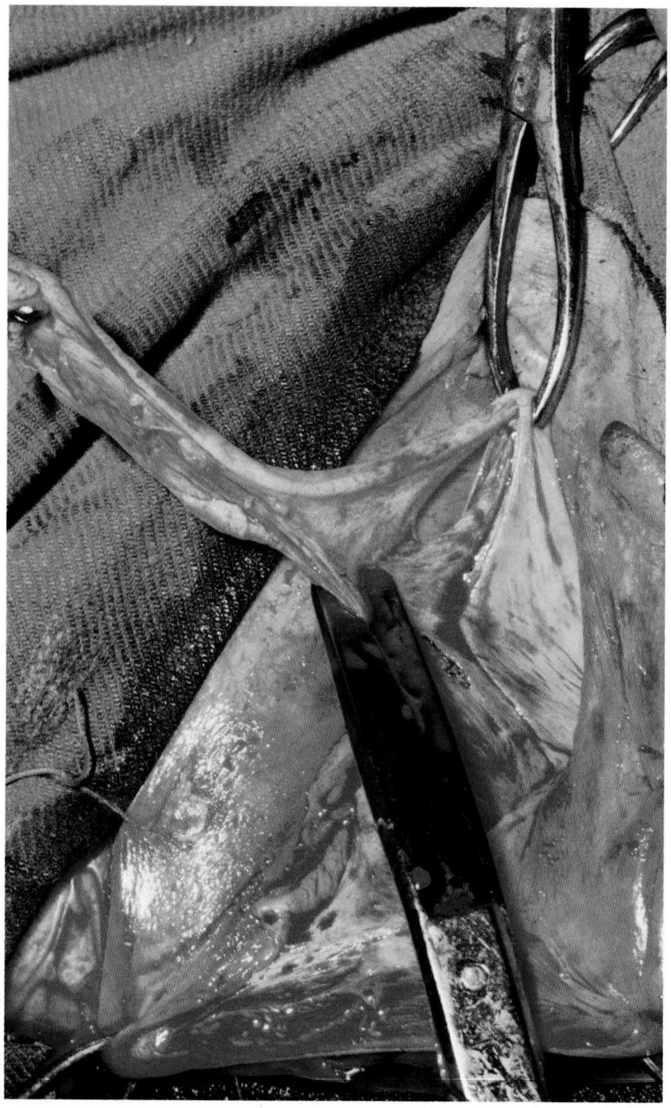

92 Limited posterior vaginal wall repair (i)
The photograph illustrates a considerable degree of rectocele and perineal deficiency. The raw area in the lower part of the illustration is a relieving episiotomy made at the beginning of the operation.

93 Limited posterior vaginal wall repair (ii)
The excess skin triangle is shown being stripped off the rectum with the aid of snips from the scissors.

94

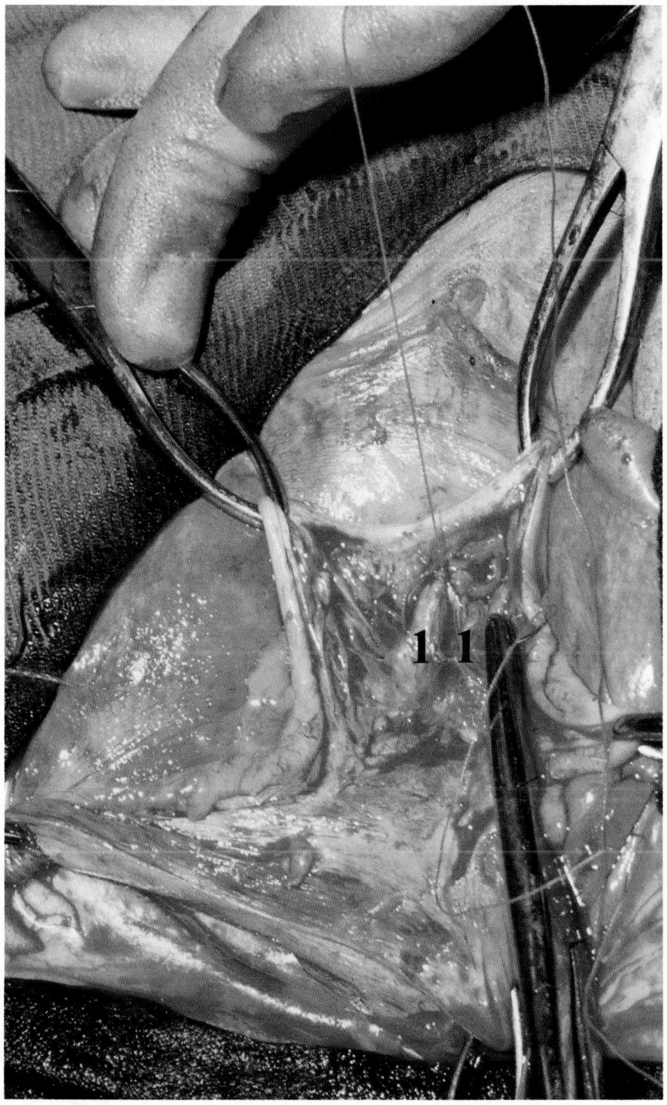

95

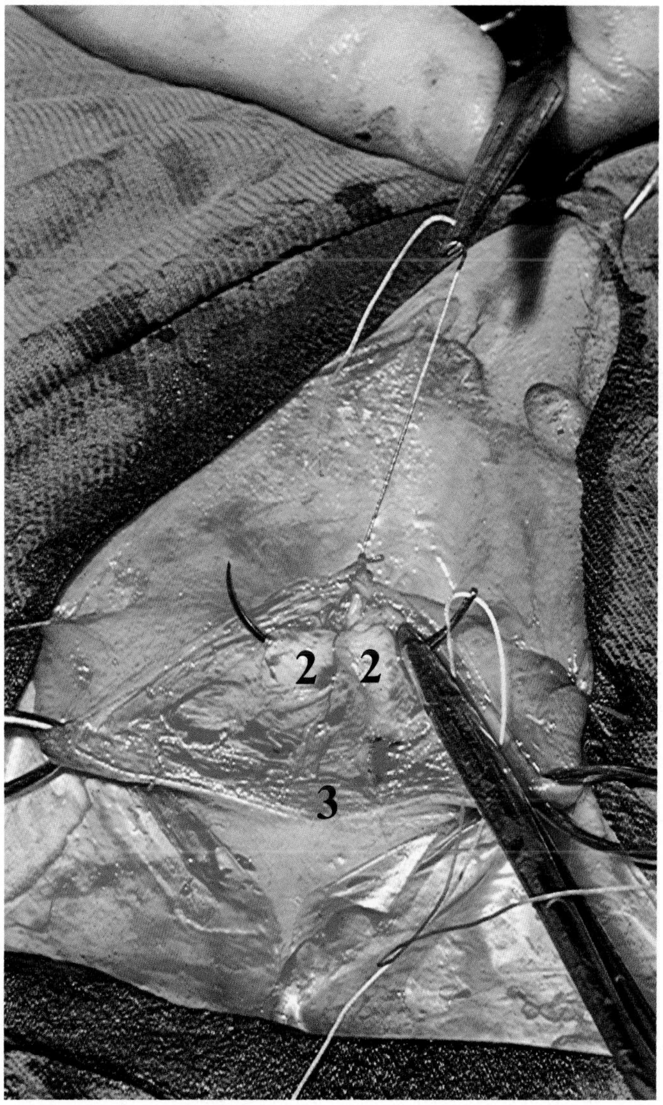

94 Limited posterior vaginal wall repair (iii)

The pre-rectal fascia is shown being approximated in the mid-line by a continuous suture. The figure 1 indicates the edges of this fascia.

95 Limited posterior vaginal wall repair (iv)

The levator ani muscles have been defined and are shown being approximated in the mid-line to reconstitute the perineum. The figure 2 indicates the bellies of the levator muscles and figure 3 indicates the fibres of the external anal sphincter.

96

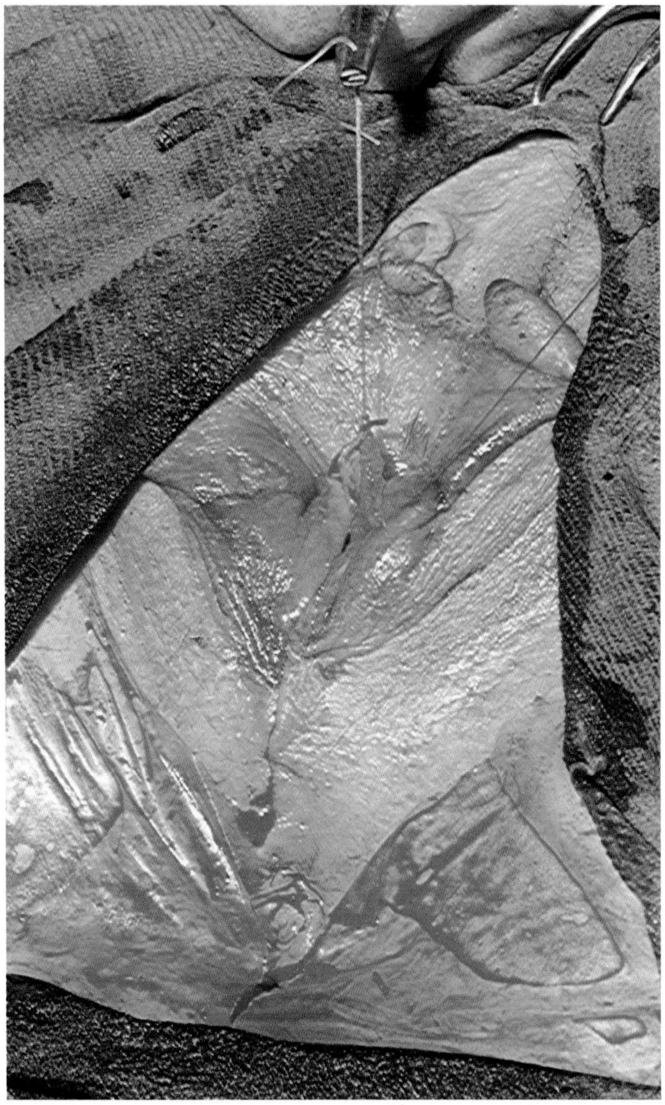

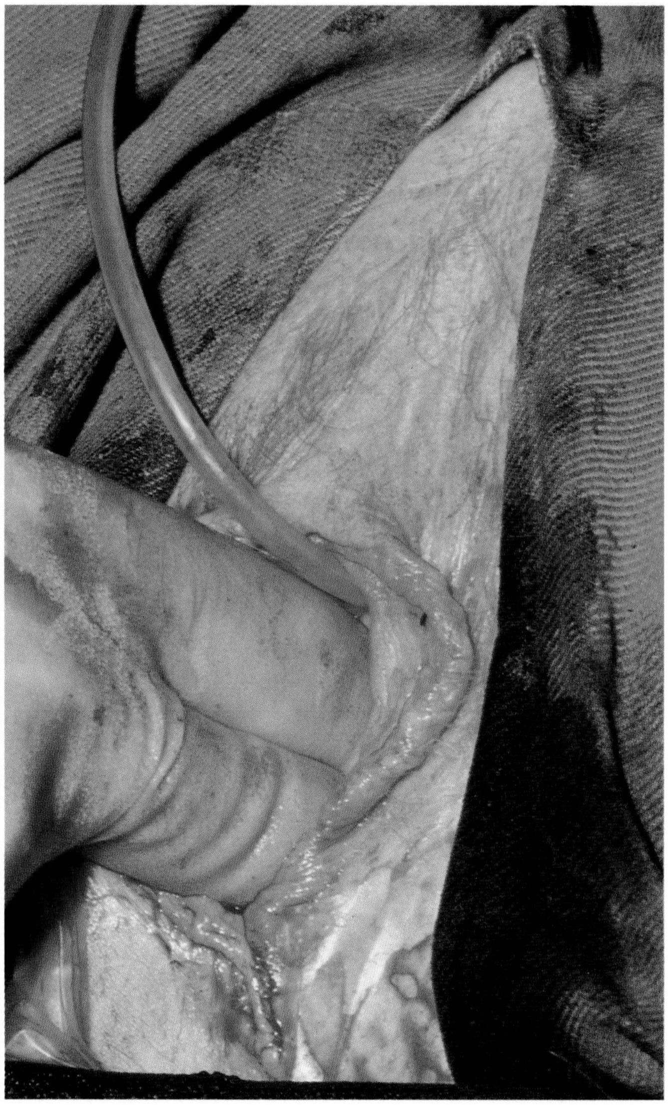

97

96 and 97 Limited posterior vaginal wall repair (v)

In **96** the perineal skin suture has been completed and is ready to tie. In **97** an estimate of the lumen of the vagina is being made. It should just accept two fingers as in this case. A Foley catheter is shown *in situ*. We prefer this because it allows the bladder to be at rest with no fear of overdistention and both surgeon and patient have no worries about urinary retention. On the other hand it could be said that it is not necessary and serves as a possible source of urinary tract infection. In practice this infrequently happens, but policy in this matter is obviously one of personal preference.

Suggested reading

1 Howkins, J. & Stallworthy, J., *eds. Bonney's Gynaecological Surgery,* p. 226–254. Bailliere Tindall, London, 1974.

2 Te Linde, R. W. & Mattingly, R. F. *Operative Gynaecology,* p. 489–504. Lippincott & Co., Philadelphia, 1970.

3 Joel-Cohen, J. *Abdominal and Vaginal Hysterectomy,* 2nd ed. Heinemann Ltd., London, 1977.

4 Feroze, R. M. (1977). 'Vaginal Hysterectomy', *British Journal of Hospital Medicine* **17** 1 69–76.

9: Post-hysterectomy prolapse

Post-hysterectomy prolapse refers to the condition where hysterectomy has been done previously. It does not mean that it is the cause of the prolapse. Re-examination of case notes sometimes indicates that there was some prolapse in the first place and in these perhaps a vaginal hysterectomy and repair would have been more appropriate, but a certain number undoubtedly develop at a later time and presumably have the same aetiological factors as any other prolapse.

Apart from the fact that the patient cannot understand why she has a prolapse of the uterus when she has no uterus, these cases present some problems for the surgeon also. They are generally elderly, they have had the condition for some time (since they did not think they could have prolapse) and their tissues are frequently atrophic. The elements of prolapse encountered are cystocele and sometimes urethrocele with mid or high rectocele and varying amounts of low rectocele and perineal deficiency. The very fact that a hysterectomy has been done usually means that there is no vault prolapse. The vault has been narrowed and drawn upwards to varying extents. In most cases the utero-sacral ligaments are fixed to the vault, thereby approximating them even if they have not been stitched together. Enterocele is therefore not common, although it does occur. The most puzzling aspect for the inexperienced surgeon is the absence of a cervix which normally serves as the focal point in all vaginal surgery.

The operation required is an anterior vaginal wall double-layer repair with a similar procedure on the posterior wall, and including any necessary perineorrhaphy. The skin is lax and looks redundant but this can be misleading. It should not be removed until the operation is completed and the skin is ready to be closed. The skin incisions should therefore be mid-line and the edges should not be damaged by heavy forceps. Needles, instruments and sutures should be of appropriate fineness, otherwise the tissues may tear or split. The post-operative course should be rather more leisurely and gentle than in straightforward prolapse cases where the tissues are well oestrogenised.

Stage 1: Anterior vaginal wall repair

1

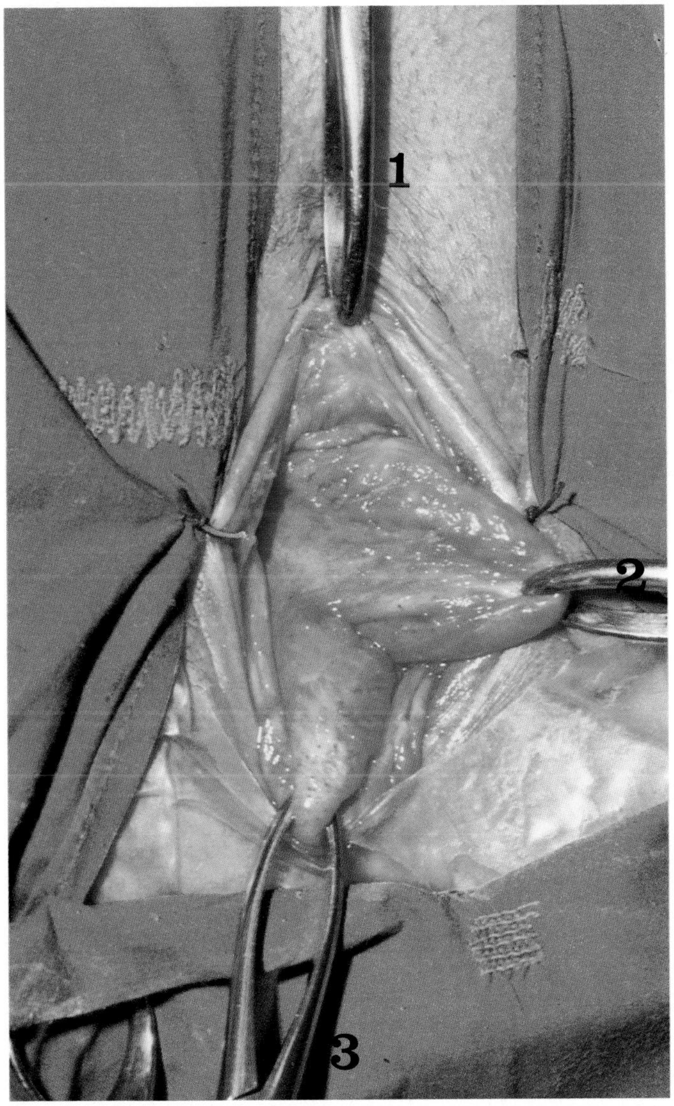

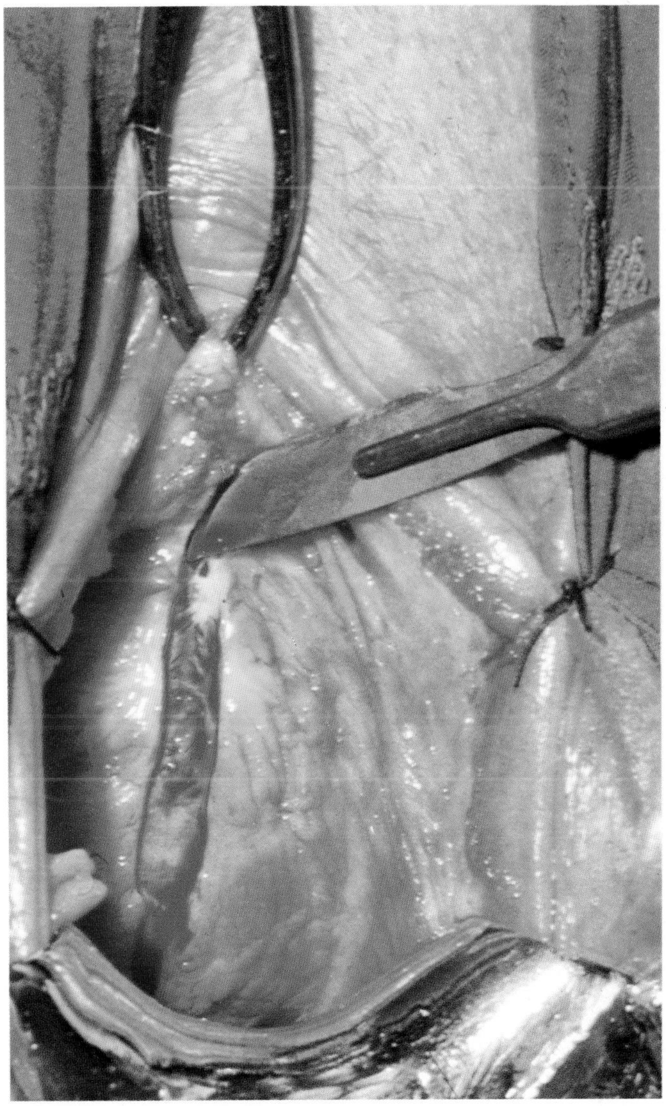

2

1 General appearance pre-operatively

The case is typical in that the skin is thin and atrophic in an elderly woman. There is marked cystocele with a good deal of posterior prolapse which continues down to the fourchette and is probably rectocele. The perineum is also deficient. Note how the vault is still reasonably well supported following the fixation of the ligaments at hysterectomy. There is no evidence of enterocele. The vault of the vagina is arrowed. Forceps (1) are applied just below the external urethral meatus, (2) display the cystocele by retracting it to the patient's left and (3) are applied at the introitus.

2 Incision of anterior vaginal wall

A mid-line incision is made in such cases because of the danger of removing too much skin. The skin itself is thin so that the incision is not carried too deeply but just sufficient to show the thinned out layer of pubocervical fascia.

3

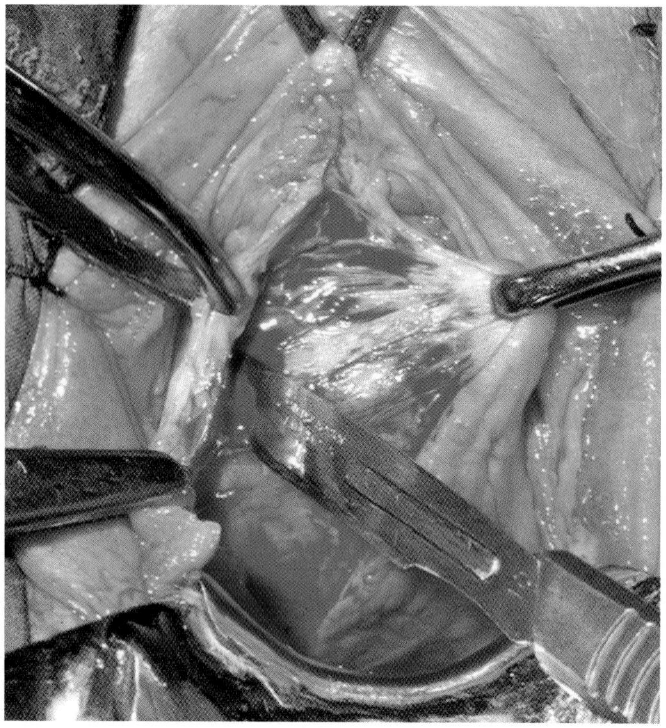

3 Definition of pubocervical fascia (right)

The thin layer of pubocervical fascia is separated from the skin on the right side by sharp dissection and then by working laterally to find a plane of cleavage between the layers.

4

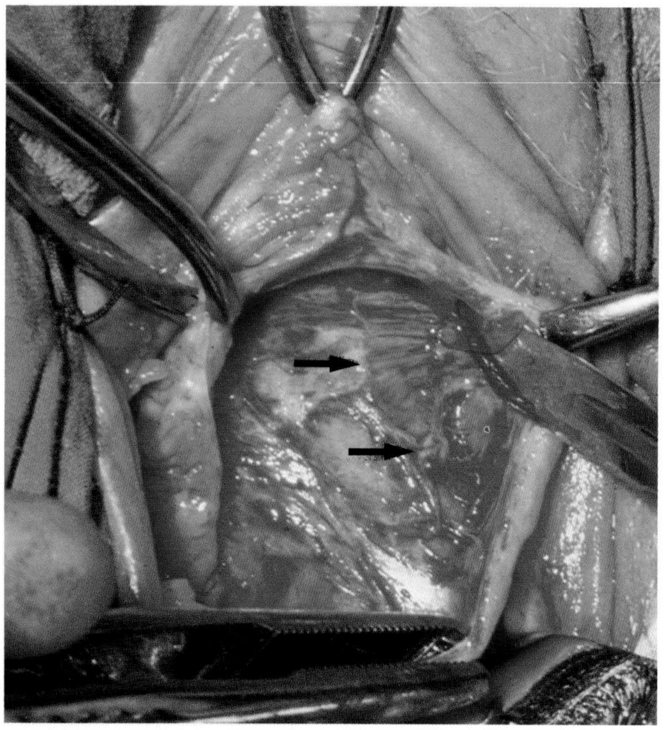

4 Definition of pubocervical fascia (left)

The same procedure is carried out on the left side. The edges of the pubocervical fascial layers are now visible and are arrowed.

5

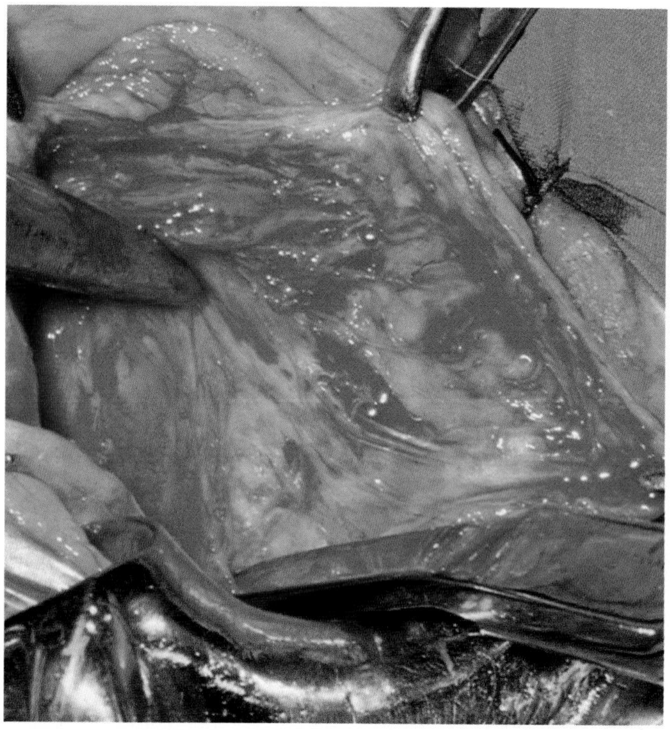

6

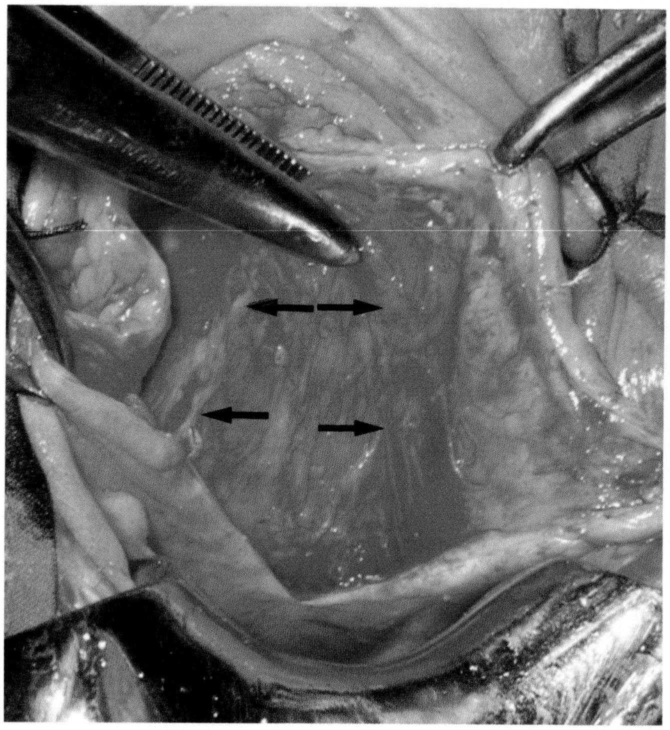

5 and 6 Exposure of pubocervical fascia

When the plane of cleavage has been established it is easy to separate skin from pubocervical fascia and this can be carried as far laterally as required. In **5** the blunt scissors points are making occasional snips to free the layers and in **6** the left leaf is well defined with the plane of cleavage clearly shown. The right edge is also clearly seen and both are arrowed.

7

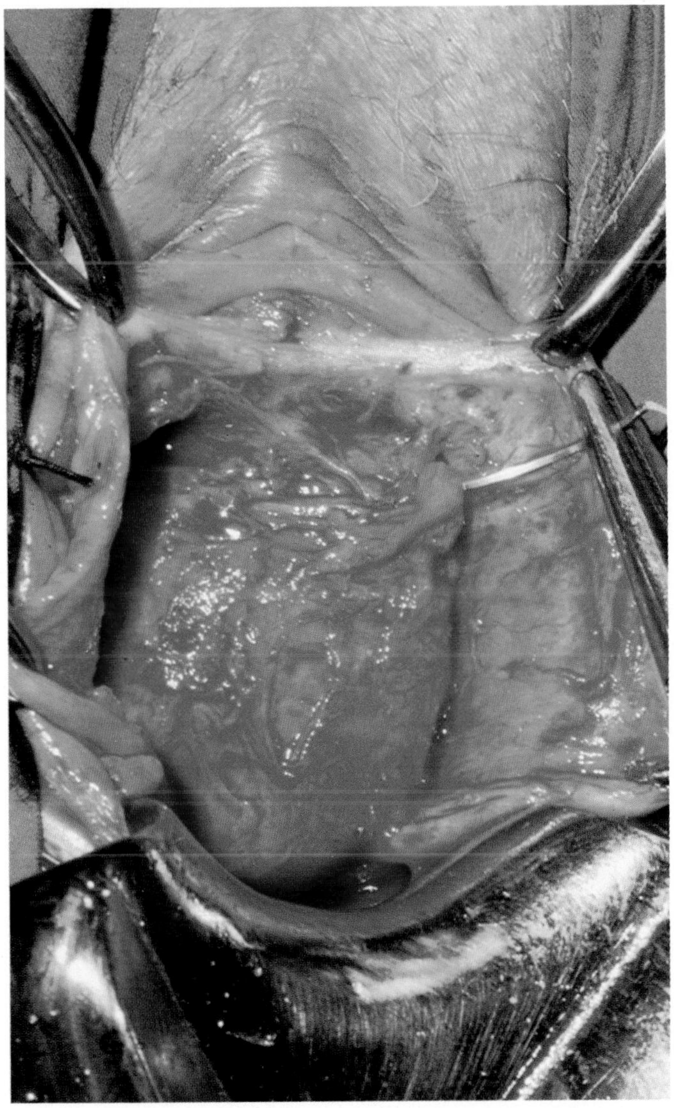

8

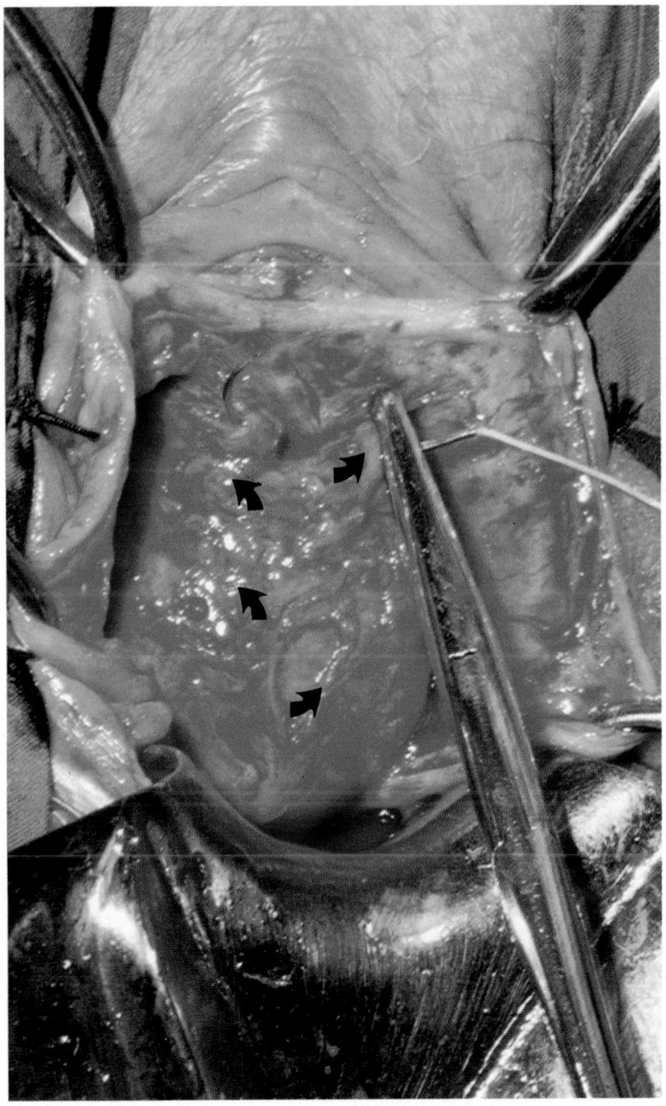

7 Approximation of pubocervical fascia (i)

The edges of the two leaves of the pubocervical fascia stand out and the next step is to suture them together. In this photograph the needle (loaded with a PGA No. 00) is shown picking up the left edge; a continuous suture is being inserted.

8 Approximation of pubocervical fascia (ii)

The edge of the right leaf is taken up on the needle in placing the first stitch. Both fascial edges are prominent and indicate the correct line of approximation. The edges are arrowed.

9

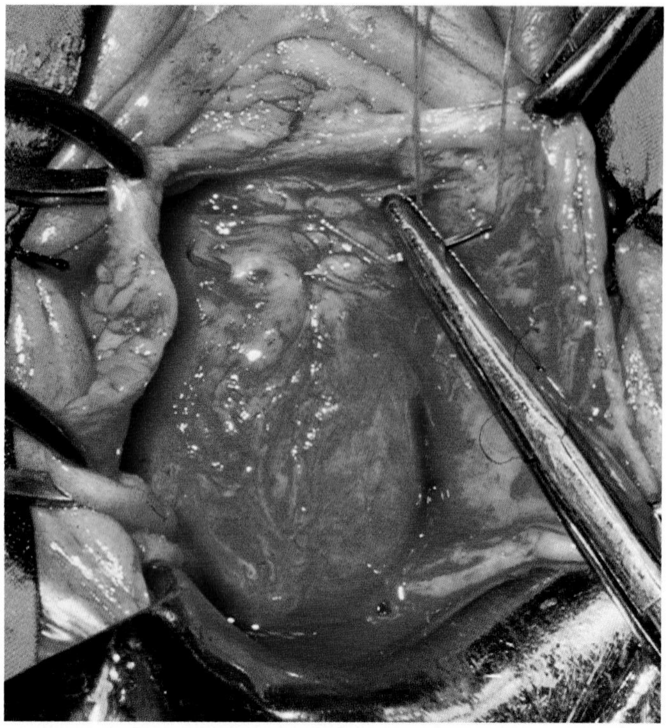

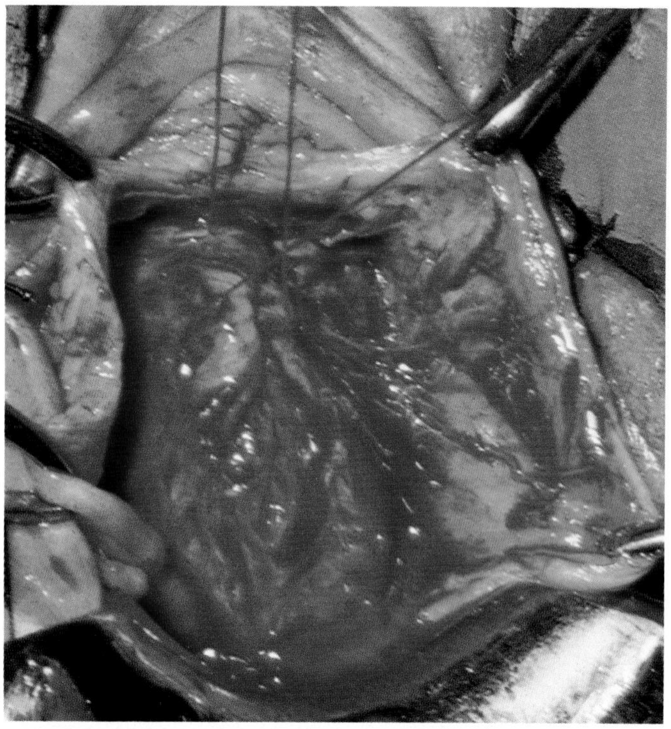

10

11

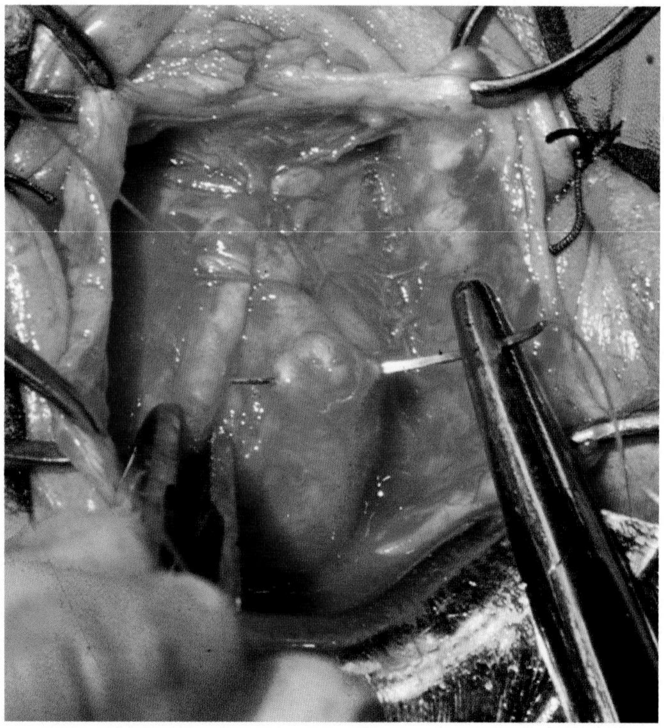

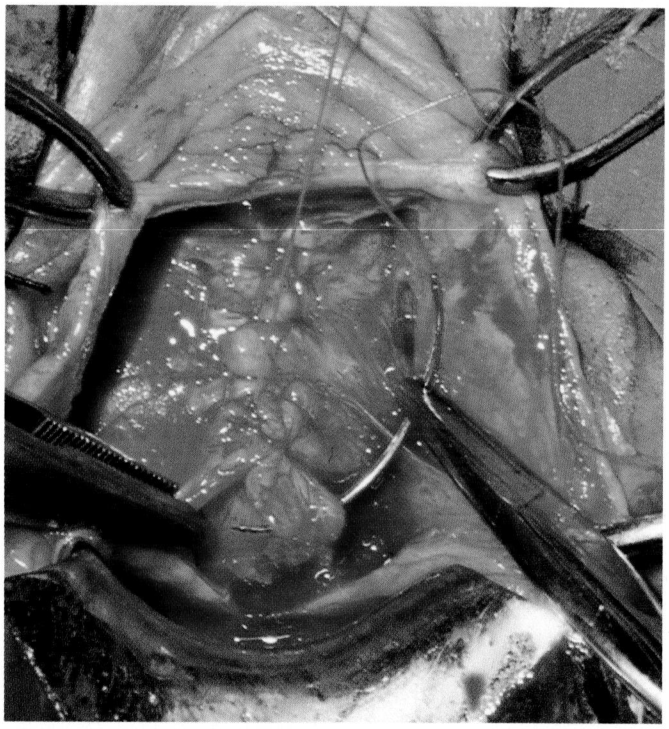

12

9–12 Approximation of pubocervical fascia (iii)

Closure of the gap between the two edges of pubocervical fascia continues with stitches placed at intervals of 0.5 cm in the length of the anterior vaginal wall. In **9** the second stitch takes up both layers and in **10** the third stitch is being run up tight. Figure **11** shows the amount of tissue that is available for suture on both sides and the depth that can be obtained without detriment to the bladder. Figure **12** shows the final stitch being placed very close to the vault. The skin incision was carried right to the vault and the apex can be seen just above the blade of the Auvard's speculum.

13

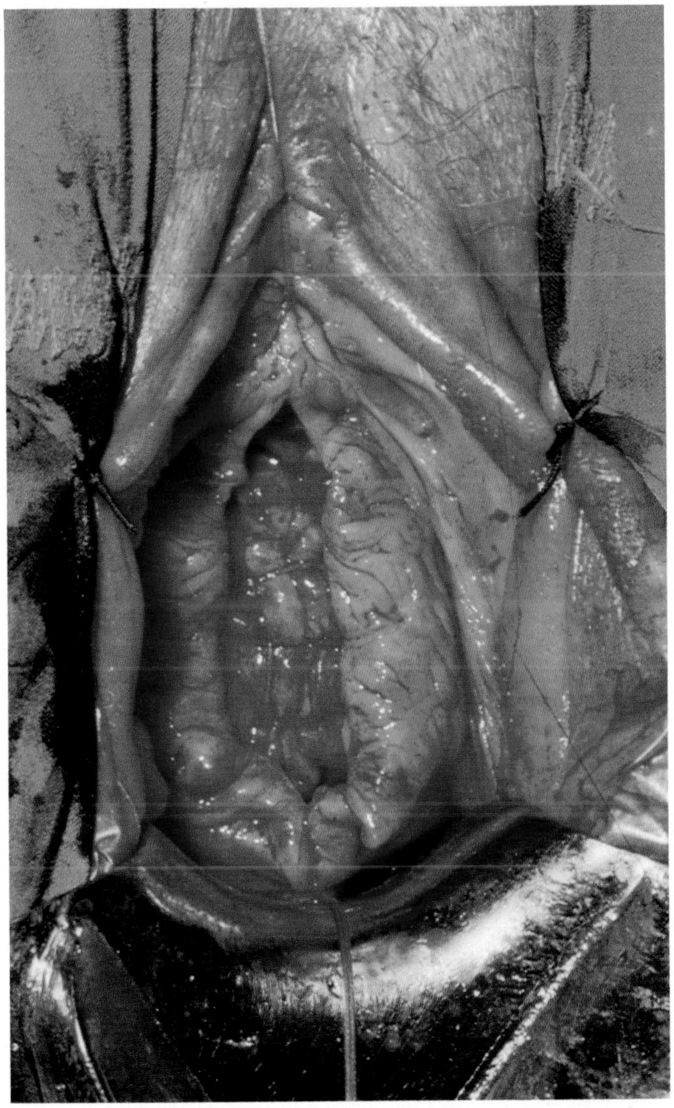

14

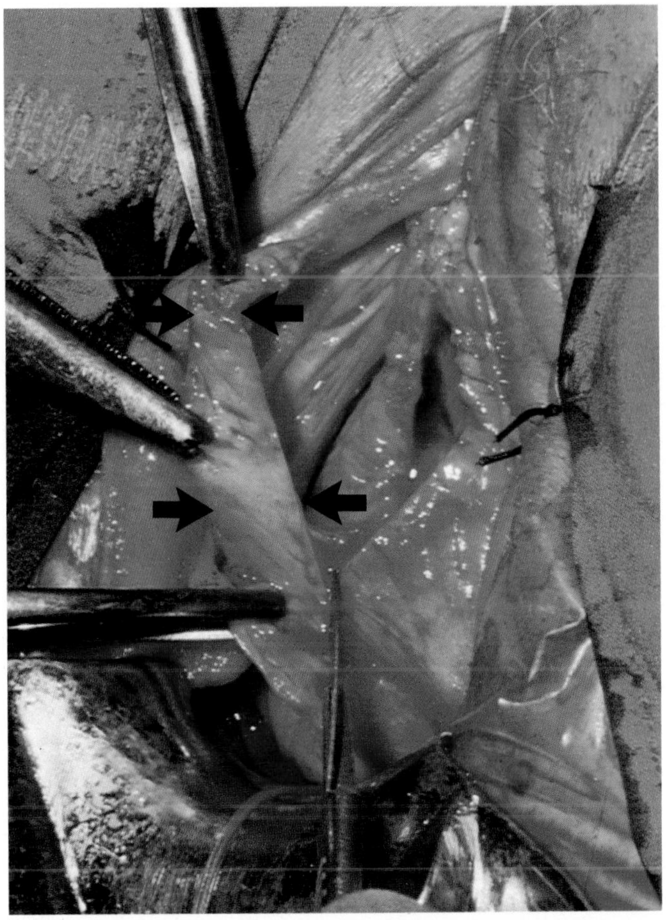

15

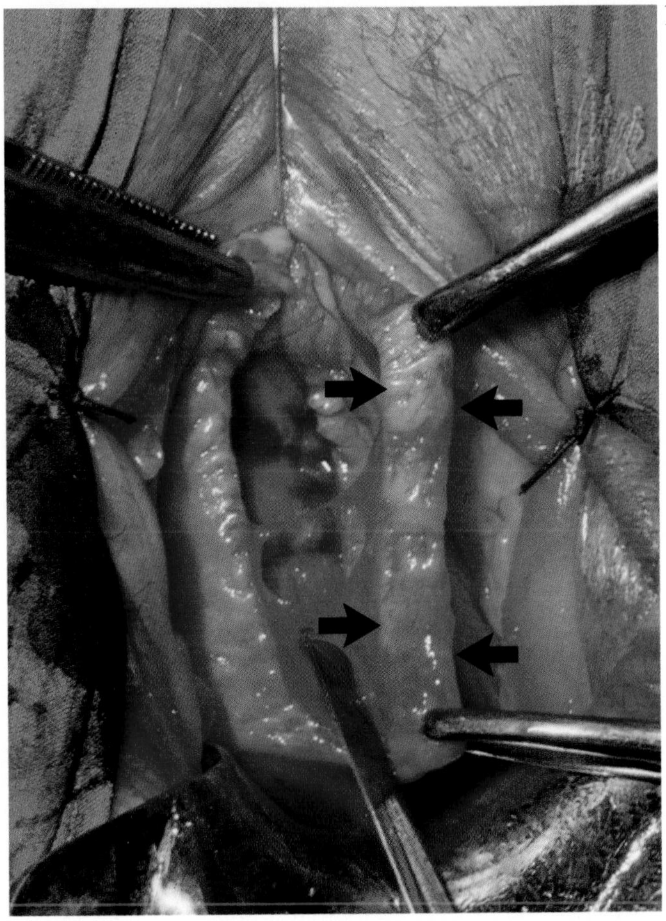

13 Pubocervical fascia reconstituted

With the pubocervical fascia reconstituted the next step is to close the skin. There is of course an excess, but as emphasised in the introduction it is not as much as expected. By bringing the two skin edges into apposition in the mid-line it is easy to find out how much has to be removed from each side.

14 and 15 Removal of excess vaginal skin

If the scalpel is used it leaves a smooth edge for subsequent suture and in this case a band of only 1 cm of vaginal skin is removed from each edge as shown. The edges are kept taut with forceps during the excision. The arrows indicate the redundant strip of skin being removed on each side.

16

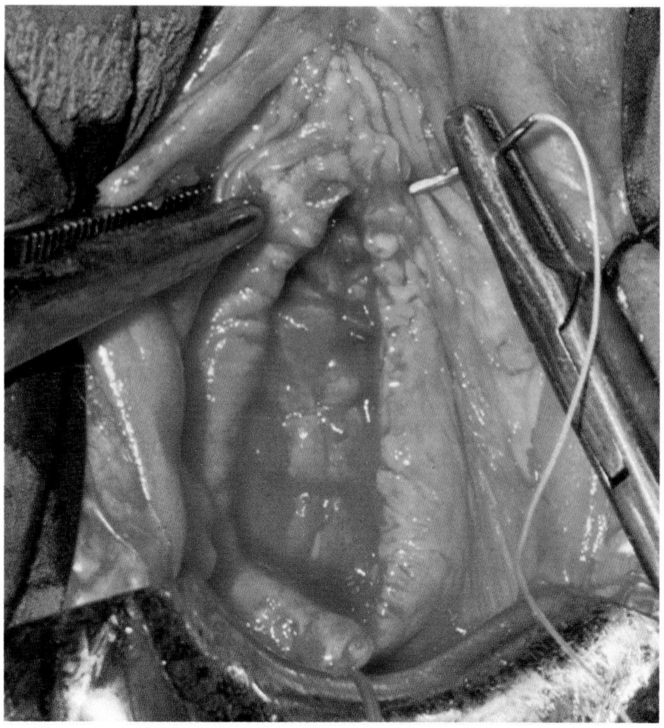

17

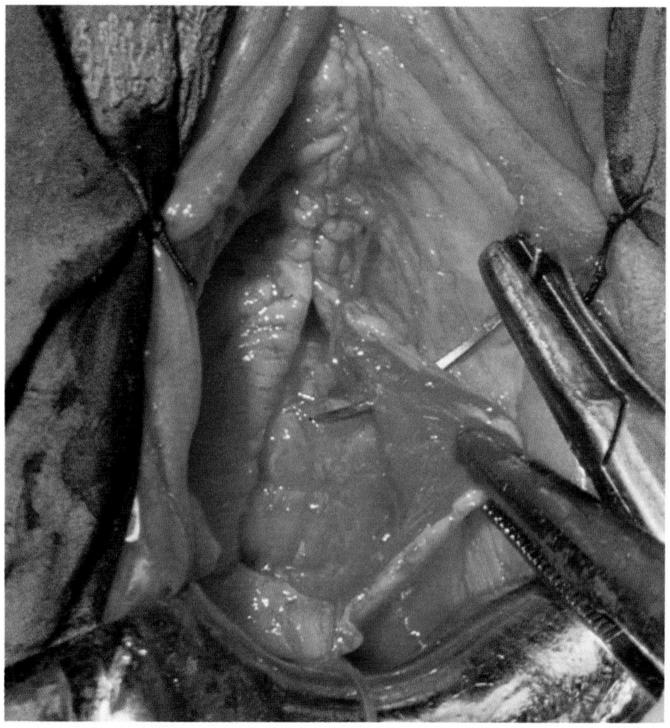

18

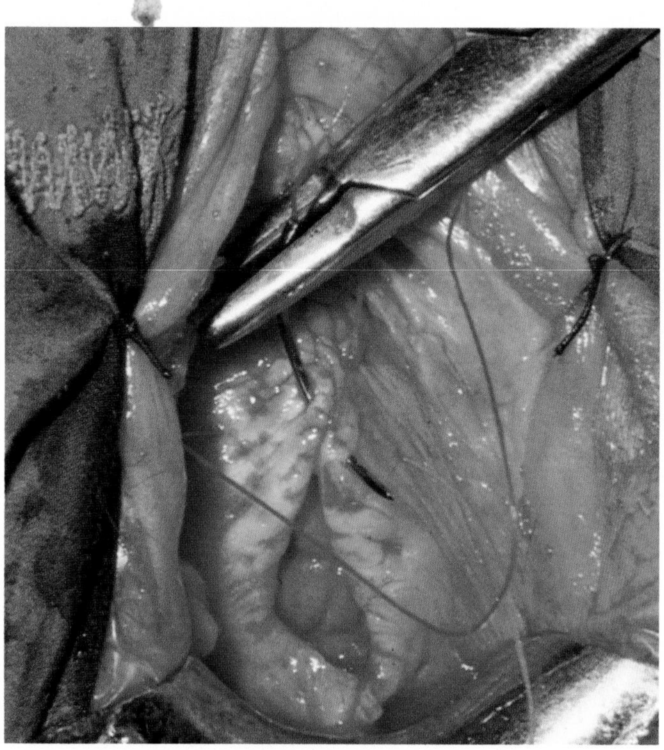

19

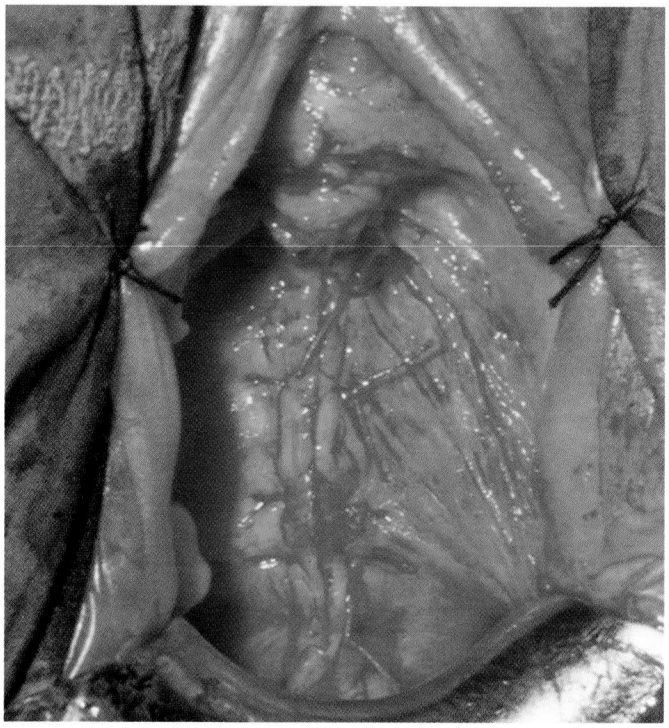

16–19 Skin closure of anterior vaginal wall

With the excess skin removed the skin opening is now ready to be closed. The reconstituted pubocervical fascia is supporting the bladder and urethra satisfactorily and when the skin is closed it will give further support besides eliminating any dead space between the layers. Suture of the anterior vaginal wall skin is by interrupted vertical mattress sutures of PGA No. 0 on an atraumatic needle. Various stages of the procedures are shown by the illustrations. In **16** the first stitch is being placed; in **17** and **18** the two sequences of the mattress stitch are shown. The completed closure of the anterior vaginal wall is shown in **19**. This method of suture gives a neat appearance with absence of slackness or pouching of the skin and the wound is quite dry.

Stage 2: Posterior vaginal wall repair

20

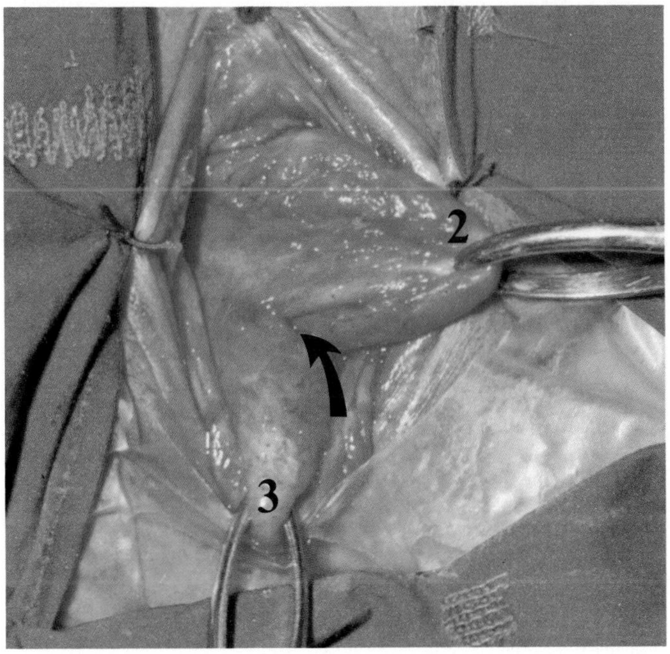

21

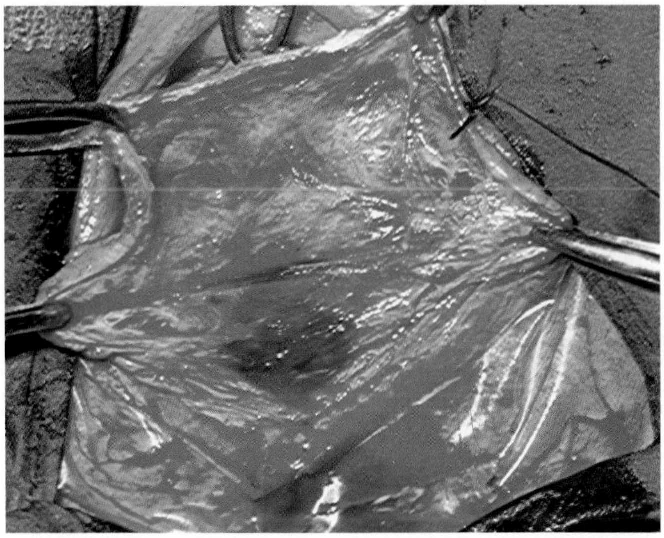

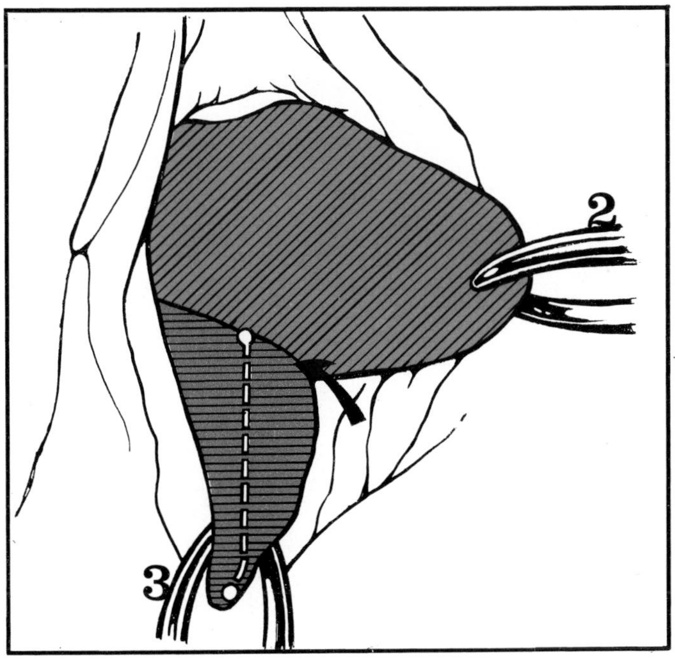

22

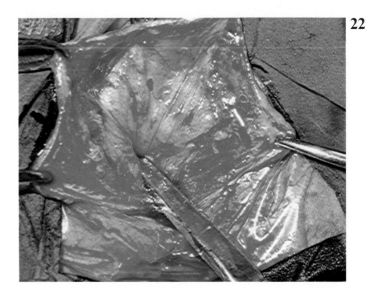

20 Incision of posterior vaginal wall for repair of high rectocele

To allow reorientation the vaginal defect is again shown. The anterior part of this defect, shaded in red, has just been repaired (**1**–**19**). The area shaded green and representing the high rectocele is now to be repaired.

The first part of this procedure involves a longitudinal incision between points as marked, the incision being continued to the perineum. It is carried out in exactly the same way and in the same depth as anteriorly. The curved arrow indicates the position of the vault.

21 Incision of posterior vaginal wall

Forceps (1) denotes the vault in the mid-line. The lax skin edges are taken up in Littlewood's forceps and held open to display the structures beneath.

22 Exploration of posterior vaginal wall incision

The skin is dissected laterally on each side with the scissors to expose the rectum with its investing fascia and to look for evidence of enterocele. The rectum covered by lobules of fat is clearly seen in the centre of the picture and there is no evidence of enterocele.

If at this stage of the operation there is any doubt whether the bulging structure is rectum or not, the operator should put on an extra glove and make a rectal examination, discarding the glove immediately he establishes the diagnosis. This is an obvious and quick way of dispelling any doubts.

23

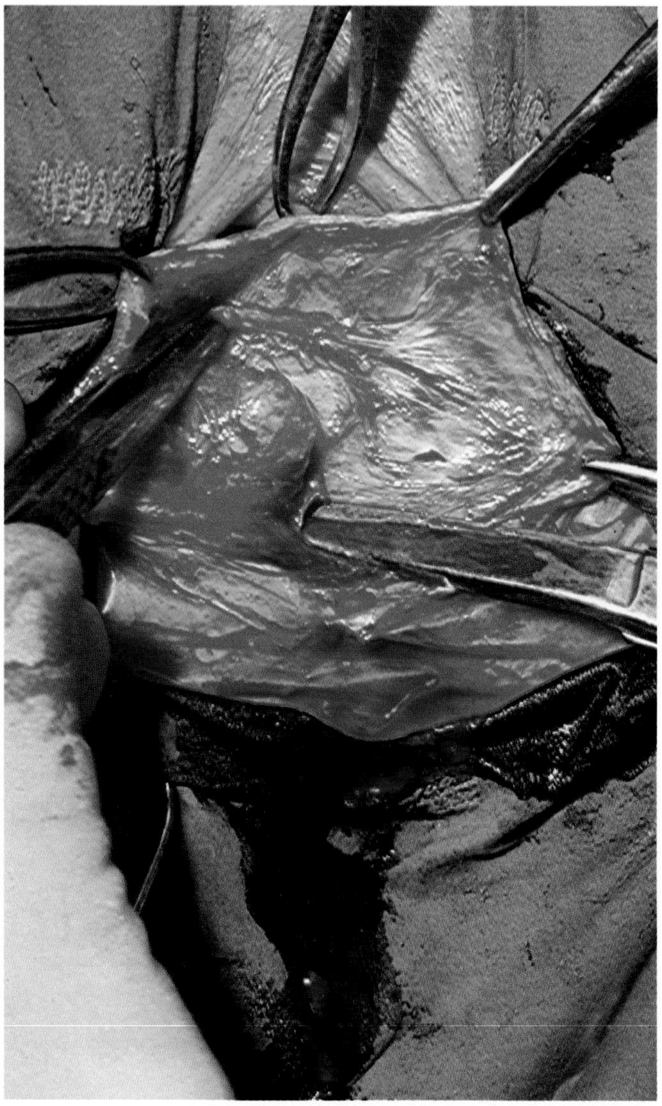

24

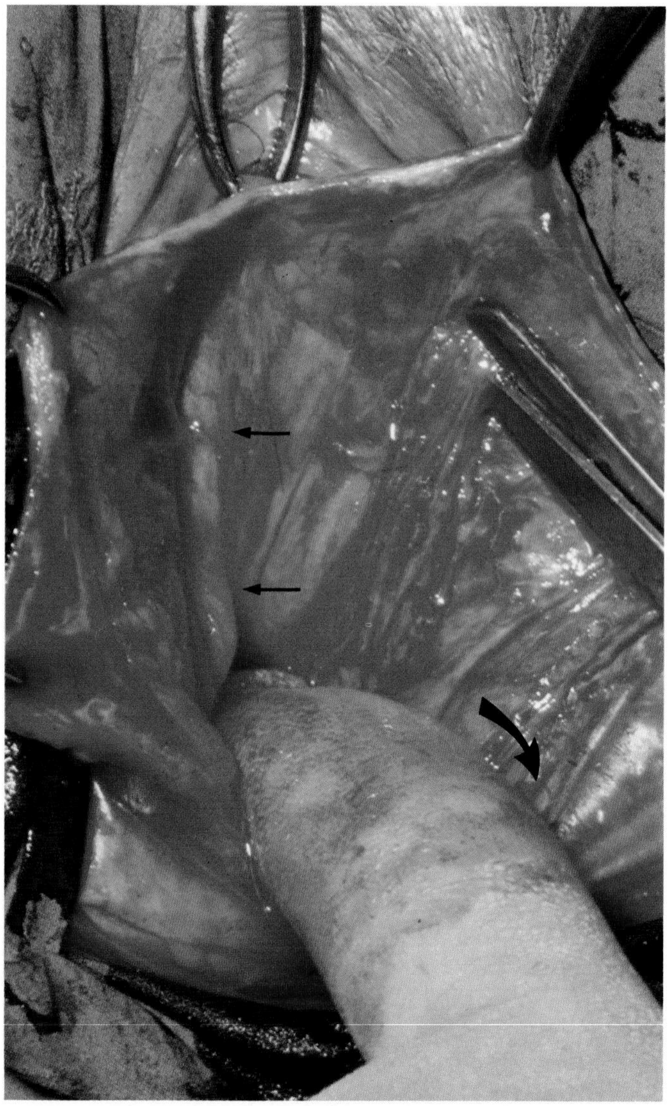

23 Mobilisation of rectum

With the scissors points and largely by blunt dissection the rectum is mobilised towards the mid-line and the lateral rectal fascia sought laterally. The rectum has an immediate investment of fat and areolar tissue and in seeking the fascial layer it is necessary to keep close to the undersurface of the vaginal skin.

24 Definition of pre-rectal fascia

By keeping close to the skin layer a plane of cleavage soon becomes apparent and the pre-rectal or para-rectal fascia can be raised and rolled medially as in this photograph. The same procedure has already been carried out on the patient's right side and the ridge of the fascial edge can be seen (arrows). The left forefinger depresses the rectum and keeps it clear of the operation field. The thick arrow shows the line of movement in this manoeuvre.

25

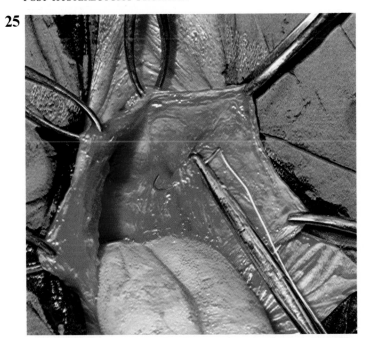

26

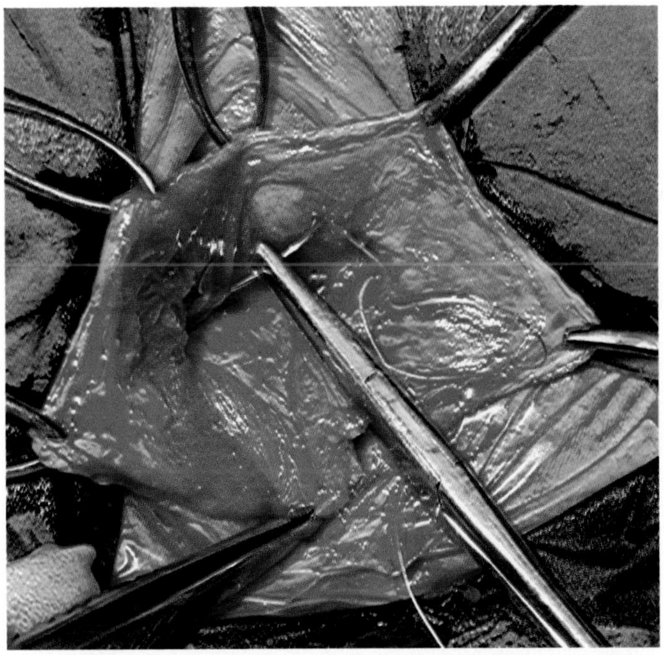

27

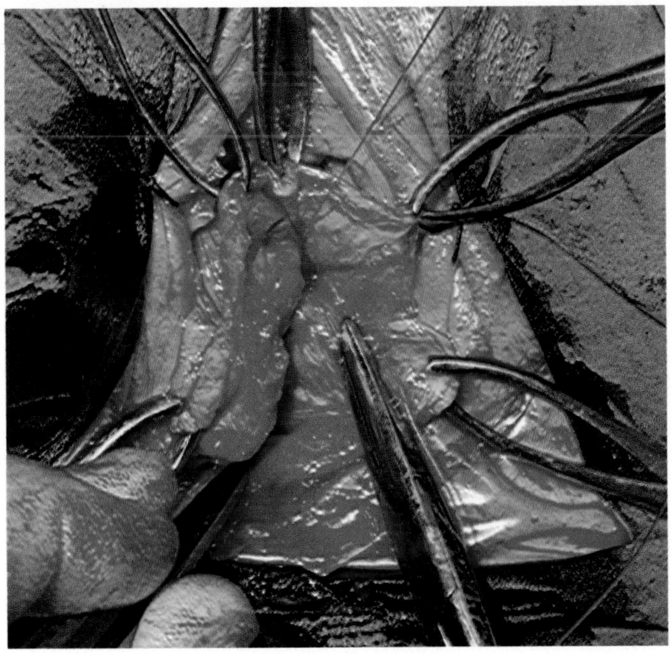

28

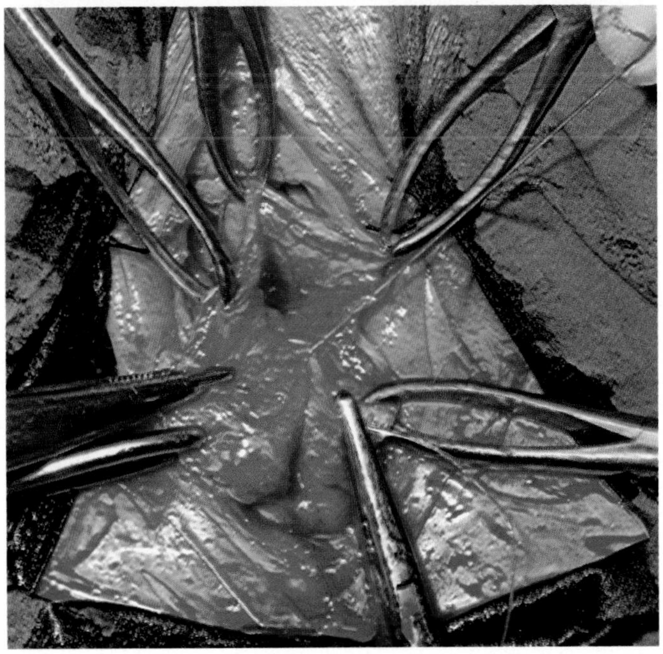

25–28 Reconstitution of pre-rectal fascia

The two layers of the pre-rectal fascia are approximated by a continuous suture of PGA No. 00 carried on a round-bodied needle. In **25** the first stitch is being placed through the edge of the thin left leaf of the pre-rectal fascia and in **26** the opposite side is taken up. Approximation proceeds down the vaginal wall with stitches 0.5 cm apart. There is clearly a good bulk of tissue at this lower level and the rectum has good anterior support as seen in **27** and **28**.

29

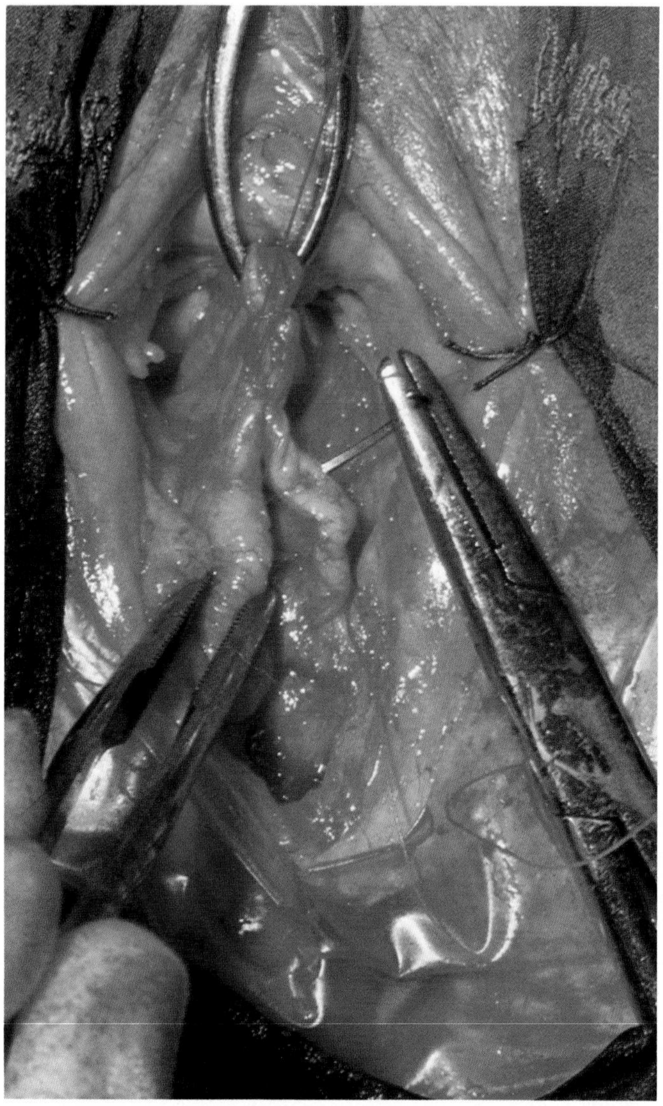

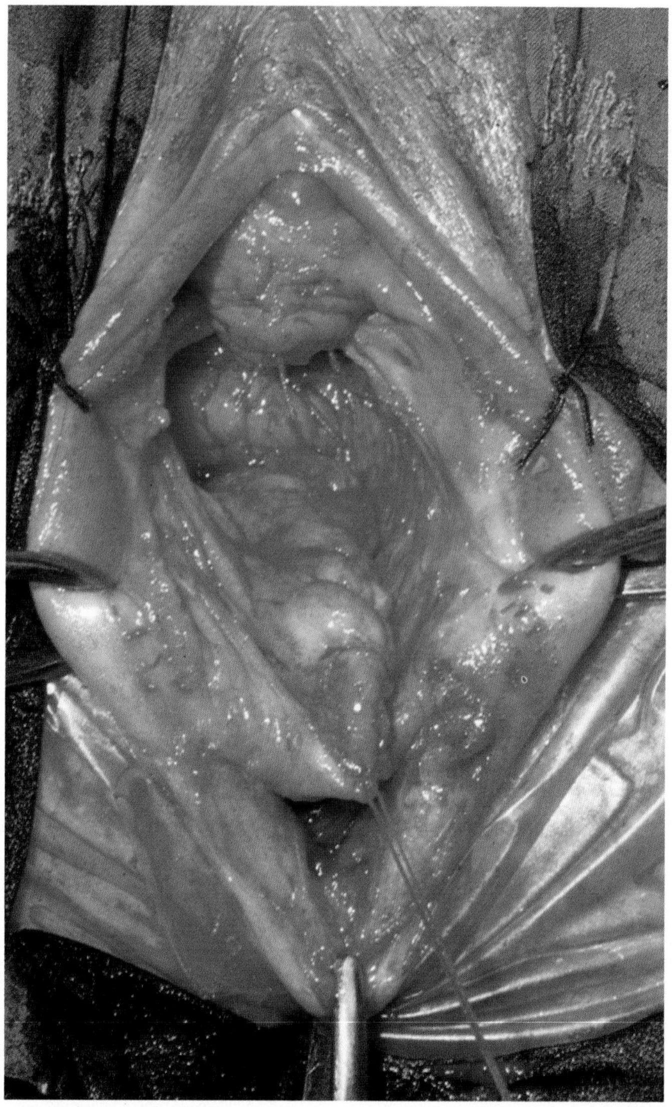

30

29 and 30 Skin closure of posterior vaginal wall

The skin is being closed in this instance by a continuous PGA No. 00 suture on a fine atraumatic needle. A continuous stitch has been chosen to avoid undue suture material in the wound because the tissues are atrophic and poor. Interrupted sutures would no doubt have done equally well.

Returning again to the question of excess skin, there was in fact no need to remove any from the posterior wall skin edge in this case, and had one done so the vagina would have been narrowed too much.

Figure **29** shows the suture soon after commencing and **30** when tied at the level of the hymeneal ring. When dealing with the rectocele it was obvious that there was perineal deficiency also, and the skin incision has been left open where it runs on to the perineum.

31
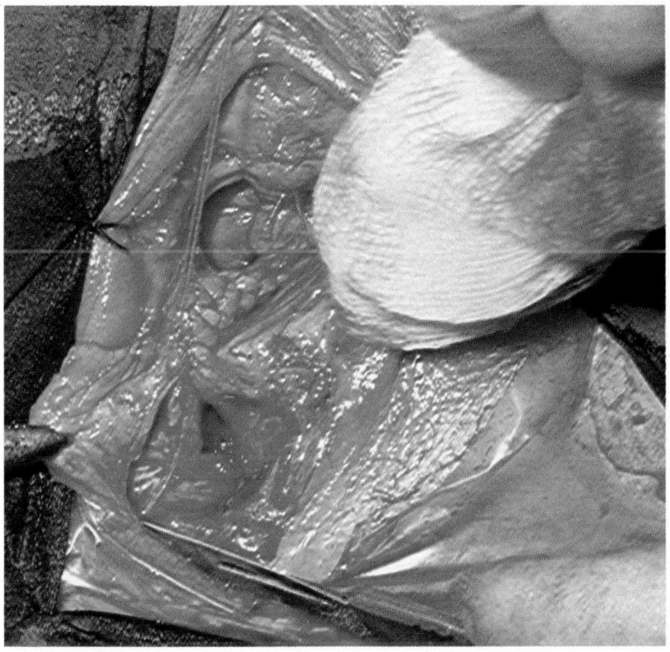

32
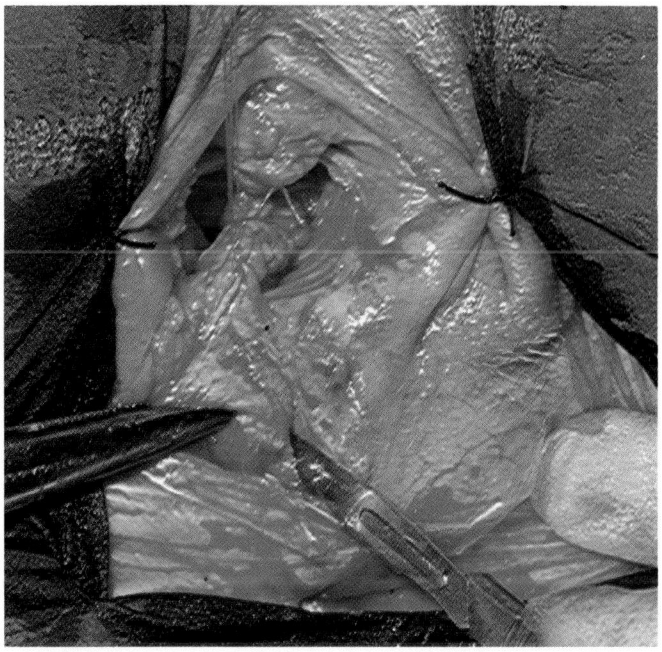

33
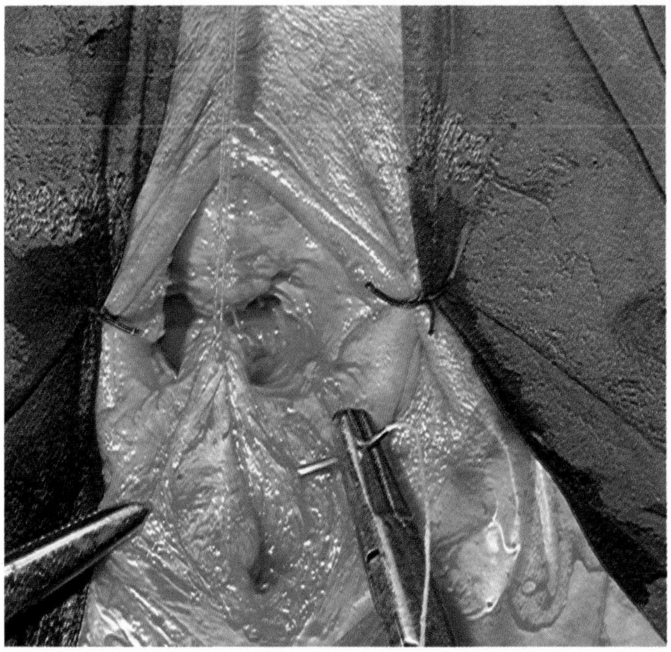

34
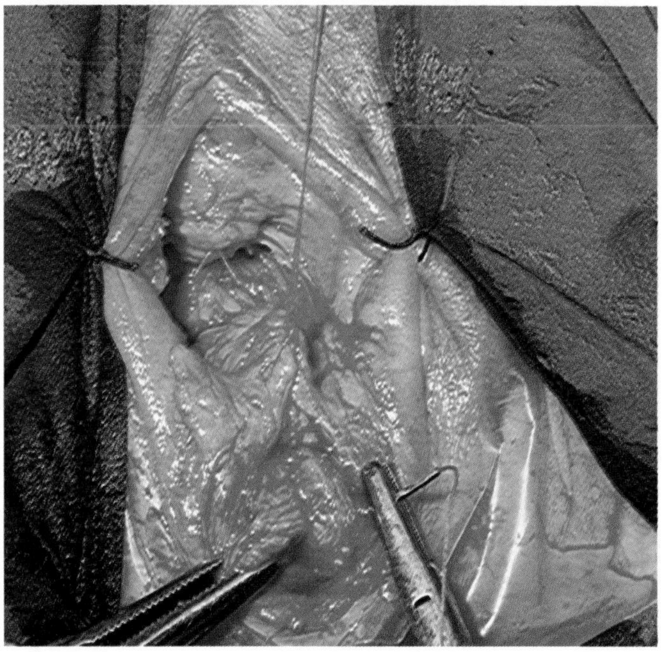

31–34 Definition and approximation of levator muscles

Holding up the lower edge of the closed vaginal skin with the uncut suture, the perineal defect is shown and the need for reconstruction is obvious. This is effected by defining the medial borders of the levator ani muscles on each side and stitching them together in the mid-line.

In **31** the skin is being freed from the patient's right levator muscle and in **32** the same is being done on the left. Figure **33** shows the two muscle bellies transfixed by a deep PGA No. 0 suture and **34** shows a second suture being placed.

35

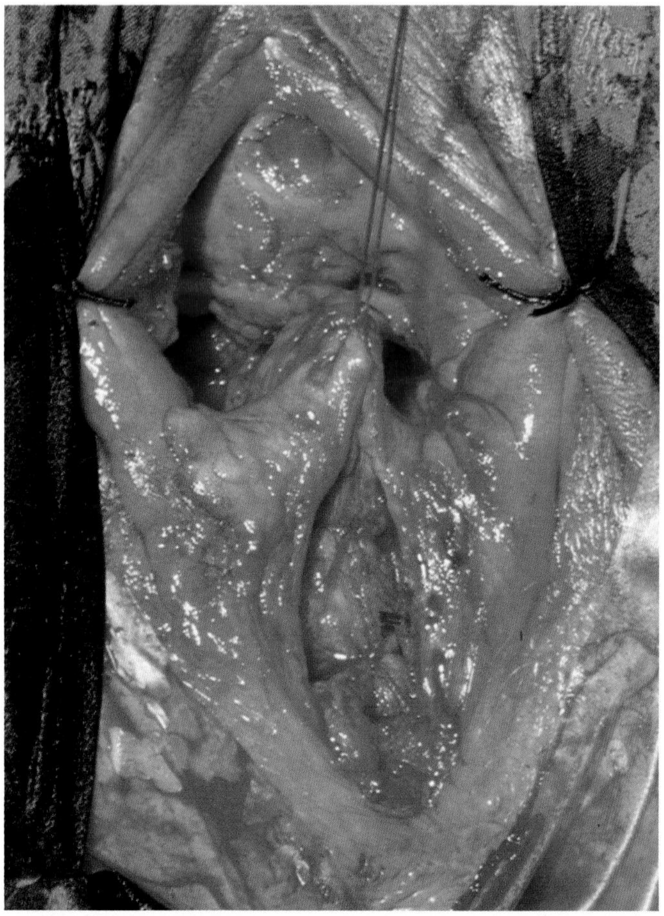

36

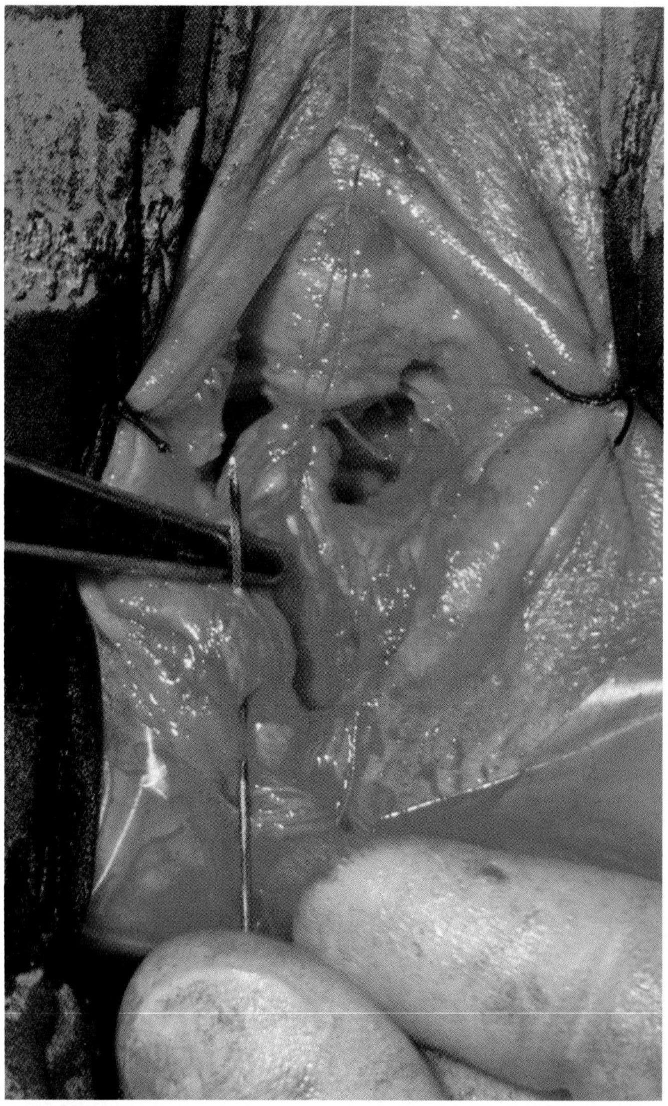

37

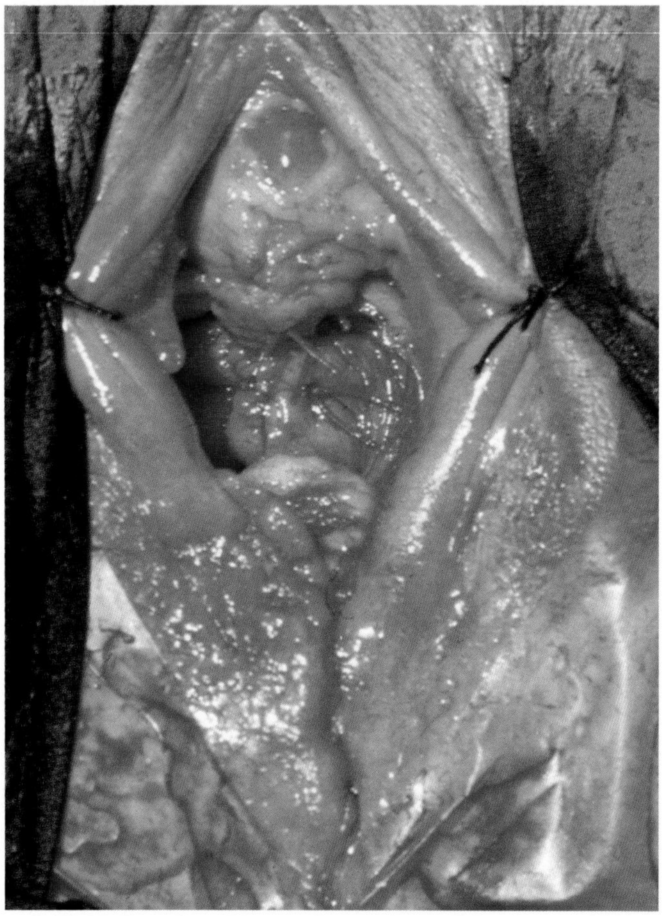

35 and 36 Closure of perineal skin

The skin is closed by a continuous subcutaneous PGA No. 00 suture on a straight triangular pointed needle, taking a good bite of subcutaneous tissue to give wide approximation of the deep skin edges. Figure **35** shows the incision ready for closure with the long posterior wall suture holding it taut; and **36** shows the skin closure continuing and emphasises the amount of subcutaneous tissue taken up by each stitch.

37 General appearance post-operatively

The perineum is well supported, the vaginal lumen is adequate and uniform and the suture lines are quite dry.

Stage 1: Preparation of fascial straps

1

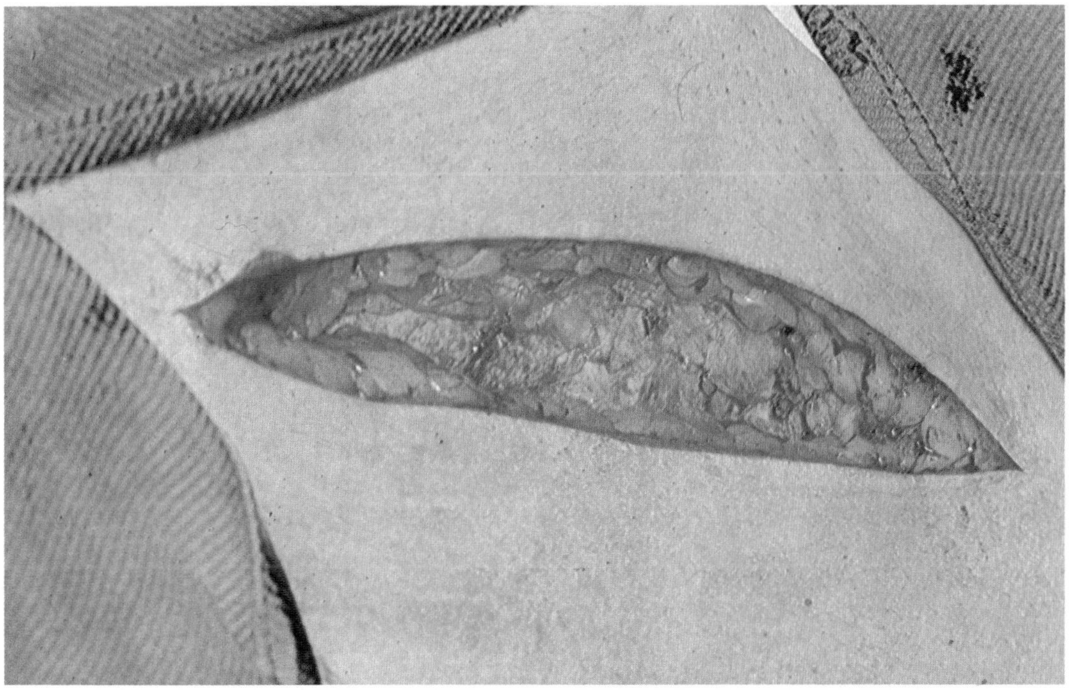

2

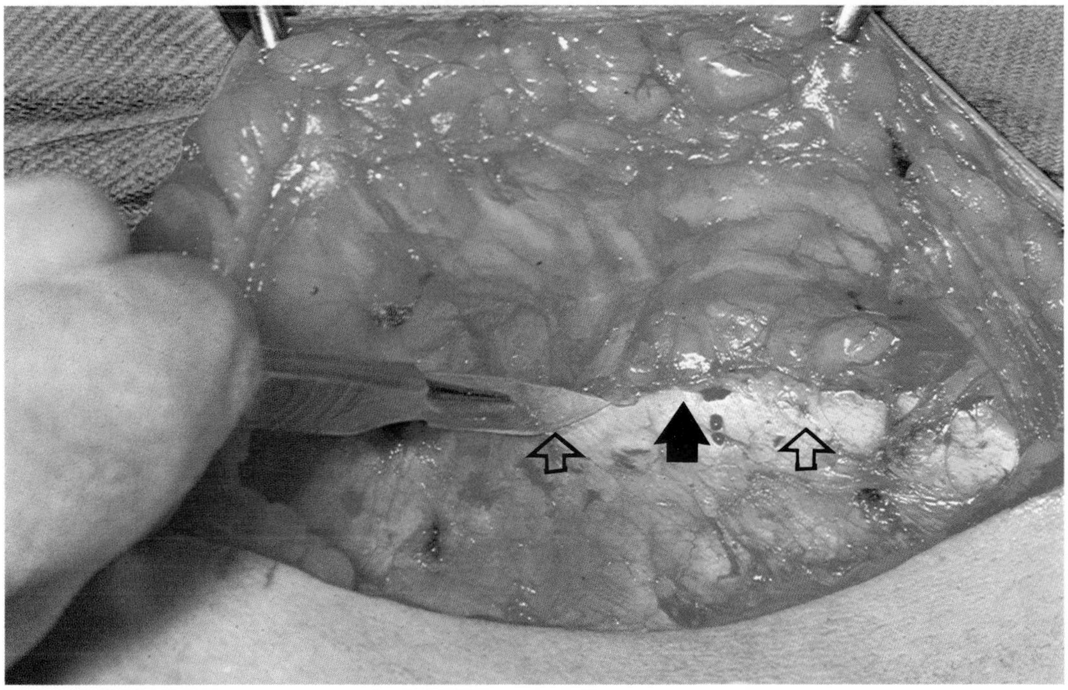

1 Lower abdominal transverse incision to abdominal aponeurosis

The length of the skin incision need not be more than 10 cm and the superficial fascia is incised down to the rectus sheath in the mid-line only. It is neither necessary nor wise to make a wide approach since blunt dissection will provide adequate access without the risk of immediate or later bleeding; note the extent of the incision which lies 4 cm above the level of the pubic crest.

2 Freeing abdominal aponeurosis of fat

Using the scalpel with a lateral pushing action the fat is cleared downwards off the rectus sheath as far as the upper border of the symphysis pubis and the pubic crest. A natural depression is felt just medial to the pubic tubercle on each side sufficiently wide to accommodate a finger's breadth along the pubic crest. These are the base areas to which the prepared straps will remain attached. The dark arrow indicates the symphysis pubis; the clear arrows show the approximate position of the pubic tubercles.

3

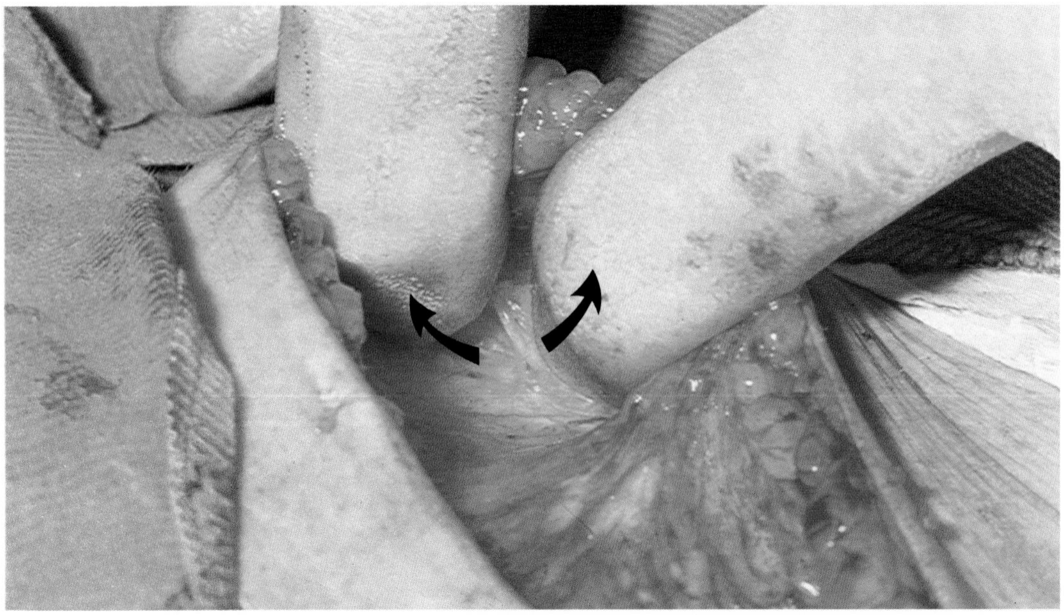

4

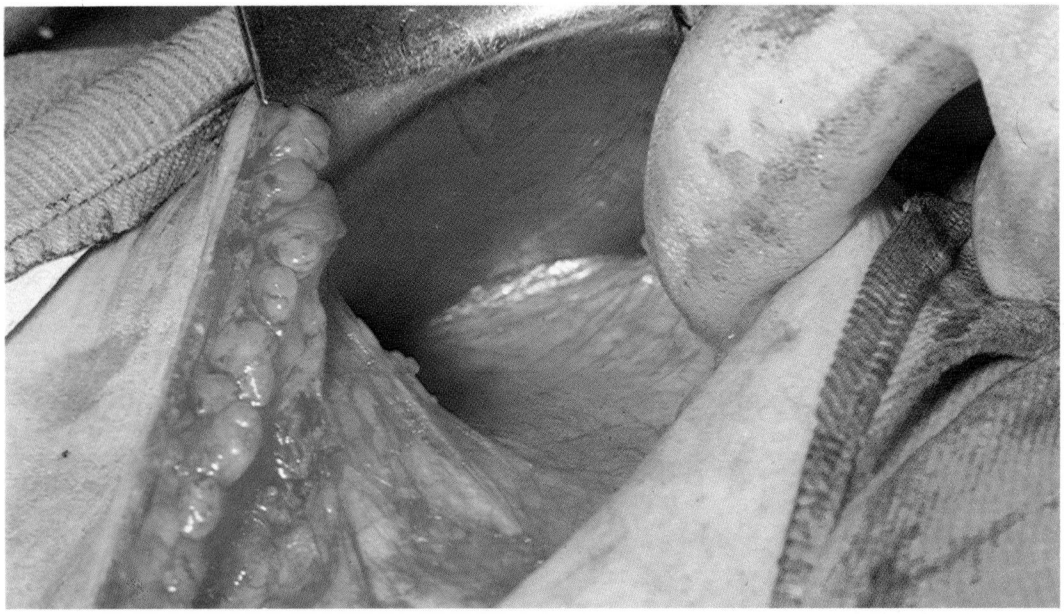

3 and 4 Preparing tunnel over rectus sheath (right)

Using the index fingers of both hands the superficial fascia is first drawn back towards the lateral part of the wound. Keeping the tips of the fingers close to the aponeurosis the fat is peeled off the lateral rectus sheath in an upwards and outwards direction to produce a tunnel which just accommodates two fingers. There should be no bleeding but small vessels coming through the rectus sheath may be seen to stretch across the tunnel and are sealed with diathermy and cut lest they subsequently be torn. The line of the tunnel is over the lateral half of the rectus sheath, as it is from there that the strap will be cut.

A Doyen's retractor is inserted into the lower end of the tunnel and drawn upwards and laterally to display the lateral part of the rectus sheath. Note that the skin, superficial fascia and the deep fascia are still attached to the rectus sheath medially, and there is no need to disturb the tissue layers in this area. By employing a blunt displacement type of approach rather than a cutting one the incidence of haematomata in the loose fatty tissues is greatly reduced and the wound and disturbed area is very much smaller. The number 1 indicates the undisturbed tissues attached to the rectus sheath medially.

5

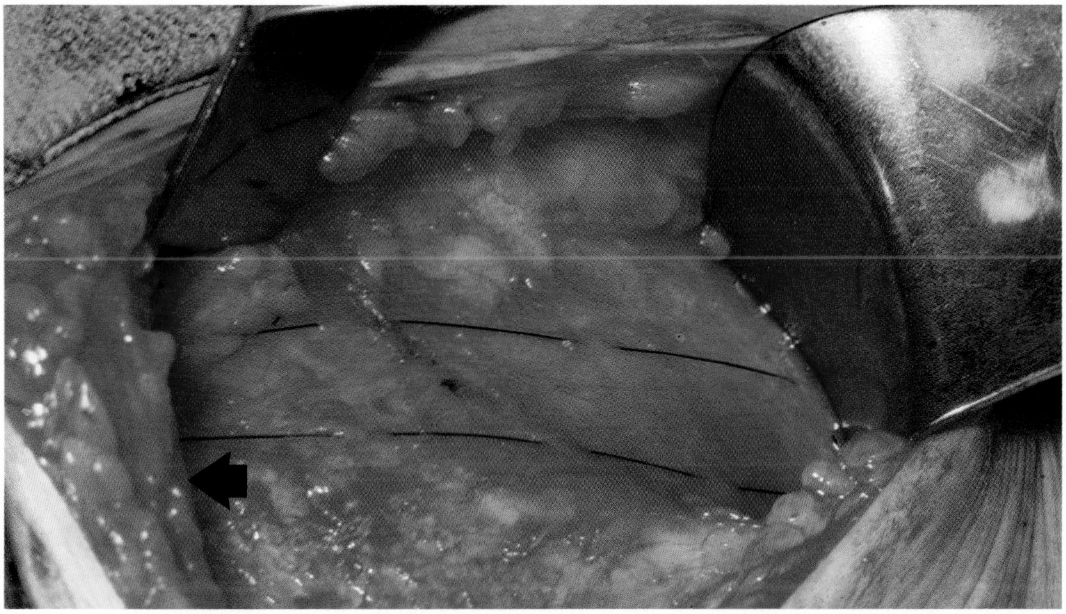

6

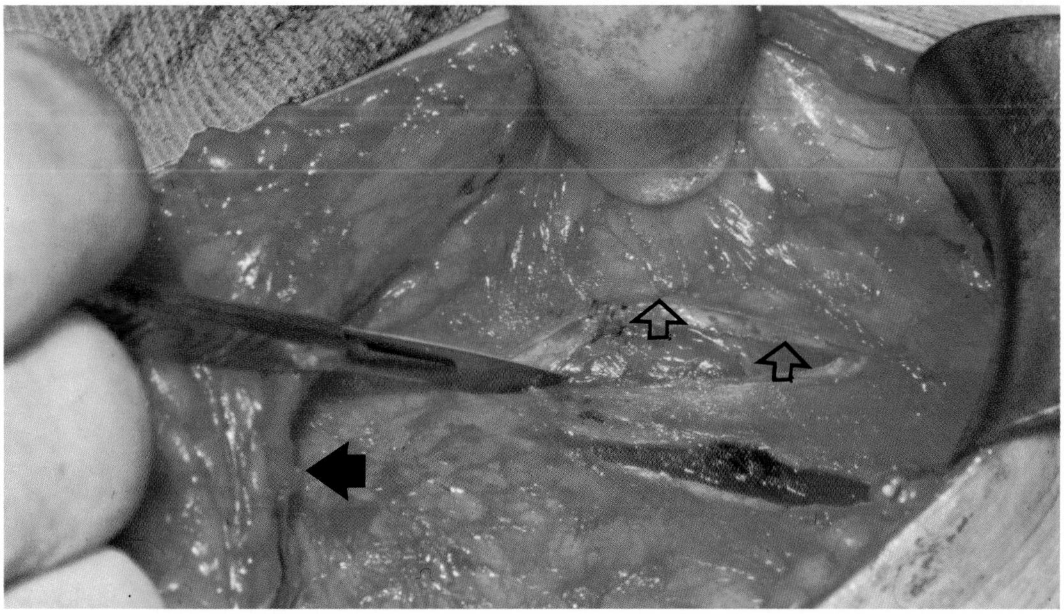

5 Planning fascial strap (right)

A dark coloured thread has been attached to the rectus sheath to demonstrate the outline of the fascial strap required. It is at least 1 cm wide and should be uniform throughout. The upper end will be detached but the lower will remain attached along the upper border of the pubic bone in the groove or area described in figure **2**. The length of the fascial strap should be 10 cm. As has already been mentioned the donor area is the lateral half of the rectus sheath, which is the strongest as it is contributed to by external oblique, internal oblique and transversus aponeuroses. All three are fused medially but laterally the external oblique is separate from the other two which remain joint and are centrally described as internal oblique. The arrow indicates the approximate area of the symphis pubis.

6 Cutting fascial strap (right)

The fascial strap which was outlined is thus made up of external and internal oblique muscle components which although joined together medially and also in the lower end of the sheath, are separate in the upper two-thirds of the planned excision. The two layers tend to slide on each other and this can make neat incision difficult. The initial incision is therefore made in the lower third of the strap for a distance of about 3 cm where the muscle planes are adherent. In the illustration the two layers are easily seen laterally but are adherent medially and therefore do not slip on each other when handled; these being indicated by the clear arrows. The dark arrow continues to indicate the symphis pubis.

7

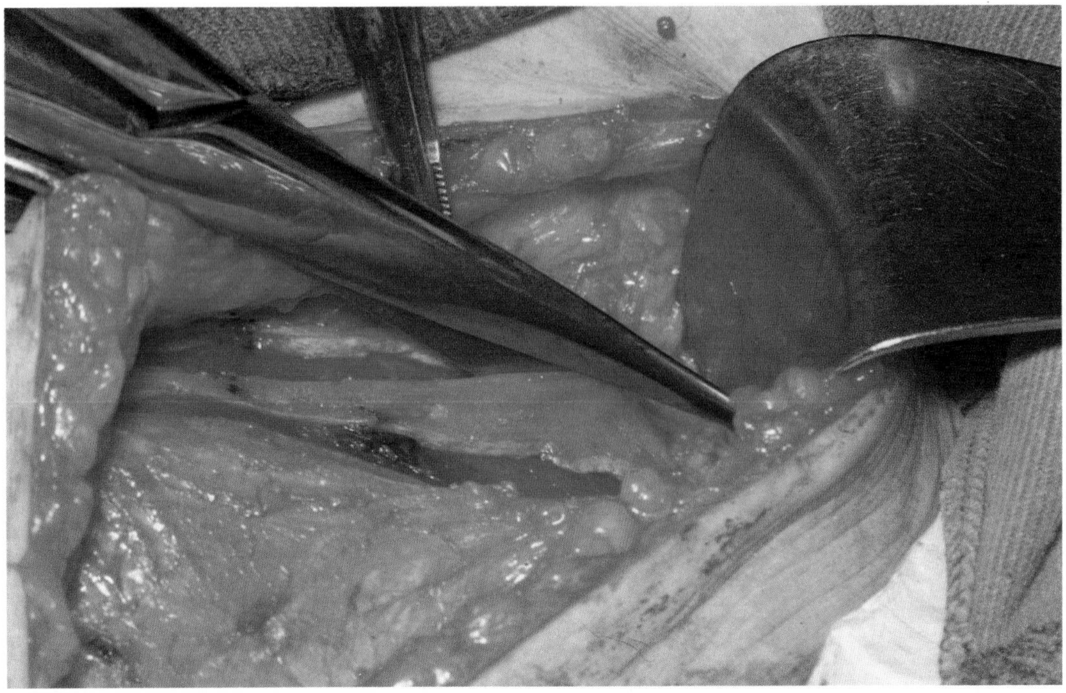

8

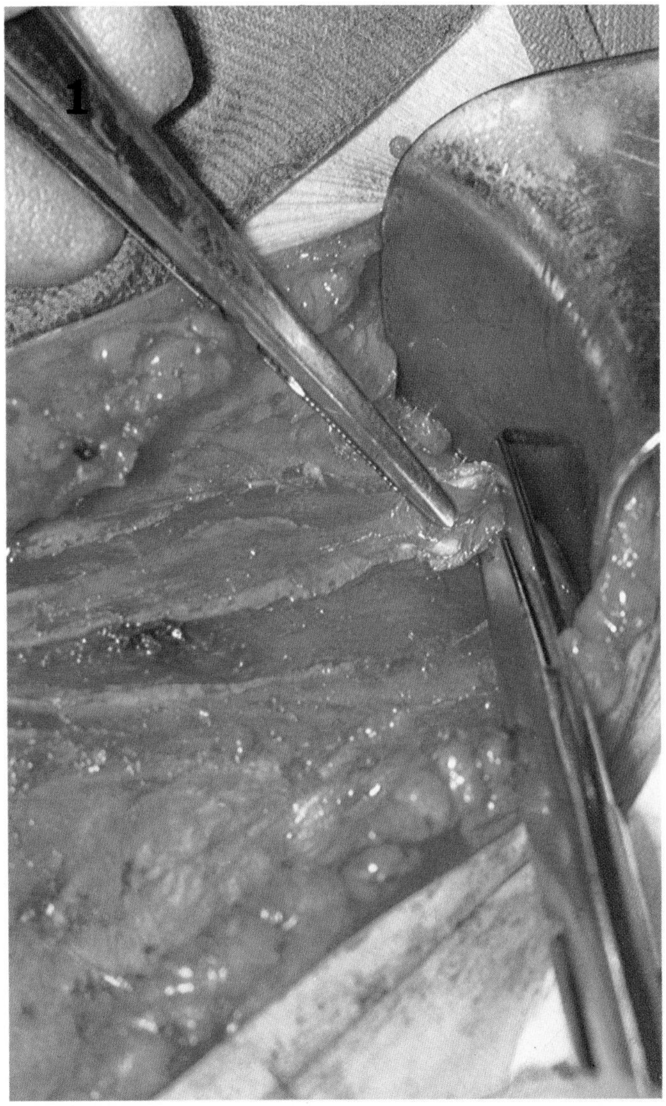

7 and 8 Cutting and detaching upper end of fascial strap (right) (right)

With straight scissors and keeping the aponeurosis on the stretch by pulling on the retractor, the fascial strap is defined and incised on the rectus muscle along the floor of the tunnel. The full length of the strap will be 10 cm. Until experienced in cutting these straps it is helpful to run a 'tacking' stitch along the centre line of the planned strap to temporarily fix the 2 layers to the underlying rectus muscle and prevent them slipping on each other during the actual cutting.

Figure **7** shows the method of excision. In **8** the fascial strap held on forceps (1) is cut across diagonally. This allows a neater closure of the gap in the rectus sheath at a later stage. The amount of tissue removed is rather critical as a width of 1 cm at least is desirable and yet the sheath must not be weakened. In fact there is no problem as long as the excised area is uniform. A wandering excision edge is bound to pose problems when closing the gap later.

9

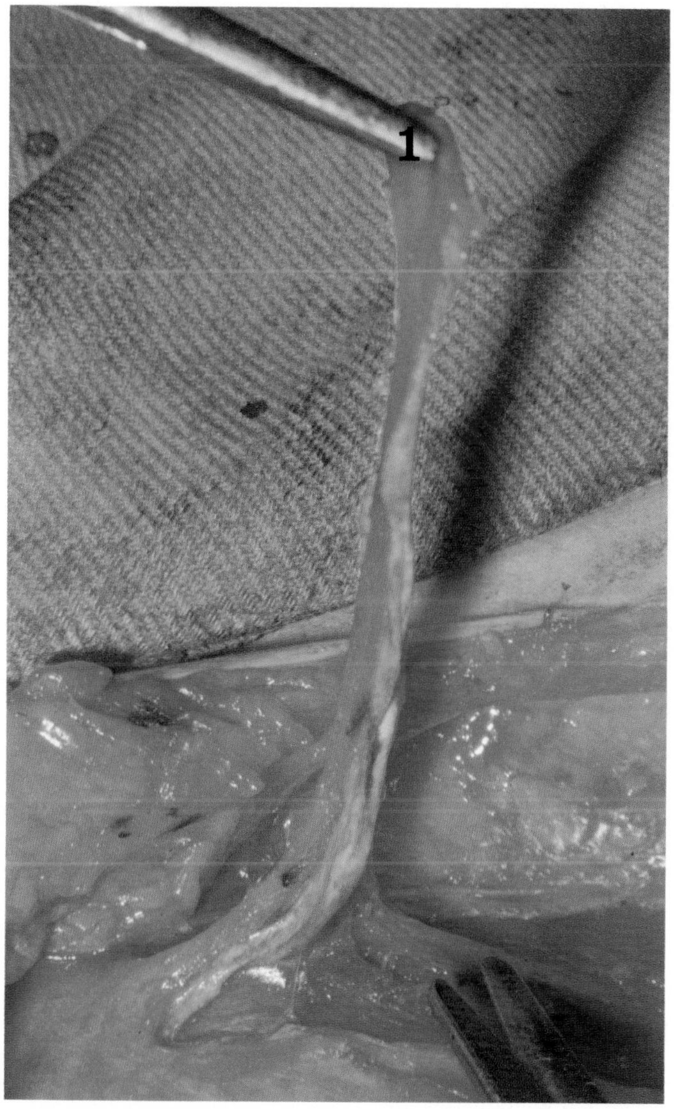

10

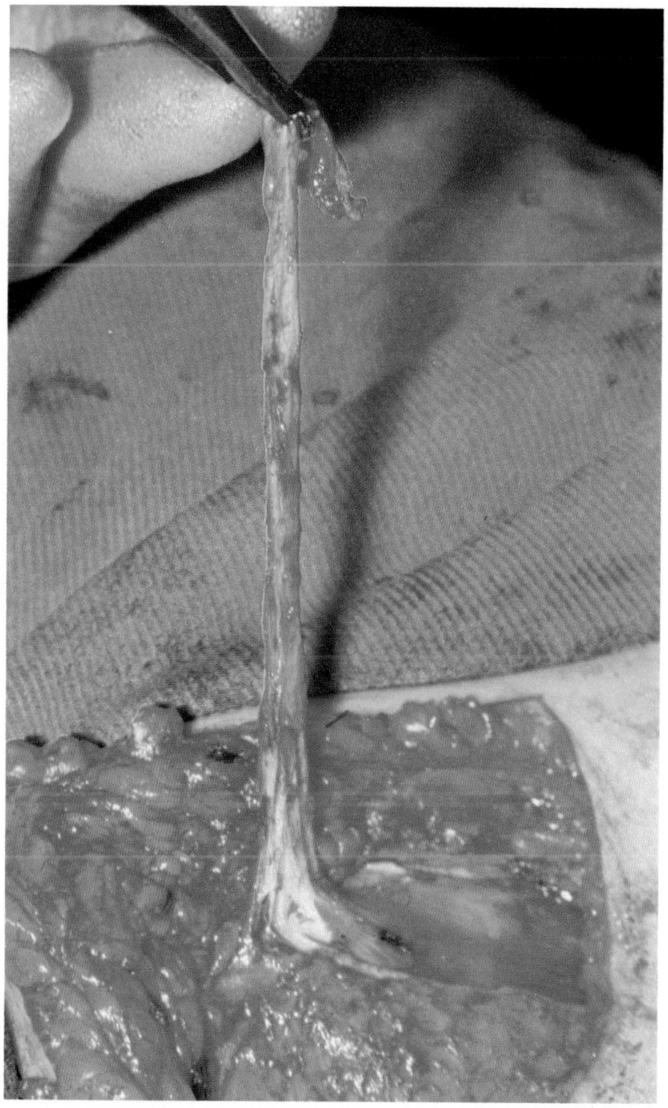

9 and 10 Elevation of fascial strap (right)

Holding its free end in forceps (1) the strap is stripped off the underlying rectus muscle using scissors where required. As it is freed downwards the defining incisions are carried right on to the pubic bone in the areas mentioned in figures **2** and **5**. In **9** the lower end of the strap is about to be separated off the pyramidalis and rectus muscles. In **10** the strap is now completely defined and free except for its attachment to the pubic crest. The underlying pyramidalis muscle is now clearly visible. Note that the strap is broadly based on the pubic crest.

11

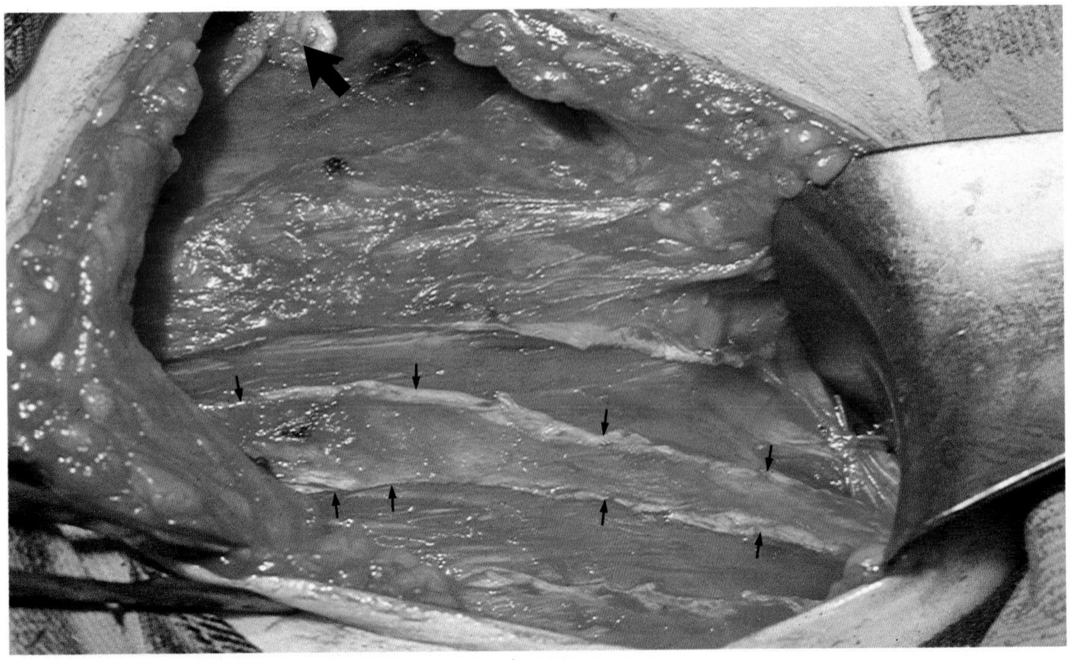

12

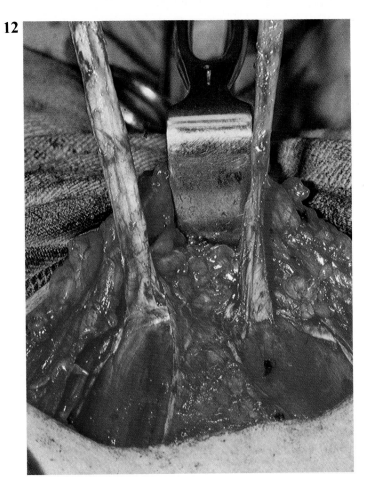

11 Preparation of fascial strap (left)

The same procedure has been followed on the left side. The retractor displays the tunnel along the floor of which the 1 cm wide strap has been cut and is awaiting detachment. The skin and fascial layers are still seen to be undisturbed medially and there is a fairly broad area of lower rectus sheath between the two straps. The detached right strap is seen in the corner of the wound. It is apparent from this illustration that the abdominal wall will have been subjected to minimal disturbance and cutting by the time the straps have been obtained. This is an important aspect of the operation. The large arrow indicates the right detached strap; the small arrows the cut edges of the undetached left strap.

12 Demonstration of prepared fascial straps

The two straps are seen to be uniform in width. They are approximately 10 cm long and firmly attached to the upper pubic border or crest. On a broad base the gaps in the sheath appear wide but it is a close view and the lateral edge on the right side is lying loosely outwards. The is a full 2 cm of intact sheath between the gaps at this narrowest point.

13

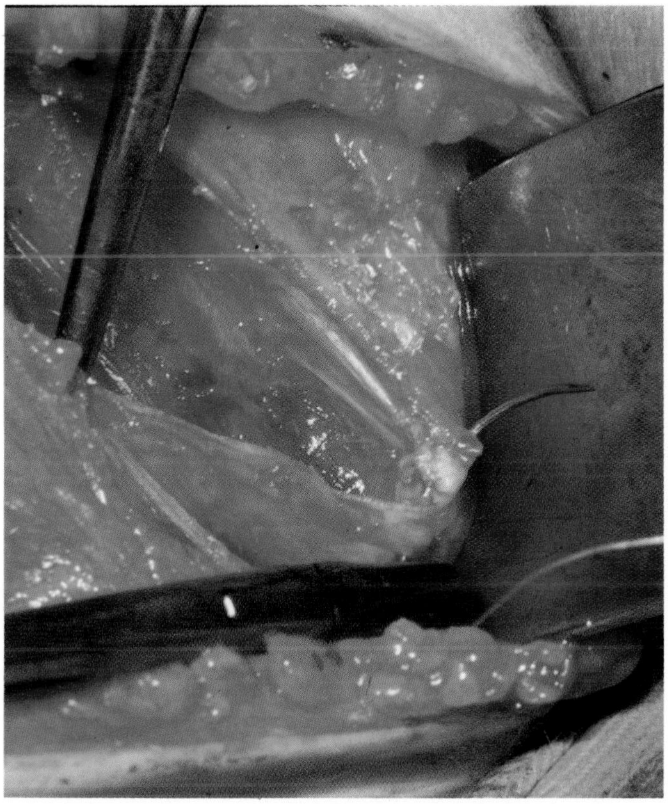

14

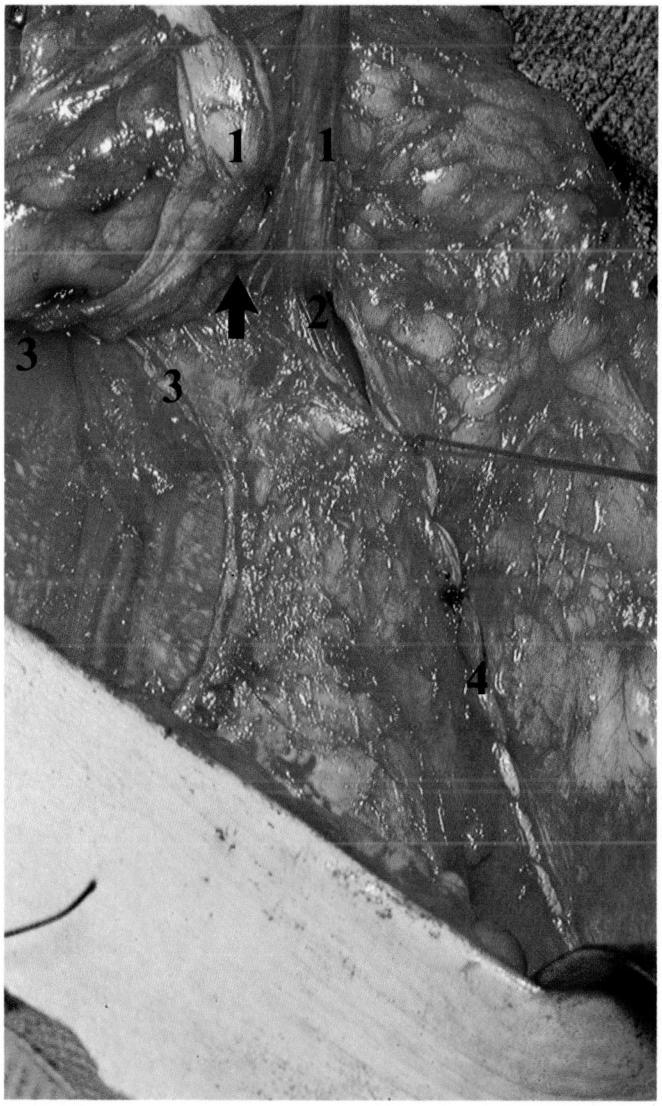

13 and 14 Closure of gap in rectus sheath (right)

The gap is closed by a continuous PGA No. 0 suture on an atraumatic needle and the initial stitch is being placed. It is important that both the external and internal oblique layers are picked up by the needle as illustrated in **13** and the oblique direction of the cut (as described in **7**) makes for neater closure. Stitches are placed near the fascial edges at a distance of 0.5 cm from each other, and in **14** approximation is completed. The edges of the fascial aponeurosis have been brought together by the continuous stitch which is tied off 2.5 cm from the pubic crest. This leaves a triangular-shaped opening over the rectus muscle where it arises from the pubis and through which the strap will be directed to the vagina. The two straps are seen and the left rectus sheath has still to be sutured. In **13** the fine arrows delineate the two layers of the rectus sheath: in **14** the numerals indicate (1) the two detached straps (2) the triangular opening (3) the edges of the unclosed left sheath (4) the closed right sheath. The thick arrow points to the symphysis.

15

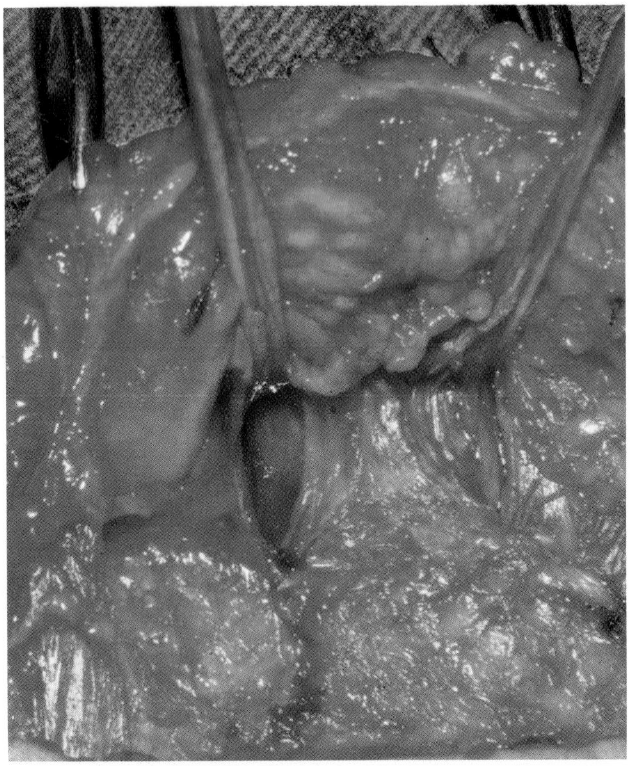

16

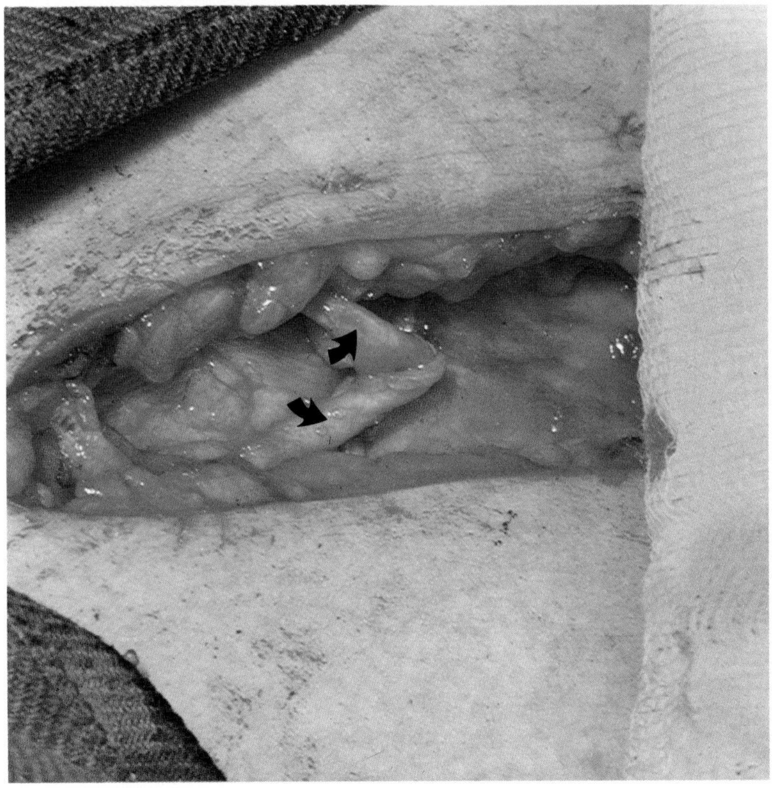

15 and 16 Rectus sheath reconstituted: abdominal wound covered.

In **15** both gaps in the rectus sheath have now been repaired with the exception of the triangular areas above the pubic crest which will be required later. Initially it was thought advisable to establish a route through the rectus muscle towards the retropubic space with a probing forceps but in the event it was apt not to be used. Probably the only circumstances in which such preparation is necessary is following a Marshall–Marchetti–Kranz operation. In these cases there is dense fibrosis retropubically and it is advisable to establish a route for the forceps. Otherwise force has to be used with risks of bladder injury.

The abdominal wound with its freed straps of fascia is left open during the next phase of the operation and in **16** a moist gauze dressing is placed over the incision while preparation is made for the vaginal part of the operation. The right side has been covered and the dressing is being rolled towards the left. The left strap can be seen curled up in the corner of the wound (as arrowed).

17
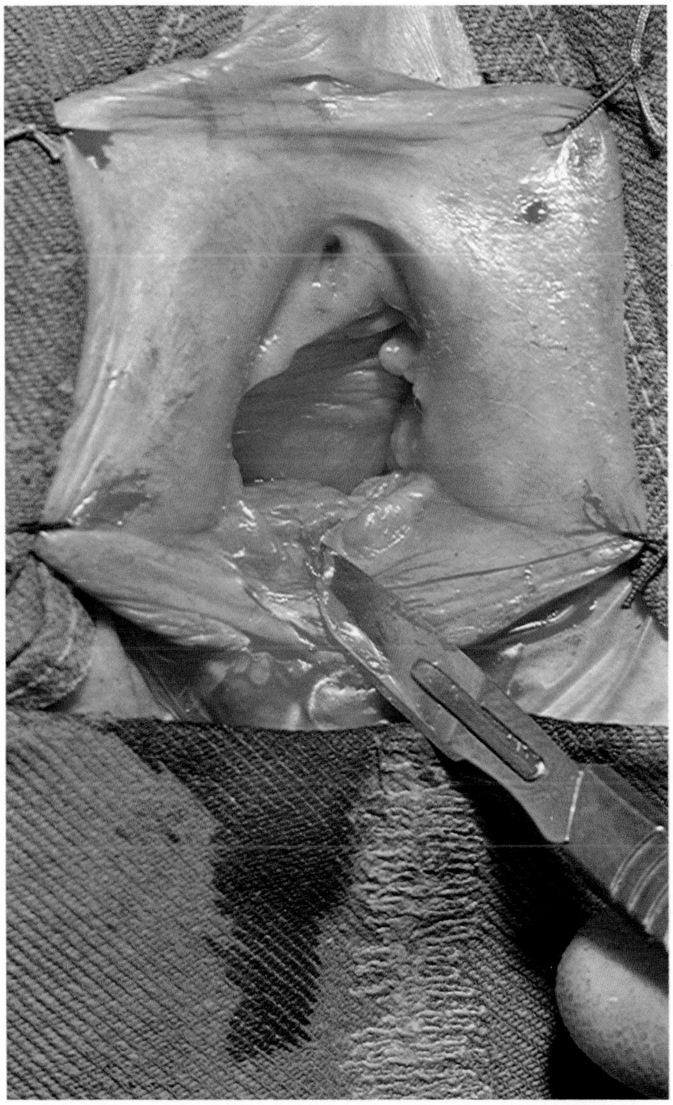

Stage 2: Attachment of fascial straps to bladder base

17 Preparation for vaginal surgery

The labia have been stitched back and the anterior wall and lower vagina are seen. As in most cases there is no cystocele and no other element of prolapse to be seen. A mid-line episiotomy is made to give better access.

18 Incision of anterior vaginal wall

A mid-line vertical incision is made in the anterior vaginal wall from above downwards. This is deep enough to cut right through the skin and into the pubocervical fascia which is usually thin in these cases. The two layers can be seen clearly. There is no question of a triangular incision as in prolapse because there is no excess vaginal skin.

18
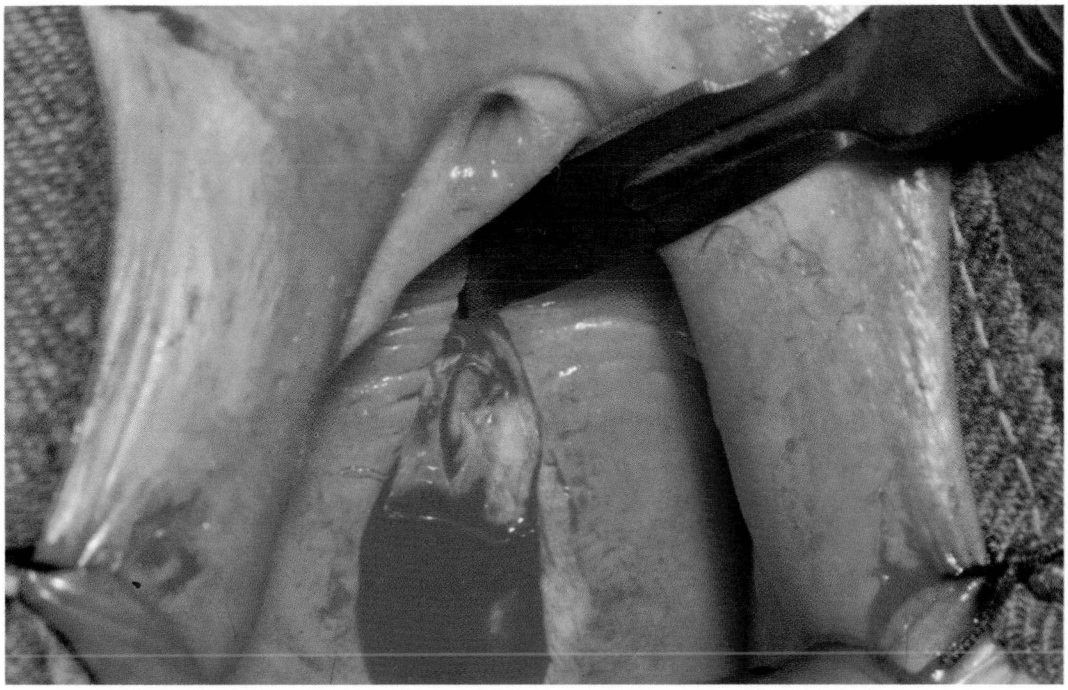

19

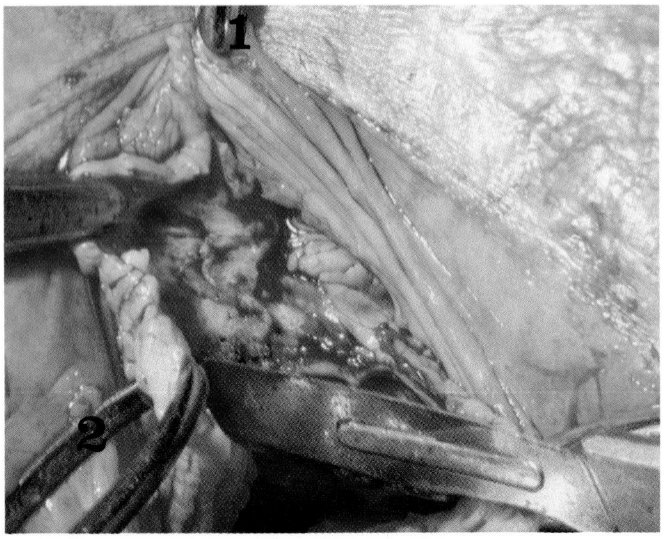

21

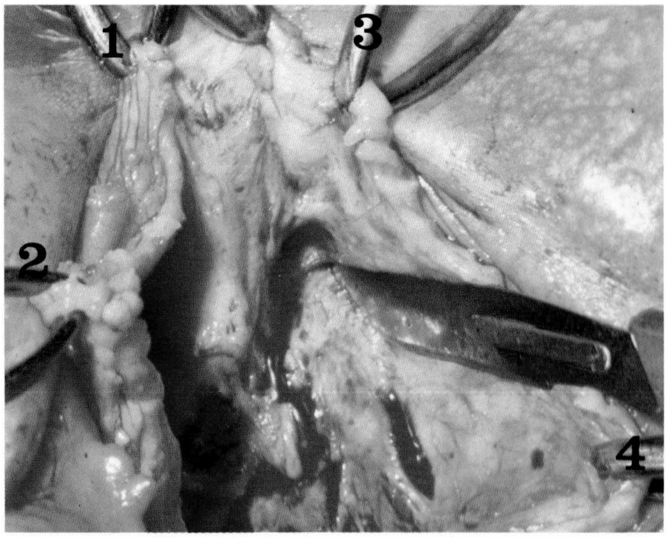

20

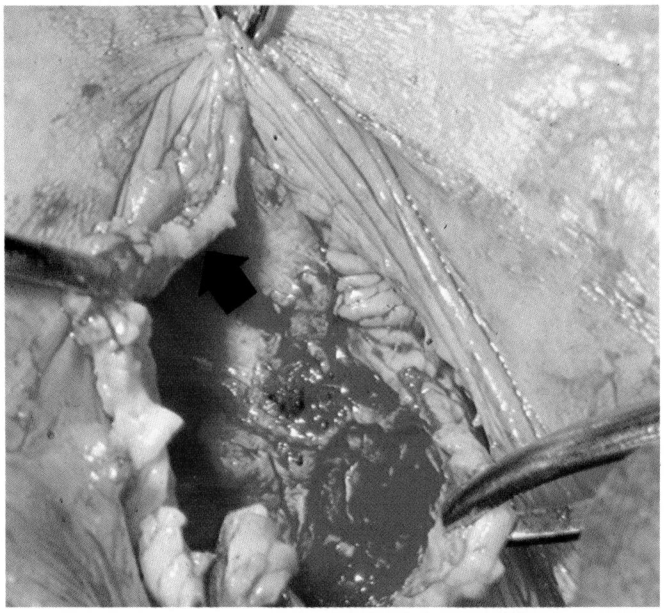

22

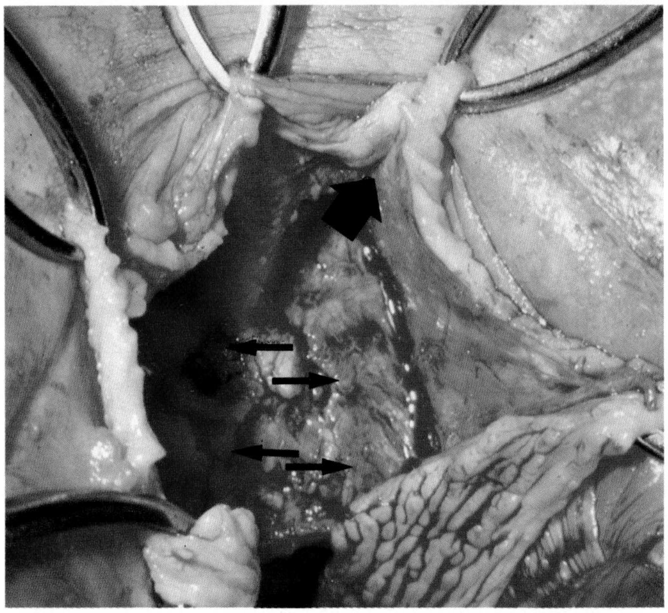

19 and 20 Separation of vaginal skin from fascia (right)

The right skin edge is held taut between the Littlewood's forceps (1) just below the urethral orifice and (2) at the level of the urethrovesical angle. With dissecting forceps and a fine-bladed scalpel the plane between the skin and the pubo-cervical fascia is sought and defined as shown in **19**. It is necessary to use sharp dissection initially but as dissection proceeds laterally the planes open up and separation by blunt dissection is easy. The sharp dissection should be done carefully to avoid buttonholing the skin.

With the skin drawn to the right, the thickened edge of the pubocervical fascia is seen in **20** and this area of separation is developed by blunt dissection until it is possible for the index finger to detect the inferior edge of the body of the pubic bone and its inferior ramus. There is a natural sub-pubic fossa at this point which just accommodates the finger tip and it is here that forceps will enter to travel retropubically to pick up the fascial strap. This point will be indicated again later, but it is identified in this figure and again in **22** by a thick arrow.

21 and 22 Separation of vaginal skin from fascia (left)

A similar preparation is carried out on the left side. In **21**, the point of the knife indicates the location of the left-sub-pubic fossa, and the blade is opening up the space between the skin and the pubocervical fascia. Forceps (1) and (2) are still on the right skin edge; forceps (3) and (4) serve a similar purpose on the left. With the skin flaps retracted the two irregular edges of pubocervical fascia are clearly seen in **22** and it is significant that the fascial layer is deficient and hardly visible centrally; the arrows indicate the fascial edges.

Dissection in this area can be vascular because there are venous sinuses just below the inferior pelvic diaphragm. Bleeding can best be avoided by keeping close to the skin layer and sweeping the fascia off it in a medial direction.

23

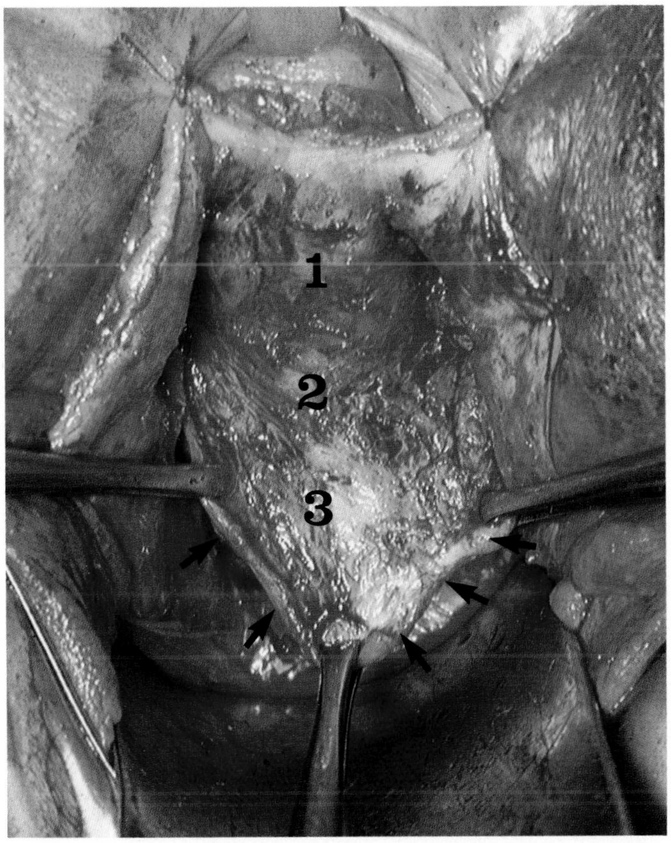

23 Exposure of urethra and bladder base

The skin edges are stitched to the labia by three fine sutures on each side to allow of access to the bladder, urethra and sub-pubic fossae. The urethra and bladder base are exposed and the general outline of the urethrovesical junction is seen. The pubocervical fascia is clearly deficient in the region of the bladder neck and its edge shows up posteriorly where the fascia covers the bladder base more completely on the right than on the left. Access to the sub-pubic fossae is just anterior to the urethrovesical junction. Number 1 indicates the urethra, 2 the urethrovesical junction and 3 the bladder base. Arrows indicate the pubocervical fascial edge.

24

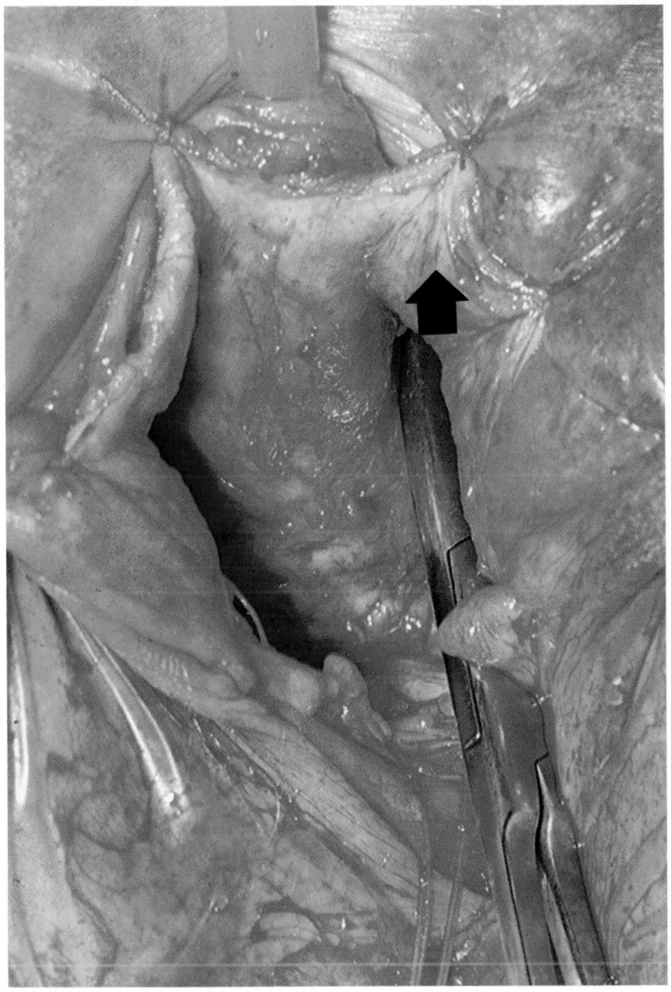

24 and 25 Preparing retropublic fascial route

To bring the fascial strap into the vaginal wound a long curved forceps with narrow shoulders (Roberts') is introduced through the sub-pubic fossa described, keeping its tip close to the posterior surface of the bone and a full 1.0 cm clear of the urethra as outlined by the catheter. It has to traverse the uro-genital diaphragm and slight pressure is needed to pierce that structure. If there is much resistance it is better to use a sharp pointed Spencer Wells forceps to penetrate the fibrous layer and make an entry point for the Roberts' forceps.

The other point of resistance is from the lower tendon-like end of the rectus muscle. In the illustrations the entry points for the Roberts' forceps are being defined with Spencer Wells forceps on each side. The arrows indicate the direction taken by the forceps.

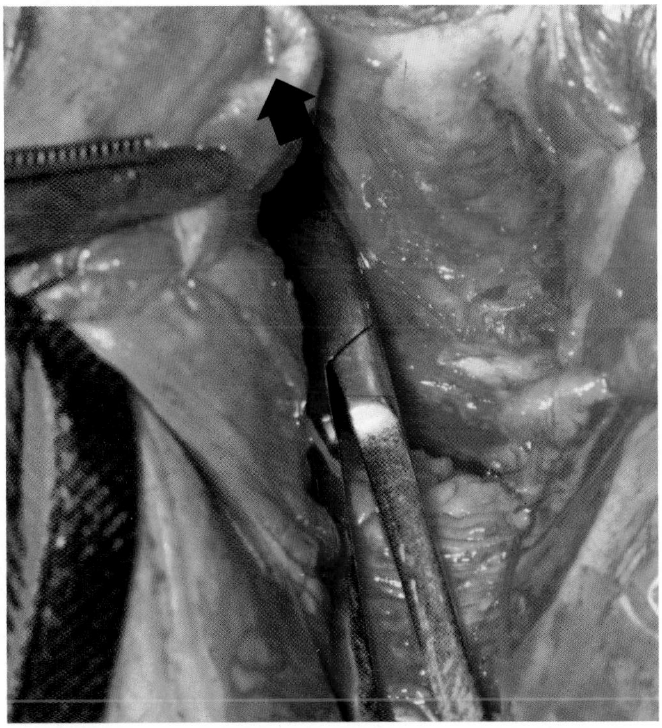

25

26

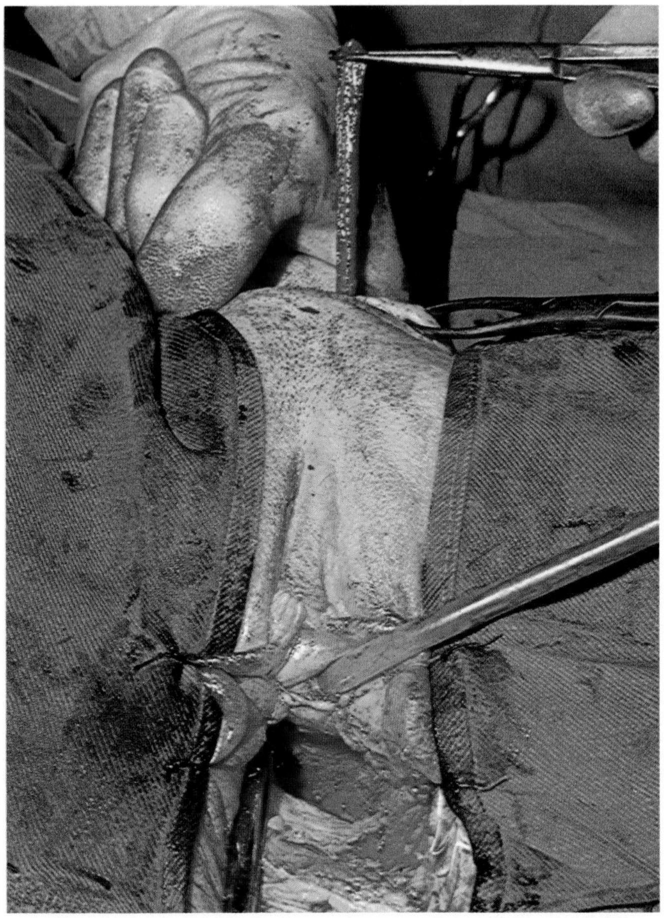

27

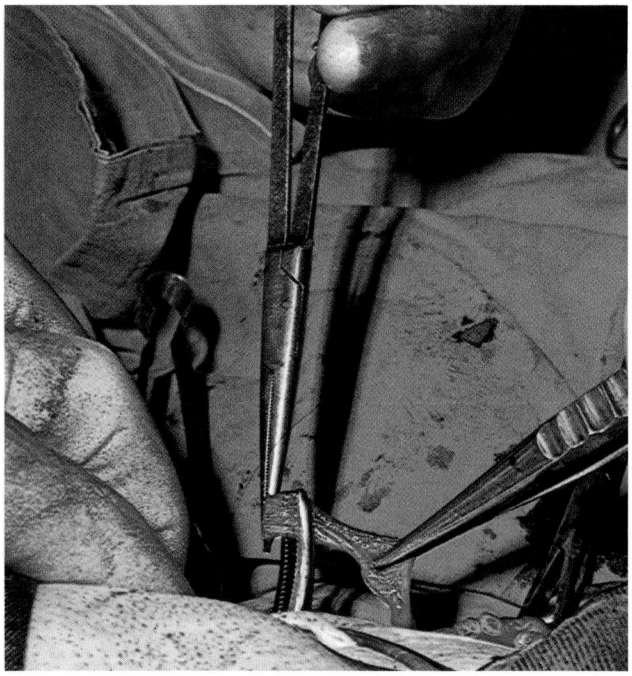

28

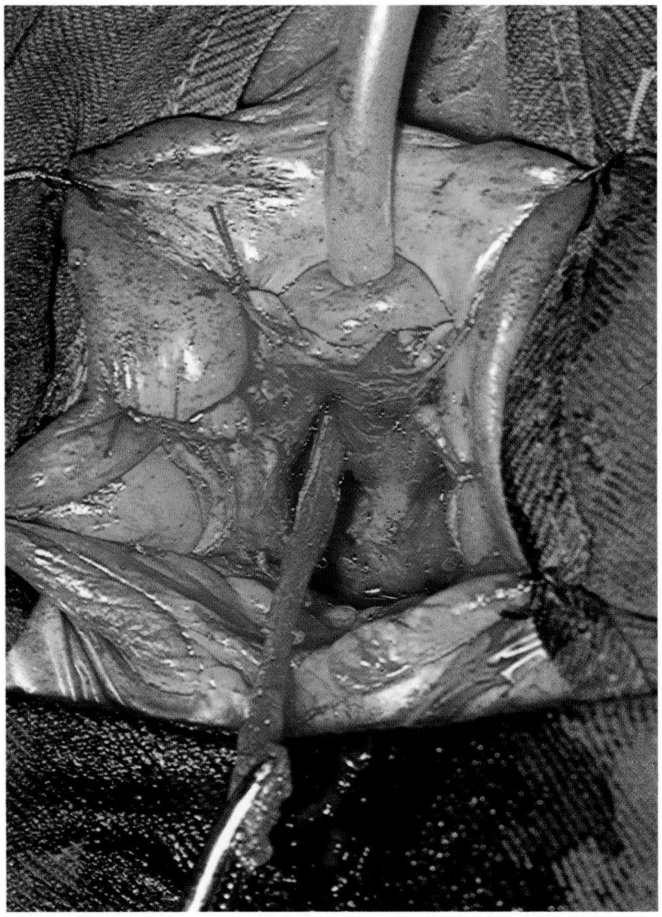

26 Retrieval of fascial strap (right)

In preparation for this step the attachment of the drapes to the pubis is freed and the abdominal wound brought into the vaginal operative field. The covering moist dressing is removed and an ancillary light focused on the abdominal wound. The joint abdomino-vaginal procedure is facilitated by lowering the operation table considerably. In the illustration the Roberts' forceps is now on its retropubic journey and has been guided past the urethra with the finger from below so that it is known to be well clear of that structure. The advancing point of the forceps is located at this stage by the index finger of the left hand in the triangular gap at the lower end of the closed aponeurosis on the right side. It is sought close to the bone and can be clearly felt through the rectus muscle which it then pierces. Note that during retrieval of the fascial bands the Auvard speculum is removed. This is necessary if the points of the forceps are to be kept on the back of the pubic bone and illustrates the vertical path that must be followed.

27 and 28 Retrieval of fascial straps on both sides

In **27** the points of the Roberts' forceps have emerged through the rectus muscle and have picked up the free end of the right strap which is held by a haemostat and supported by dissecting forceps.

In **28** the same strap has been drawn down into the vaginal operative field by the returning Roberts' forceps. It is seen to be of more than adequate length and it is not usually necessary to anchor it with forceps. The same procedure is carried out on the left side.

29

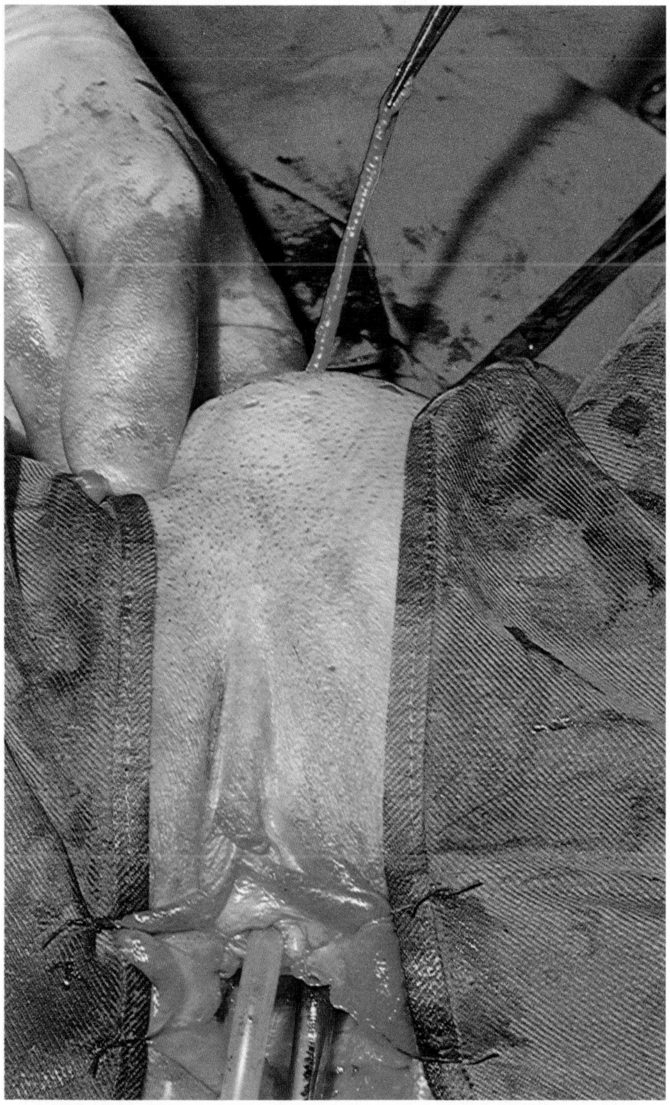

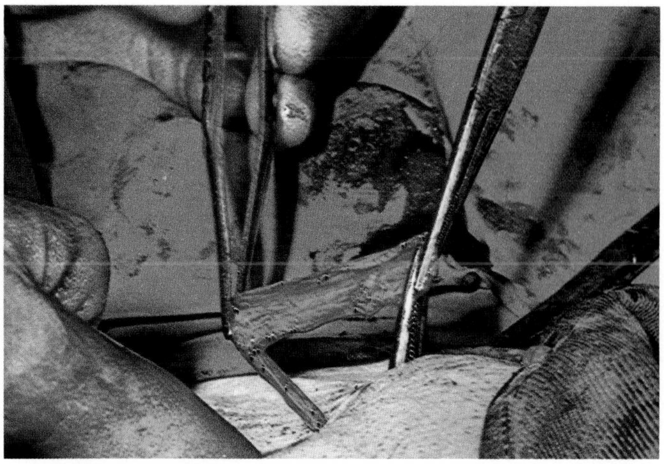

30

29 and 30 Retrieval of fascial strap (left)

In **29** the index finger of the left hand is locating the point of the Roberts' forceps and it is helpful at this stage if the assistant holds the strap taut by its free end so that the surgeon's index finger is guided into the triangular gap over the rectus muscle mentioned in **26**.

In **30** the tip of the Roberts' forceps has emerged to receive the end of the right fascial strap preparatory to drawing it down into the vagina.

31 and 32 Fascial straps in vaginal field

The two straps have been crossed over each other under the urethrovesical junction and thus indicate the cruciate nature of the planned fascial support. They are obviously longer than will be required in this particular case and that is generally so if they are 10 cm long. The length of the retropubic space, however, varies greatly and in some women with deep pelves the full 10 cm is required. These points are illustrated by **31**.

An estimate of the length of strap required is made by measuring to the lower border of the posterior wall of the bladder and then cutting off the excess. In **32** the left strap has been trimmed and the right one is in process of being shortened.

31

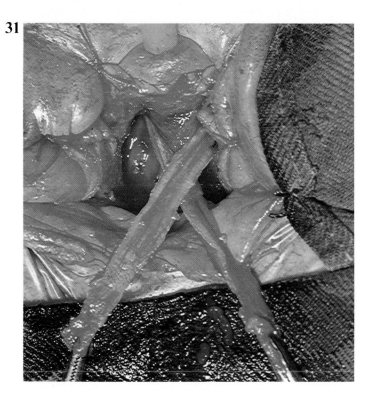

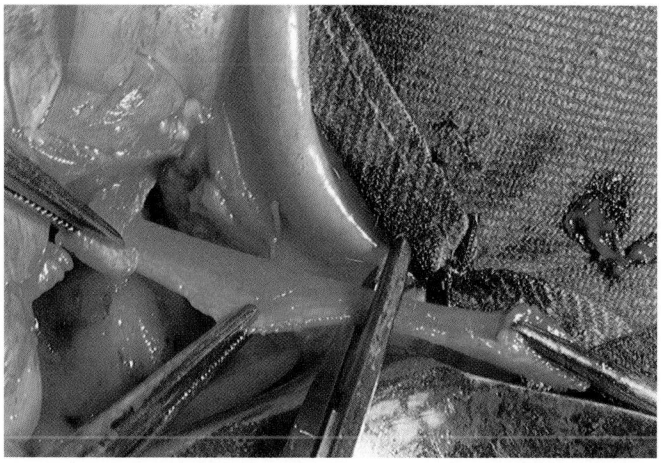

32

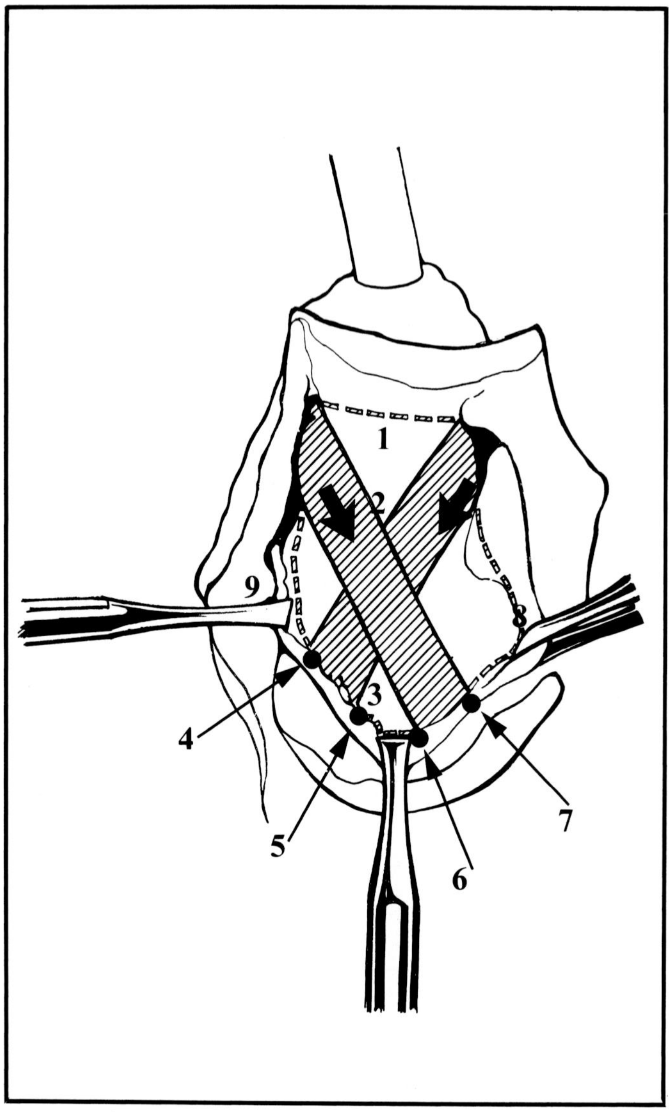

33

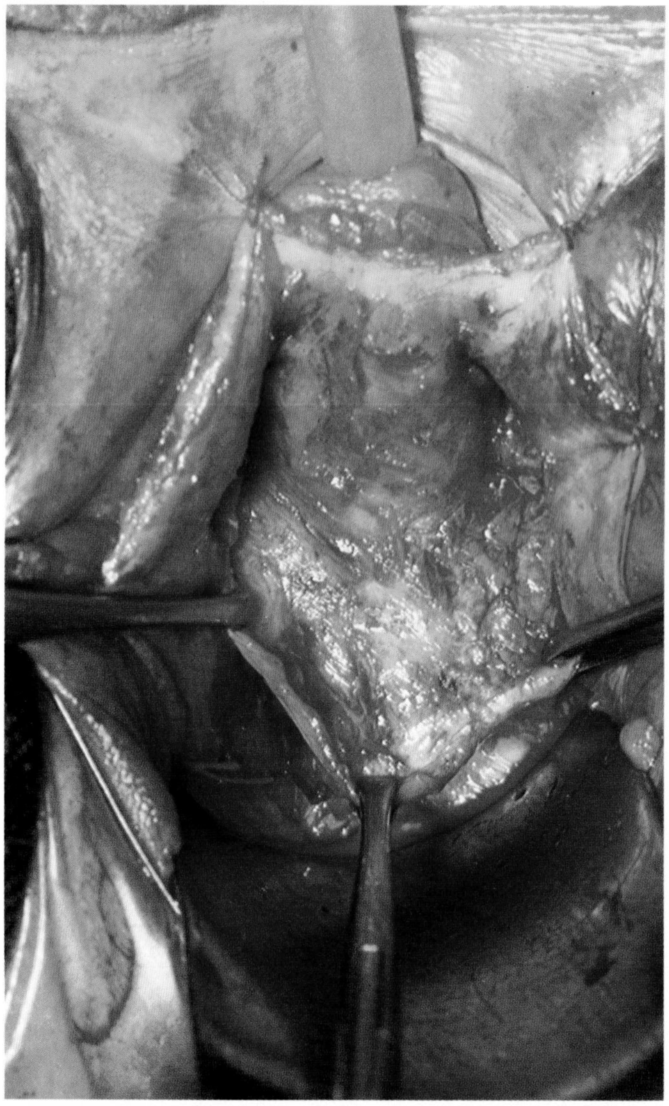

33 Planning attachment of fascial straps

The pubocervical fascia to which the fascial straps are to be attached is defined by the forceps holding it at 3, 6 and 9 o'clock. The right strap crosses over to the left and vice-versa, the cross-over point being just under the urethrovesical junction (2). This is shown on the diagram where the actual points of attachment are numbered. The patient's right hand strap is attached at points (6) and (7): the left hand strap at points (4) and (5). The straps will subsequently be fanned out laterally over the bladder base (3) to invest it as completely as possible and the points of lateral attachment are indicated by numbers (8) and (9). The final step involves suturing the medial borders of the superior limbs of the X so that the area under the urethra (1) is completely supported.

At the conclusion of these steps the whole bladder base and the proximal two-thirds of the urethra are completely covered or supported by a new investing layer of fascia. This area is outlined by the broken line in the diagram. This new fascia is looked on as a replacement for the deficient or absent pubocervical fascia.

34

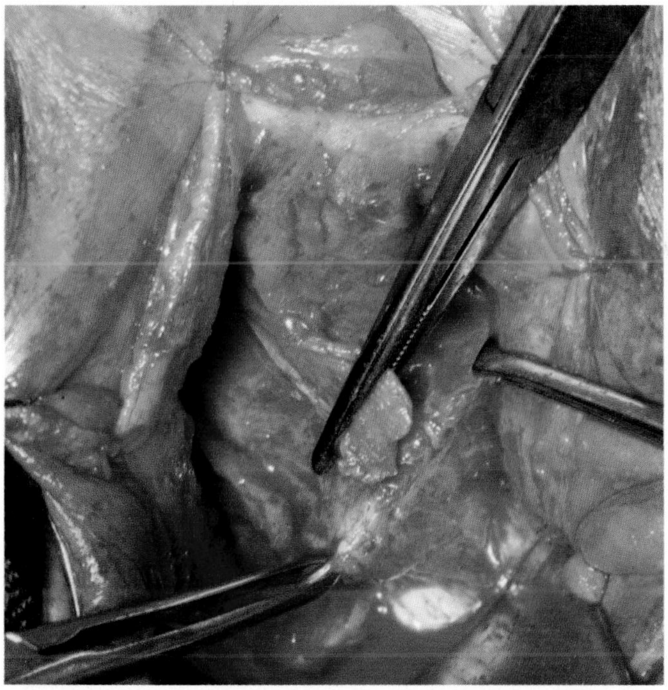

35

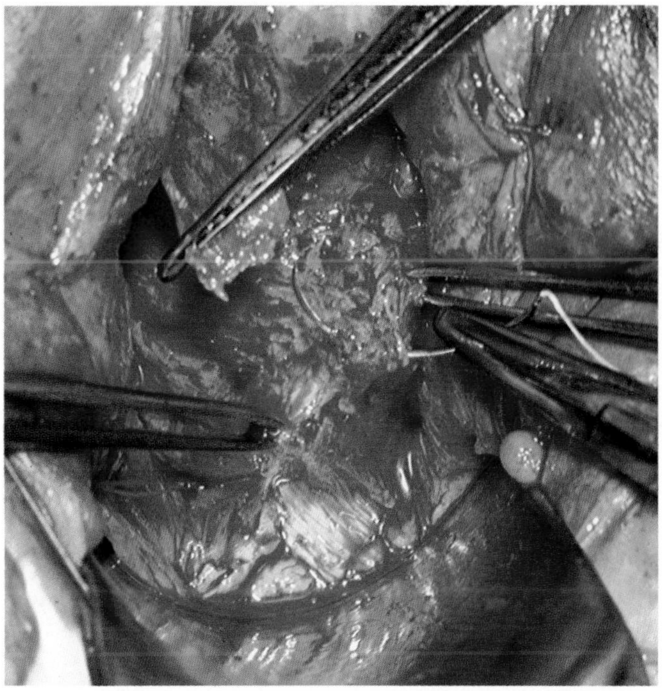

36

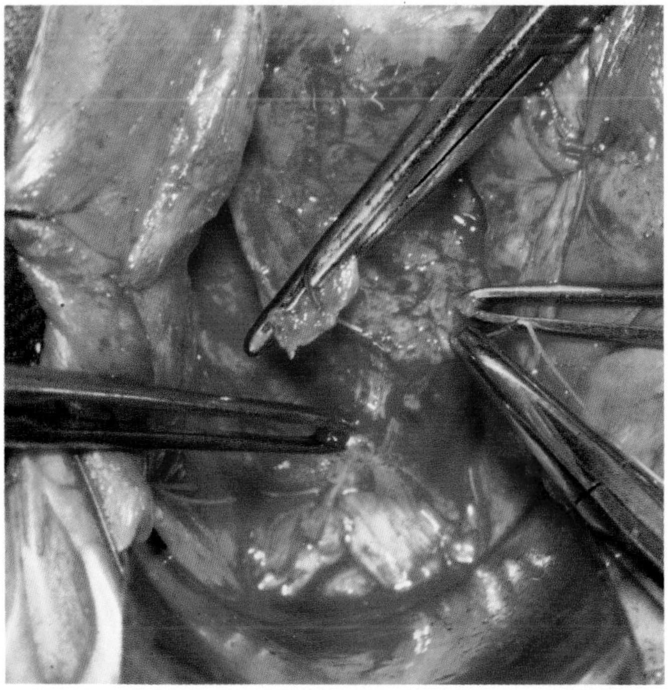

37

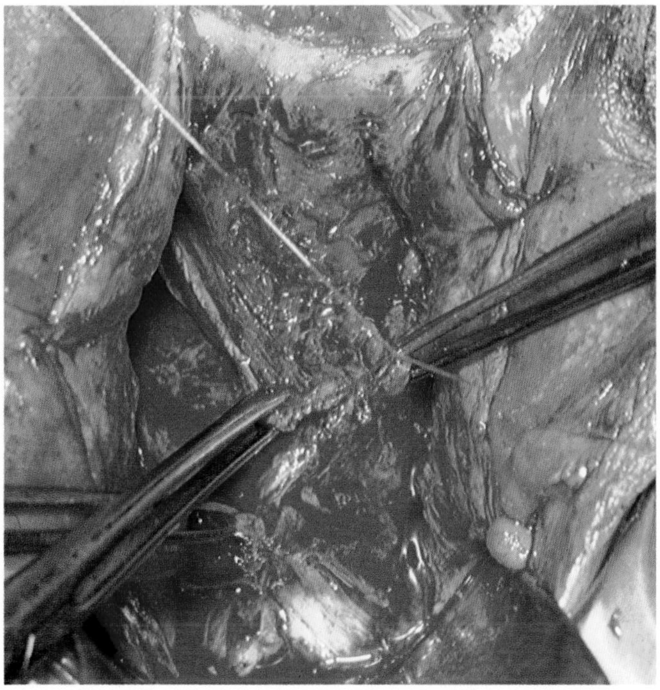

34–37 Attaching right fascial strap to bladder base

In **34** the trimmed strap is held in position ready for attachment to the pubocervical fascia covering the bladder base on the left side. In **35** the fine round-bodied needle carrying a PGA No. 00 suture picks up the pubocervical fascia with a firm bite, in **36** the end of the fascia strap is traversed and in **37** the suture is shown being tied. In the meantime the other edge of the strap is supported by forceps in the position it will occupy.

38

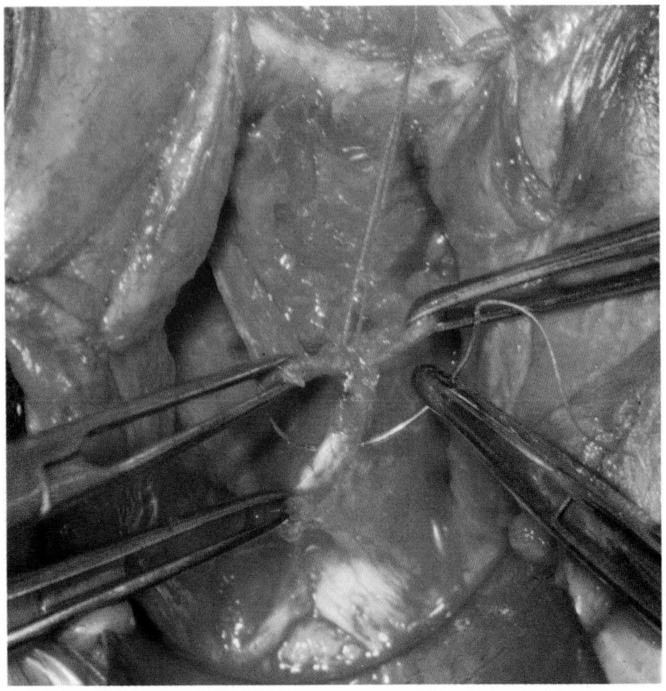

39

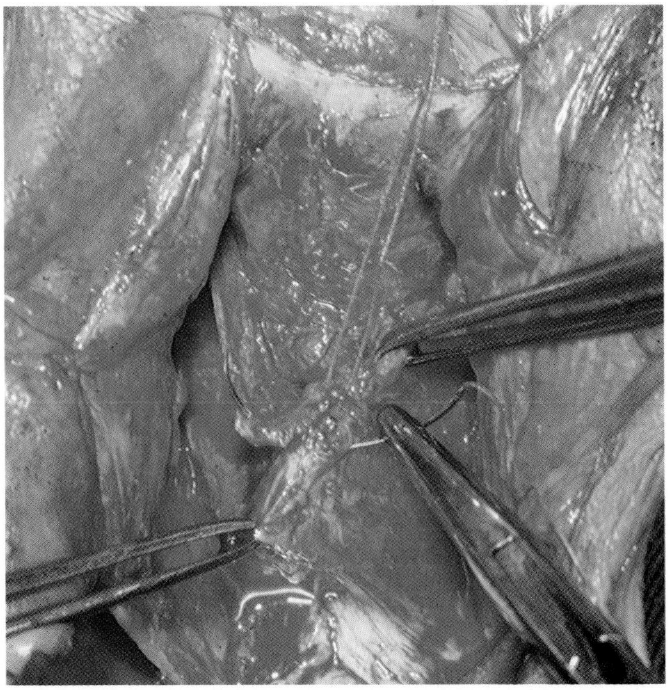

40

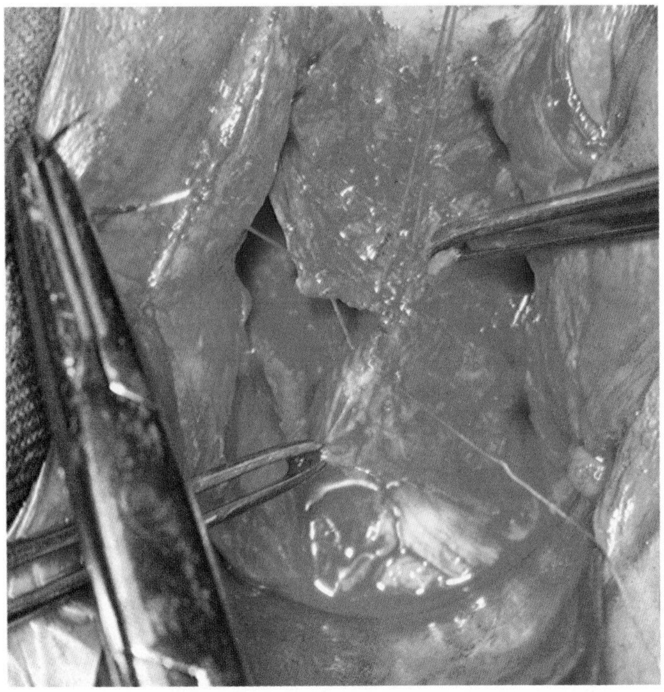

41

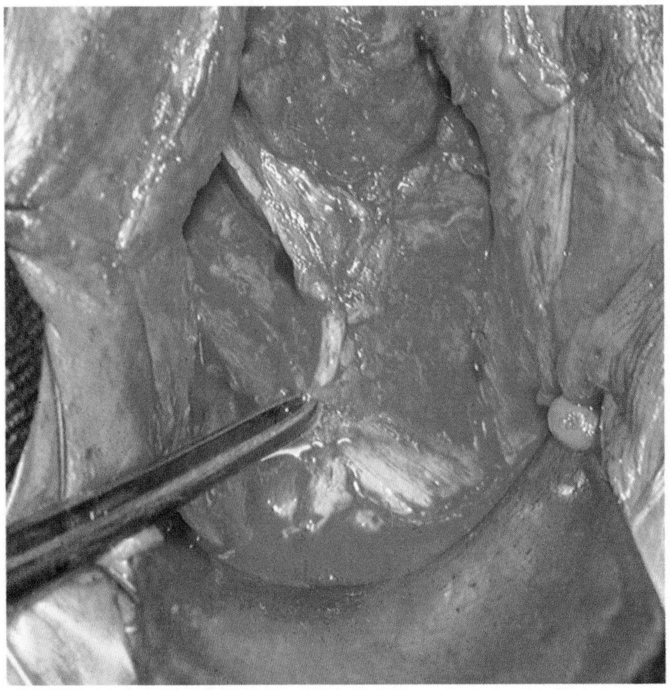

38–41 Attaching right fascial strap to bladder base

In **38–40** a second attaching stitch is inserted as in **34**, and it is so arranged as to keep the strap flat and as wide as possible. In **40** the strap is now secured in position so that it lies snugly on the bladder base without tension.

42

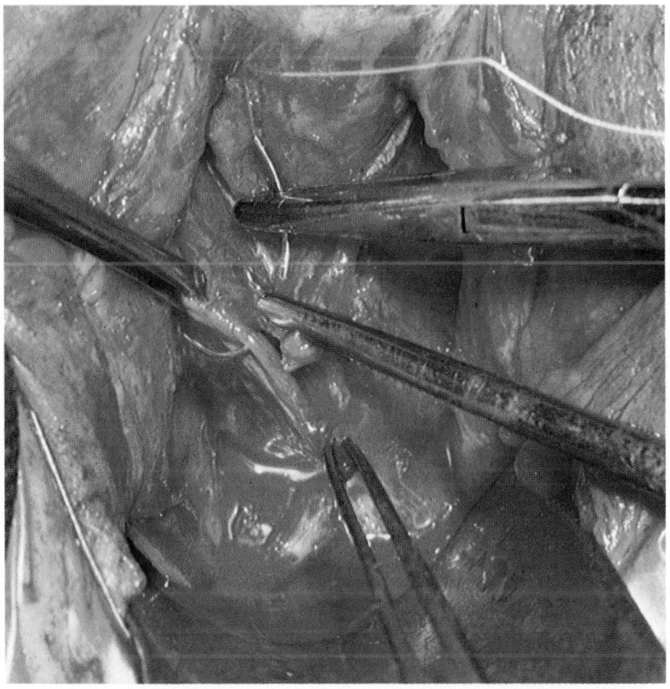

43

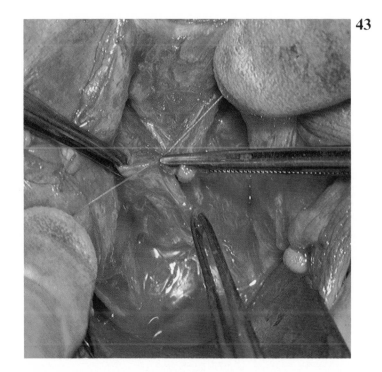

44

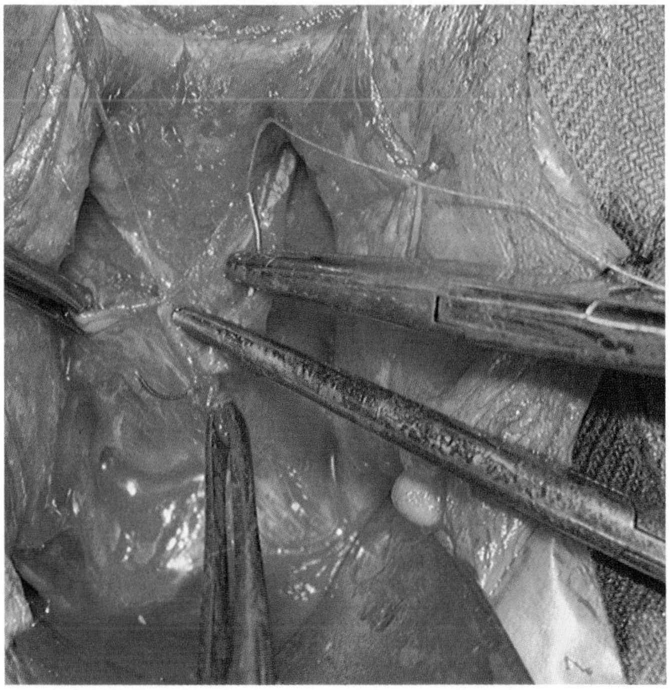

45

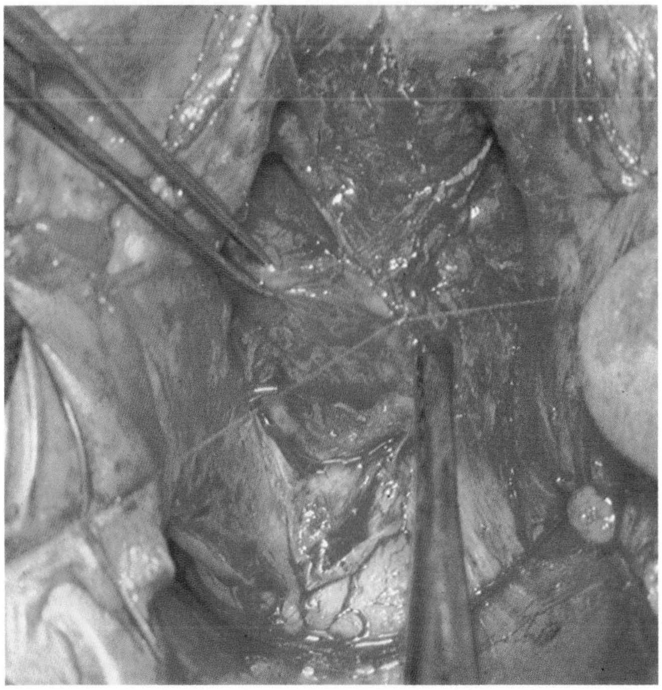

42–45 Attaching left fascial strap to bladder base

Exactly the same procedure is carried out as on the other side. In **42** and **43** the first stitch is placed and tied and the adjacent right strap can be seen clearly. In **44** and **45** the second suture is inserted in such a way as to utilise the maximum width of the strap.

46

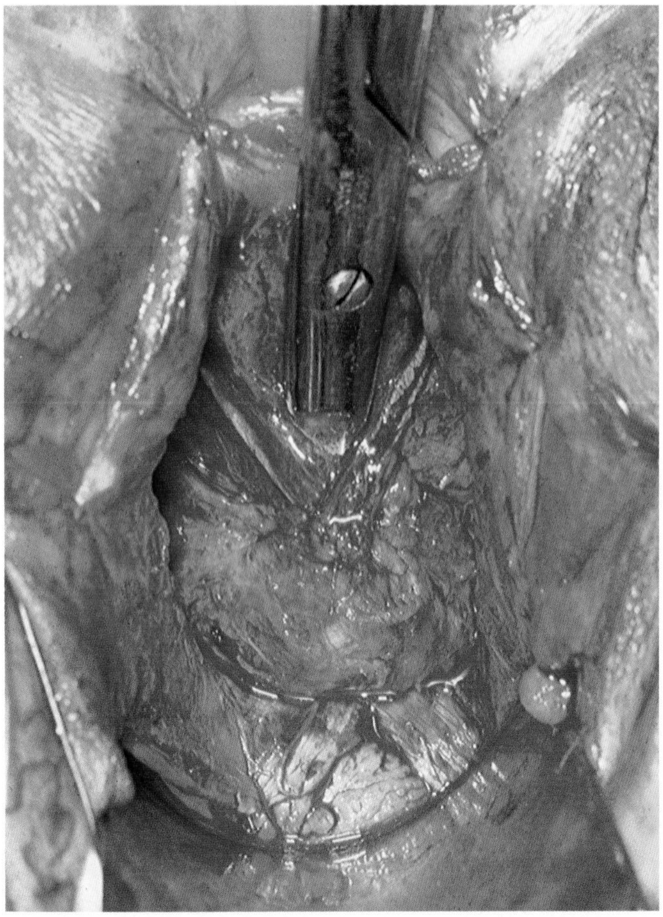

47

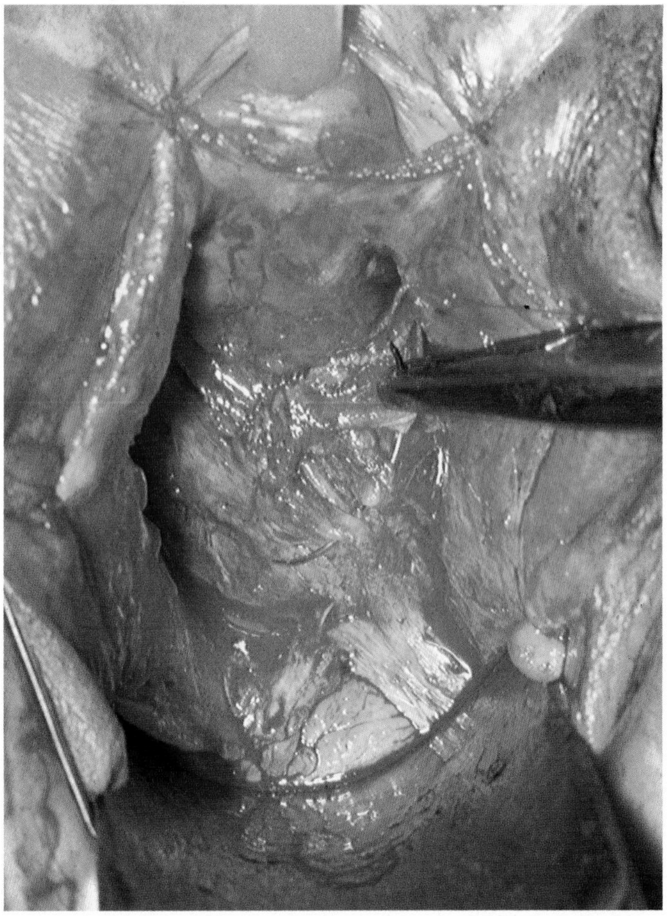

48

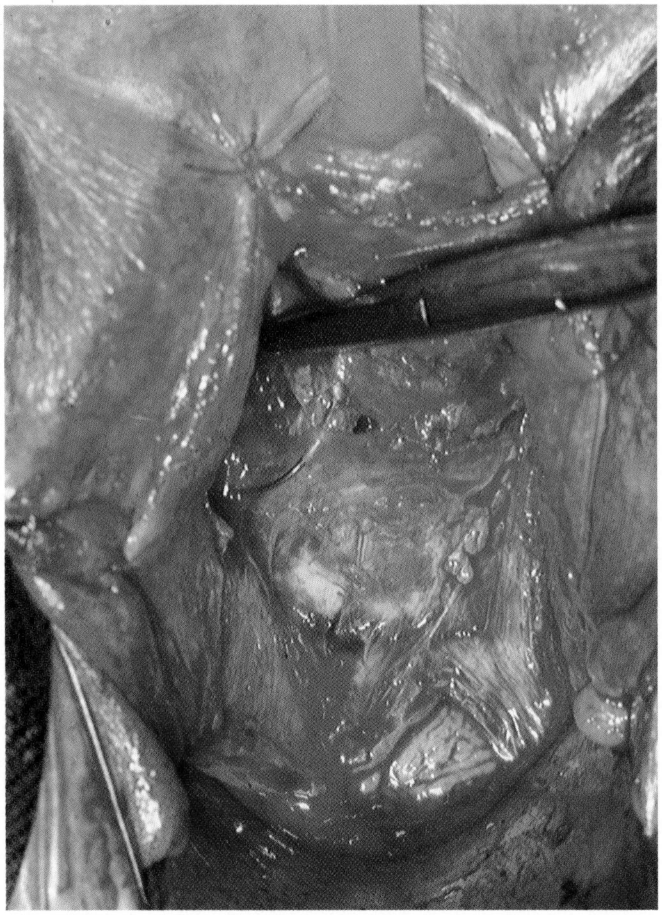

46–48 Fascial straps to bladder base

This illustrates the cruciate nature of the fascial support and elevation of the base of the bladder. There is no tension on the straps at this stage and they are attached only sufficiently firmly to keep in contact with the tissues throughout their length. The pubocervical fascia is at normal tension. The scissors are inserted underneath the crossing straps at the urethrovesical junction.

It is desirable to fan out the straps over the bladder base to form an investing layer of abdominal fascia which will replace the absent or deficient pubocervical layer. In **47** a stitch is being placed to approximate the limbs of the 2 straps over the left bladder base and in **48** the same is being done on the right side. The bladder is now seen to have an almost continuous hammock of fresh fascia to support it inferiorly.

49
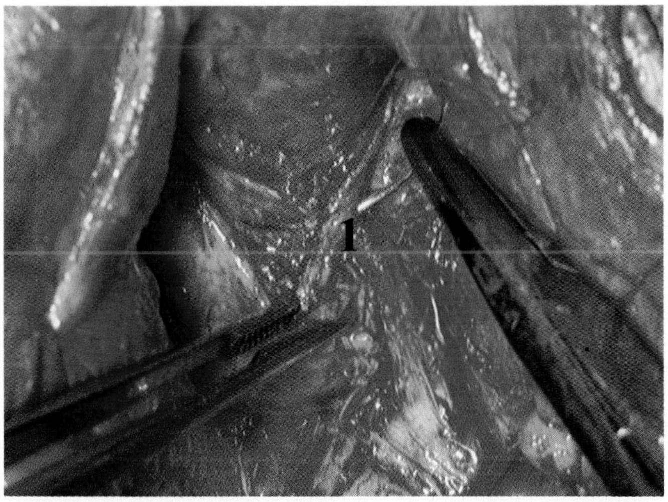

50
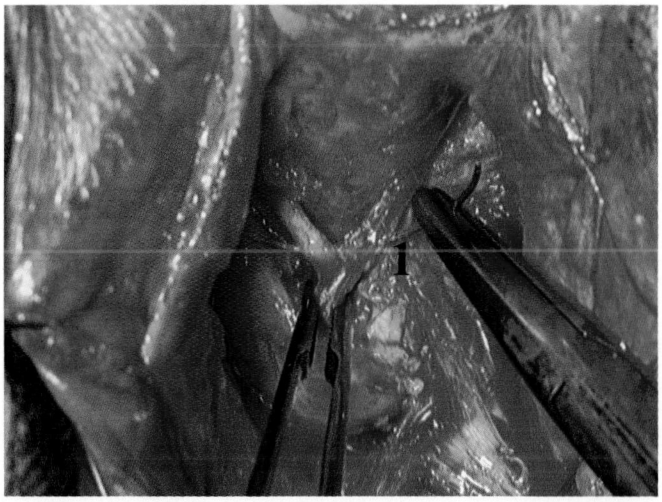

51
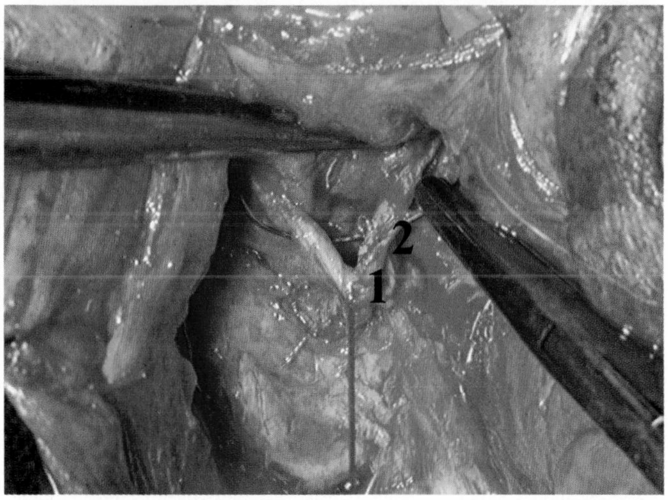

52
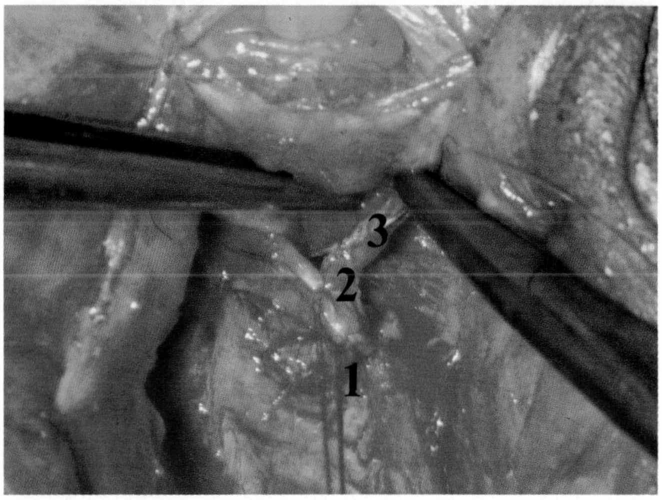

53
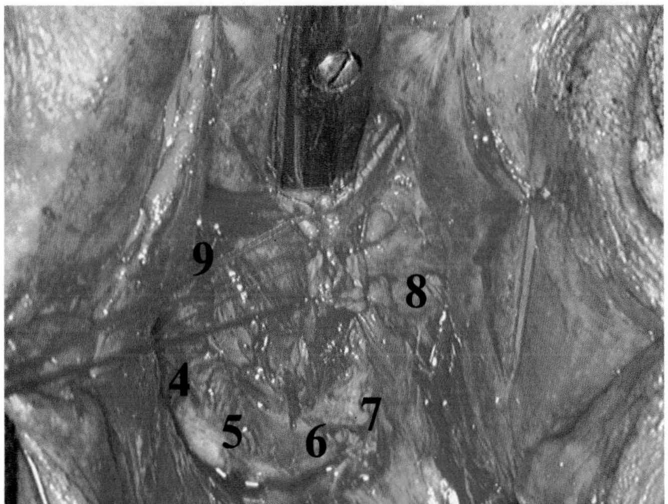

49–52 Supportive platform for urethra

In this important step the medial borders of the anterior limbs of the fascial X are stitched together by a series of interrupted sutures and PGA No. 00 is again used. The aim is to create a fascial platform which will support the urethra and restore it to its correct position without kinking or pinching it. The stitches are placed at not more than 0.5 cm distance from each other and care is taken to pick up both layers of each strap and keep the straps themselves flat on the urethra as the approximation proceeds. In **49** and **50** the first stitch is being inserted. In **51** a second and in **52** a third is being added. These stitches are numbered in sequence.

53 Completed urethral platform

Formation of the urethral platform is now complete, the straps having been stitched together at three points. Three stitches are generally about the right number. It is possible to carry the suture line further forward but that length of support is not required and it does seem that in such circumstances there is sometimes difficulty with retention of urine immediately post-operatively. The scissors have been inserted between the platform and the urethra which is displaced backwards. The urethra is seen to be supported over most of its length and is not kinked or pinched in any way. The attachment of the straps to the pubocervical fascia posteriorly is indicated by the numbers 4 to 9 corresponding to those on **33**.

54

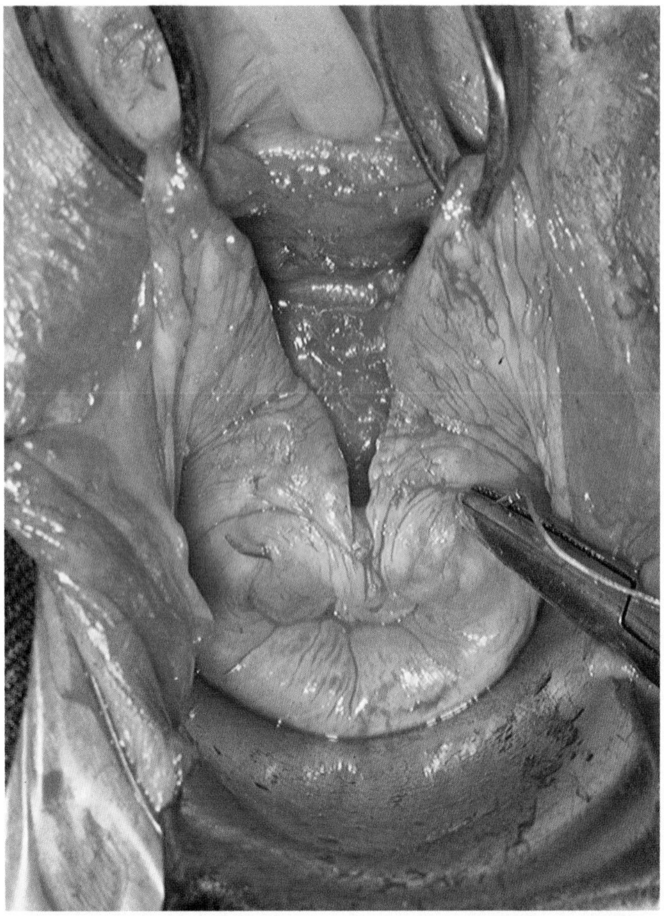

55

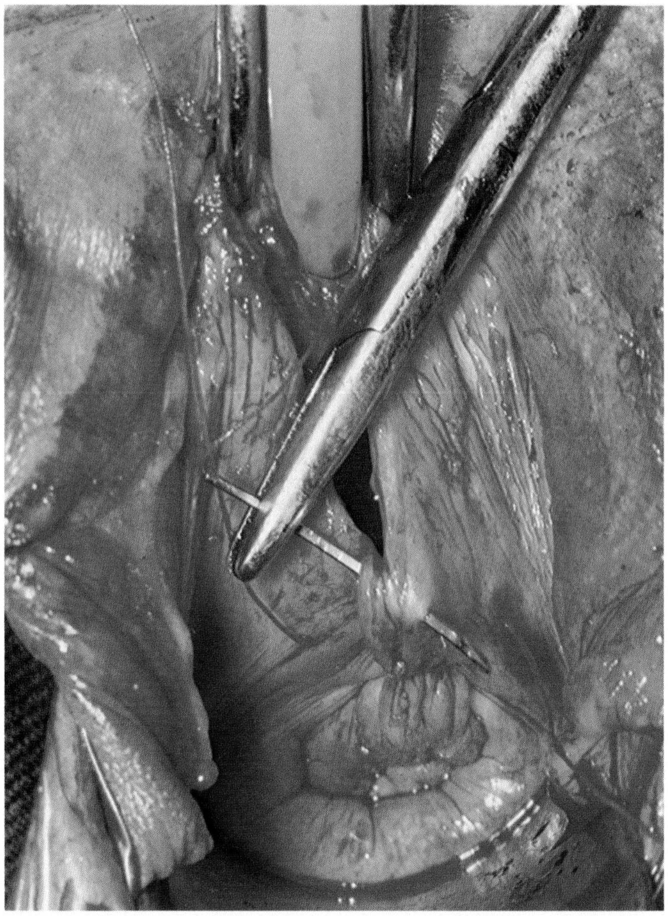

56

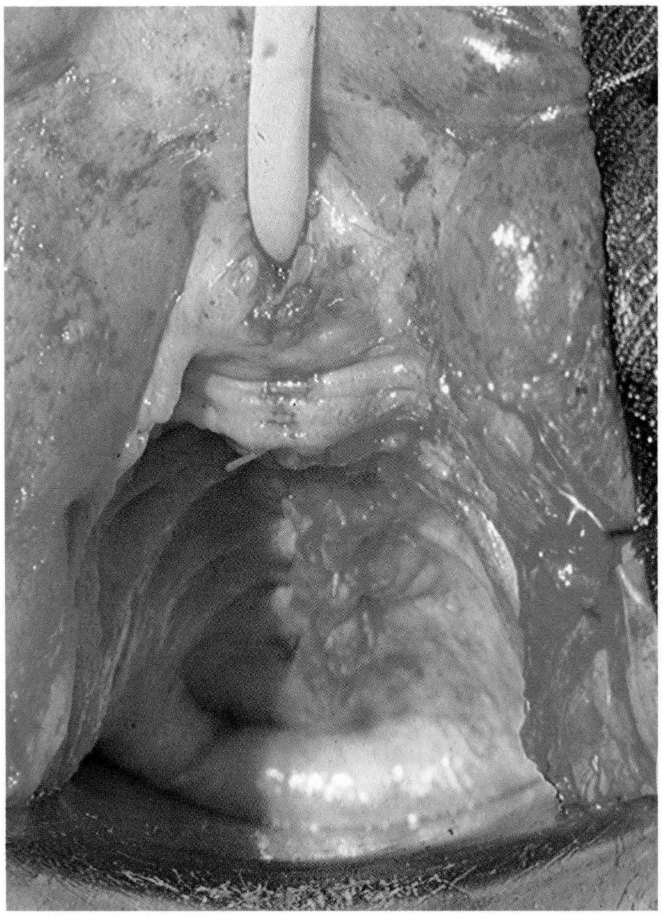

54–56 Closure of vaginal skin

The vaginal skin is closed by a series of vertical mattress sutures of PGA No. 0 carried on an atraumatic needle. In **54** and **55** the two phases of the first suture are shown, and in **56** the vaginal wall is completely sutured. The Foley catheter has been replaced by a No. 12 Sialastic catheter which is quite inert and is ideal for such cases. It is connected to closed drainage for six days. There is no narrowing of the vagina, the area is dry and no pack is used.

57

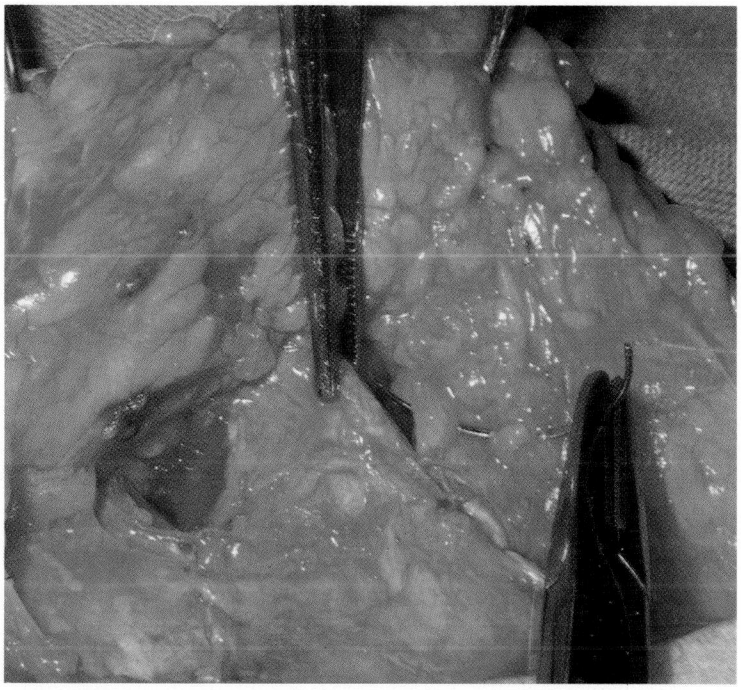

58

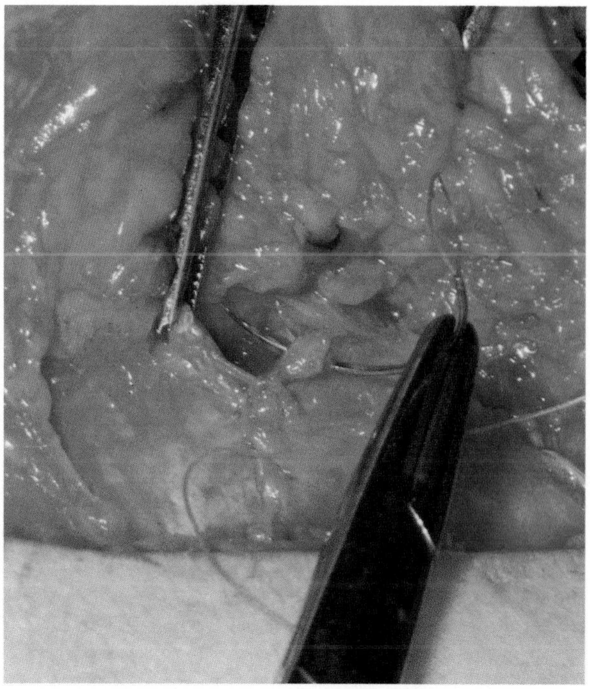

59

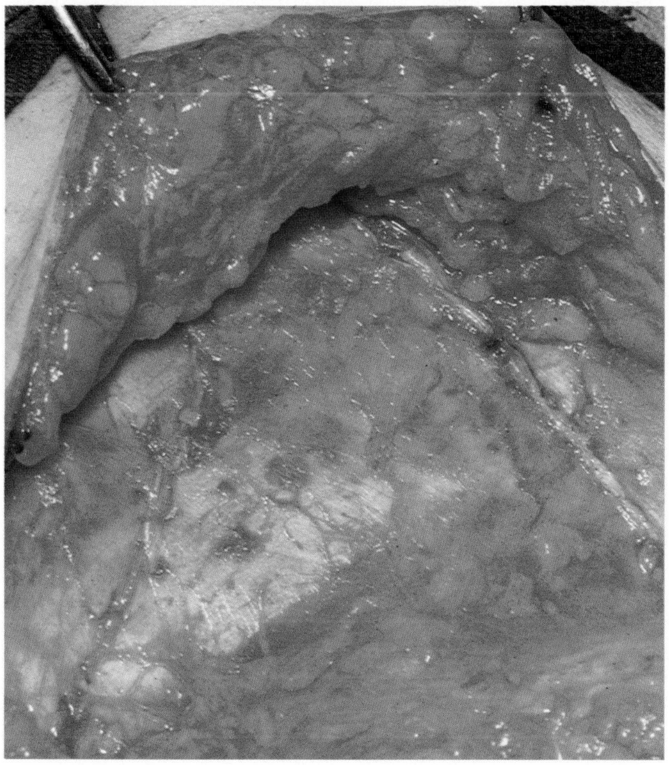

Stage 3: Closure of abdominal wound

57–59 Closure of abdominal wound

The triangular areas at the lower ends of the incisions in the rectus sheath are now closed. In **57** and **58** the right and left sides are being stitched in turn, and two stitches usually suffice. Very rarely there is some bleeding or oozing from the retropubic space but that is catered for by a Redivac drain which lies in the tunnels over the rectus sheath incisions. In **59** the triangles have been closed.

60

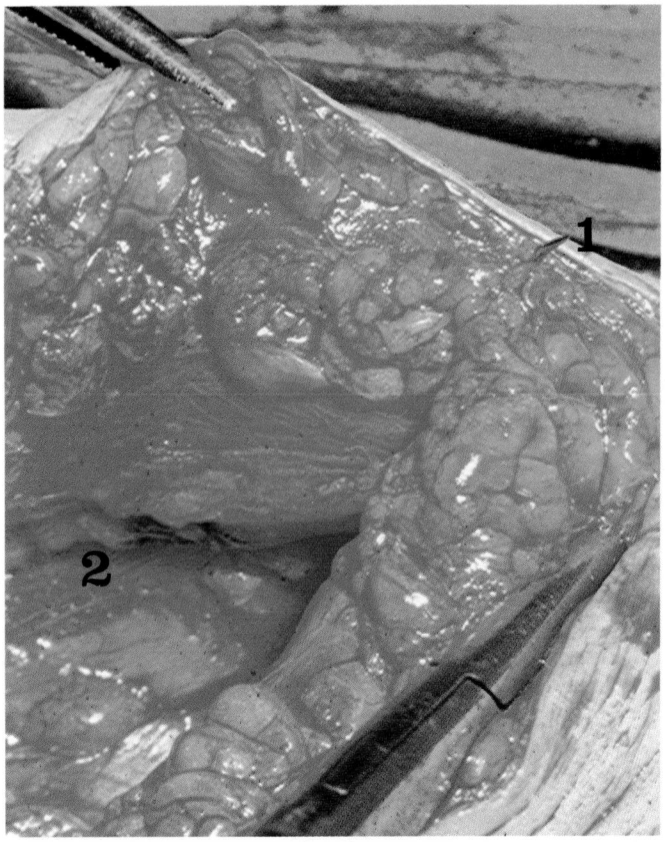

60 and 61 Closure and vacuum drainage of abdominal wound

The deep fascial layer is being sutured by continuous PGA No. 00 suture in **60** and the Redivac tube is just visible in the depth of the wound where it is placed before the suture is inserted. The skin incision is ready for closure in **61** with the Redivac drainage tube now in position. It is so placed that it lies in the tunnels over the rectus sheath and crosses just above the pubic crest so that it can drain any blood coming from the retropubic space. The numeral 1 indicates the tip of the needle; 2 shows the Redivac drain in the depth of the wound.

61

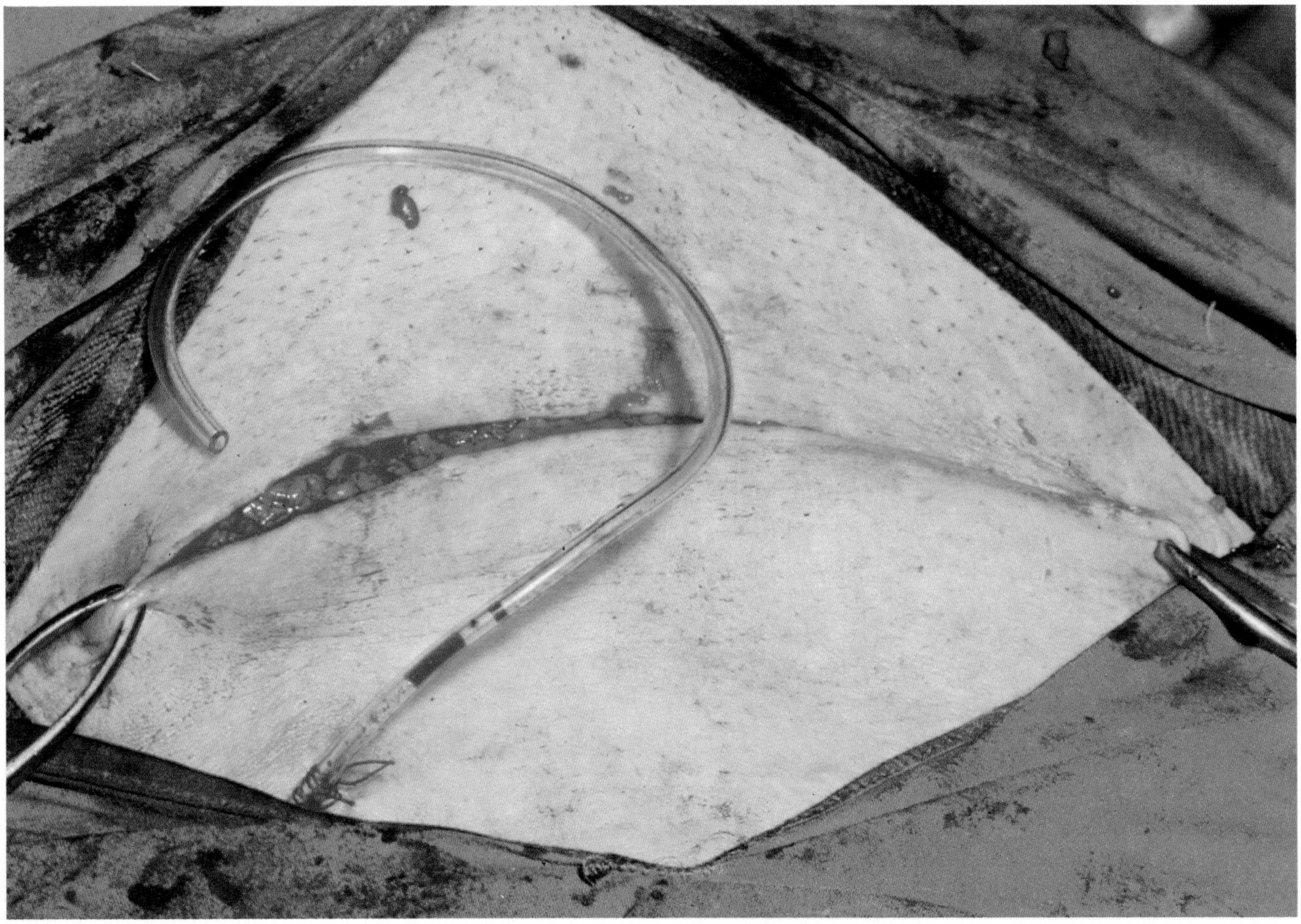

11: Vaginoplasty – Repair of a localised vaginal constriction

Even when done with the greatest possible care, vaginal operations sometimes result in narrowing of the canal. Provided the lumen is uniform and the patient is properly supervised post-operatively no great harm results; the vagina subsequently stretches to regain an adequate size. If the lumen is not uniform and if one area is appreciably narrower than elsewhere the vagina may well be restored to a satisfactory width in the lower part but it will remain narrow at the area of constriction.

Since the vault area of the vagina is roomy in any case the defect appears as an hour-glass deformity. Fibrous tissue is laid down under the constriction ring which makes it feel hard and ridge-like and it becomes tighter as the fibrous tissue becomes denser and contracts. Resulting dyspareunia or apareunia can cause much unhappiness. Some patients quickly return to the surgeon for relief but occasionally one discovers the deformity on routine examination. It is sad that some women stoically accept such unfortunate results as something which they have to bear.

It is important to know how to correct this kind of deformity because it is not all that uncommon. The treatment is not difficult and is based on two fundamental and important principles of plastic surgery. The first necessitates a simple shift or slide of vaginal skin which will eliminate the narrowing at the expense of slight shortening laterally; while the second involves the excision of the fibrous scar tissue. If the latter is not adhered to it will invalidate whatever else is done.

Diagrammatic illustration of the steps in the operation

The steps of the operation are shown in the diagrams overleaf, which are taken from an 'external' viewpoint. It will be understood that the operation is being done internally *per vaginam* and the purpose is to show how the layers are fashioned, approximated and how subsequent fibrosis at the site of the suture line is avoided.

1

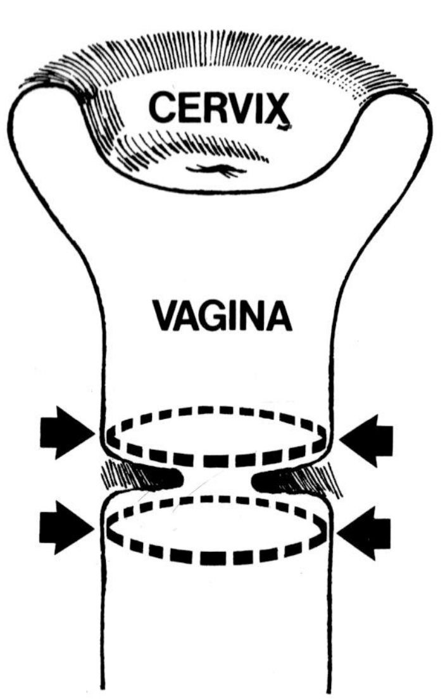

2

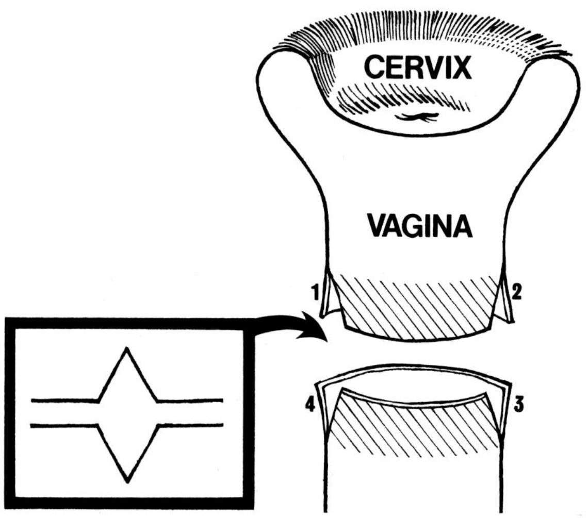

1–4 Diagrammatic representation of localised vaginal construction and its treatment

In **1** the narrowed lumen is shown and the ring of fibrosis is represented by dark shading. The interrupted lines circumscribing the vagina indicate where the incisions are made above and below the stricture which is then excised as a ring of skin with attached dense fibrous tissue. The area to be removed lies between the two sets of arrows.

In **2** the vagina is now in two separate parts or segments, the intervening part having been removed. The striped area indicates the amount of skin to be undermined or freed as a flap from both upper and lower segments. Before doing so and as a necessary part of the operation 4 vertical incisions (as numbered) 1.5 cm long through skin only are made at the most lateral points on the free edges of upper and lower vaginal segments (see insert).

3

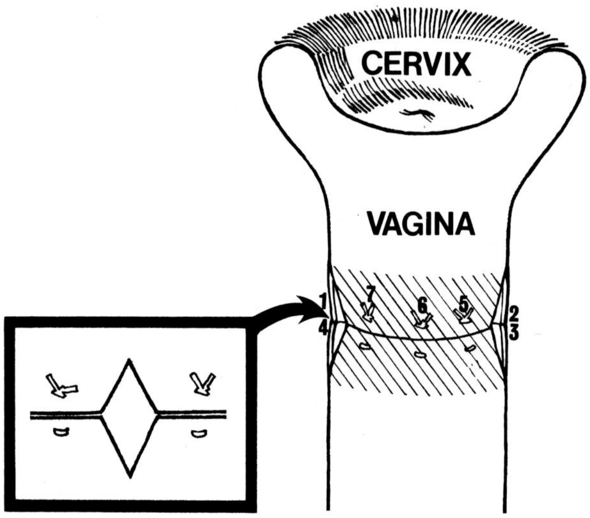

4

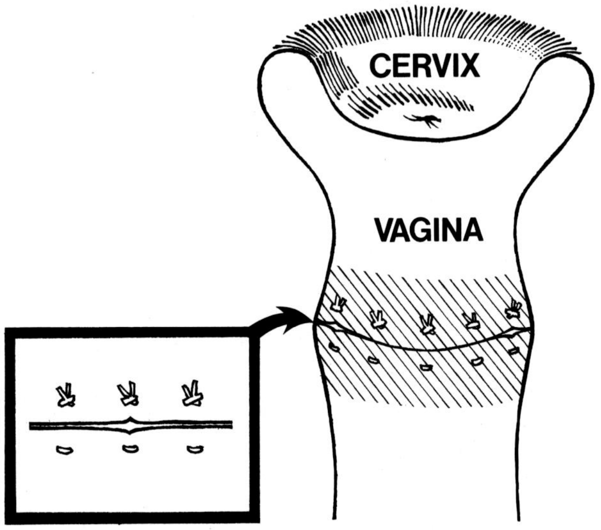

In **3** the vaginal canal has been reformed by stitching together the two segments across the anterior and posterior vaginal walls. Only the lateral aspect is left uncovered by skin where the vertical cuts are partially open and present as triangular areas with their bases in apposition on the suture line to form a rhomboid shaped raw area (see insert).

In **4** the final step in the reconstruction is to flatten out the opposing triangles by suturing the apex of the one to the apex of the other and then adding a stitch on each side of that to ensure a continuous neat circular suture line round the vagina (see insert).

5

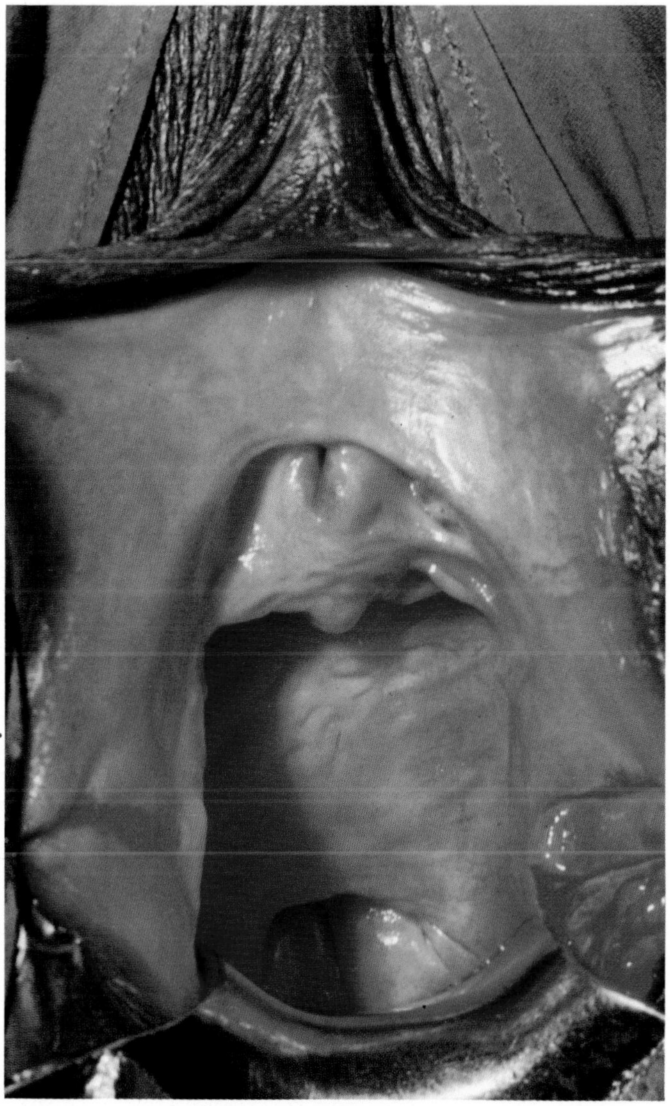

6

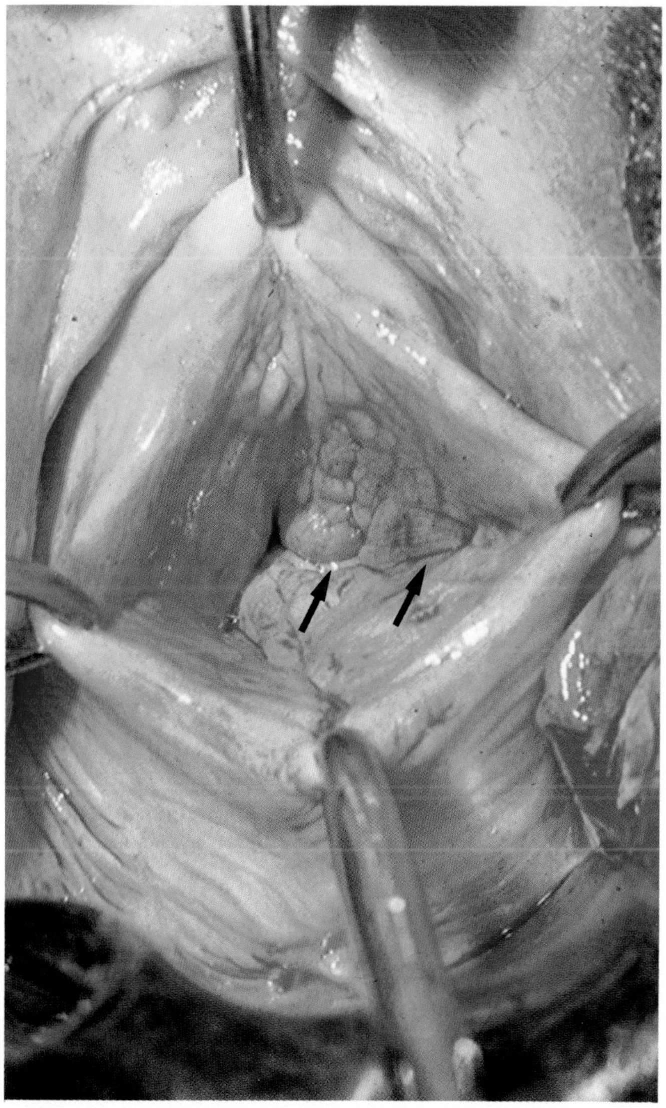

5 and 6 General view pre-operatively

The localised constriction deformity is seen at the junction of the upper and middle thirds of the vagina in **5**. The actual width of the constriction band is only about 0.5 cm but the edge is firm due to underlying fibrous tissue which has contracted to increasingly narrow the lumen. In **6** the edges of the constriction band have been picked up by a series of Littlewood's forceps which demonstrate the contraction and show the normal capacity of the vaginal canal above. This patient had multiple uterine fibroids and has just had a total hysterectomy. The transverse closure of the vault is seen in **6**. A left lateral episiotomy is seen in both illustrations and was made to give better access. The vault incision is arrowed.

7

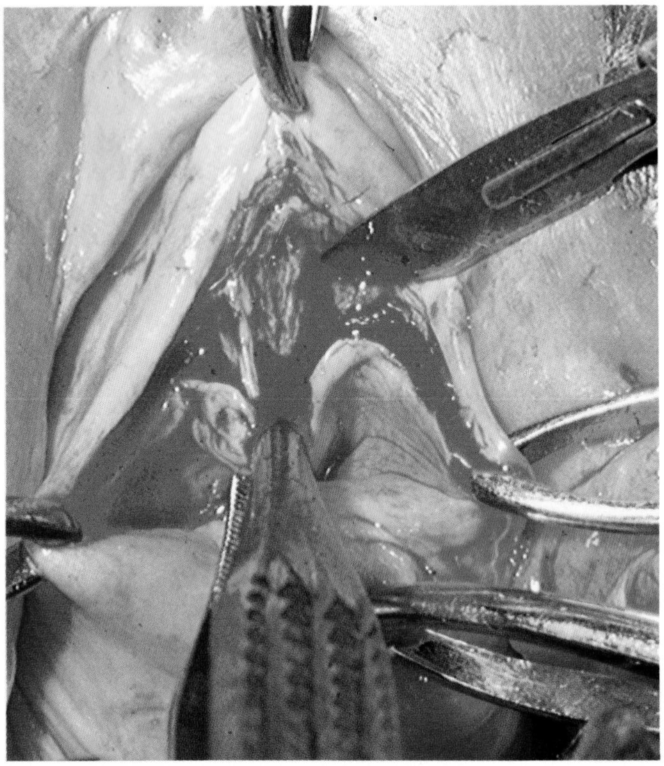

9

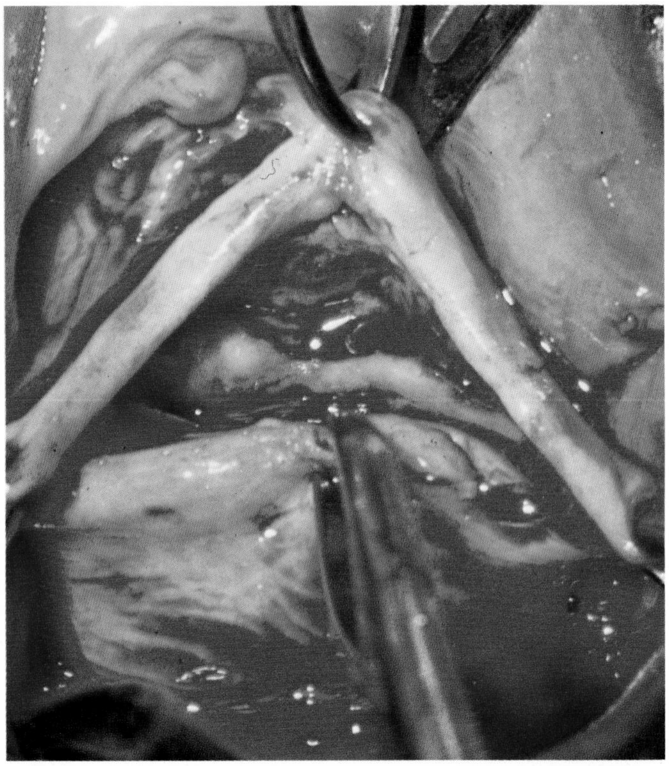

8

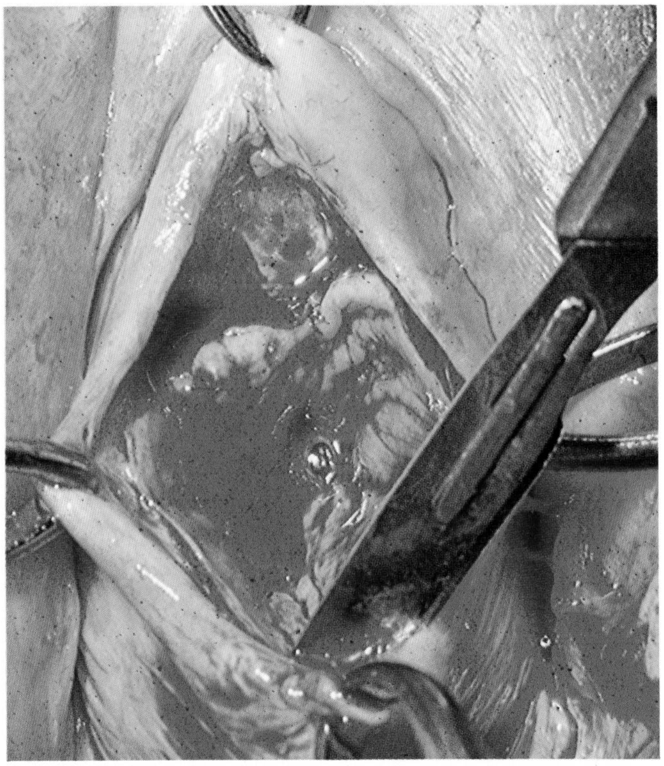

10

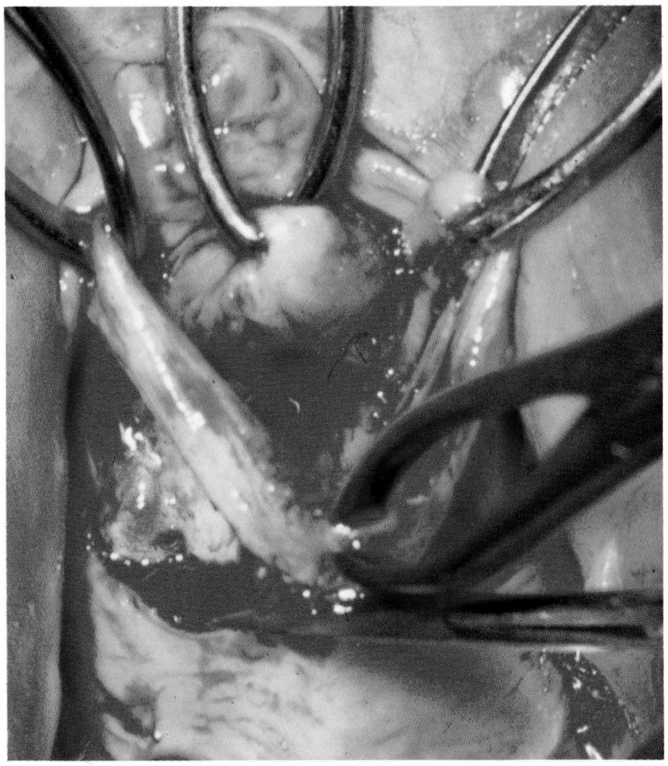

7 and 8 Circumcision of the vagina above the constriction

With the contracted ring held taut by the Littlewood's forceps a circular skin incision is made around the vagina just above it. In **7** an anterior semi-circle is made and in **8** a matching posterior one.

9 and 10 Circumcision of vagina below the constriction

The same steps are carried out in the same way below the firm constricted edge. The width of the skin hoop is about 1 cm and adequately covers the tight constriction felt underneath. The incision in all cases is taken through the skin quite boldly so that a clean-cut edge is available. The subcutaneous tissues are entered but are comparatively loose and bladder and rectum fall away from the knife so that there is no danger to them.

11

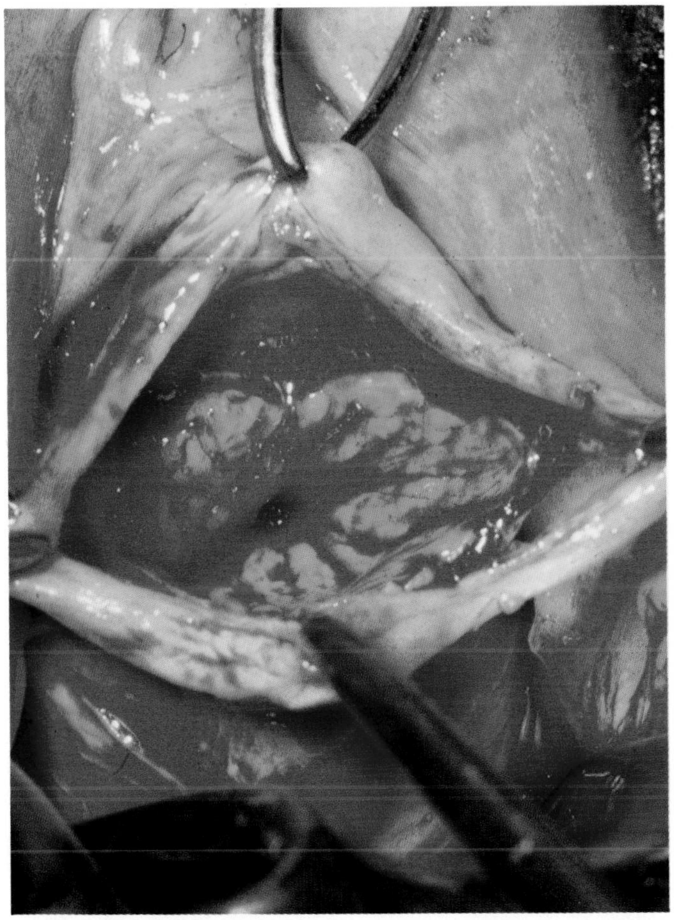

12

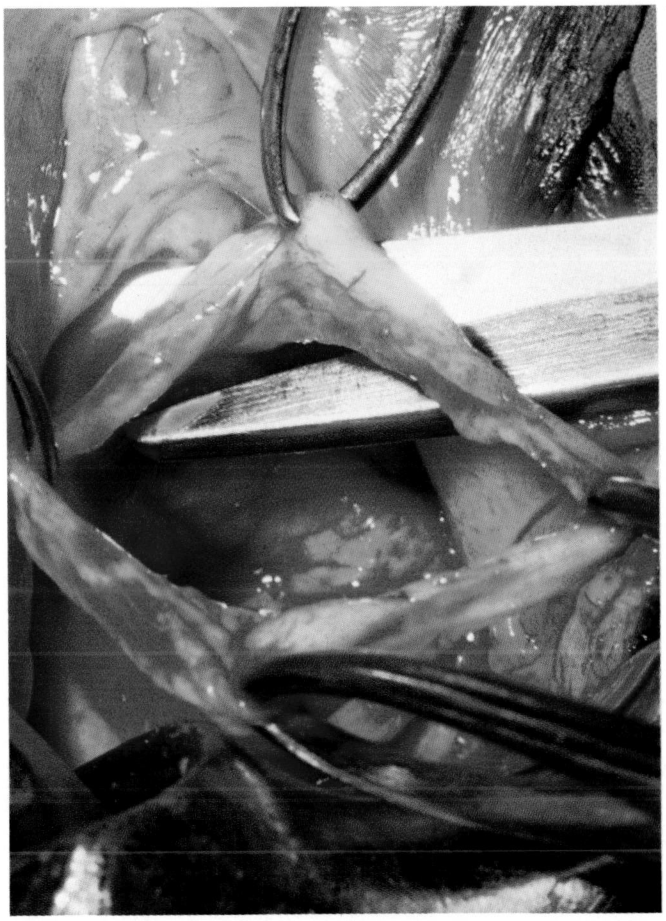

13

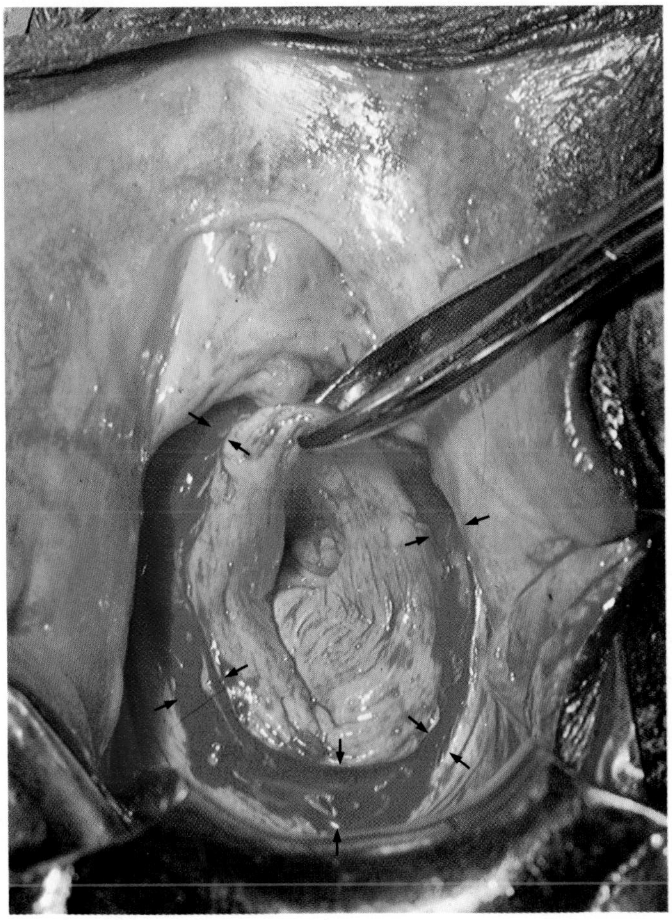

11 and 12 Displaying and excising contracted ring

In **11** the fibrous tissue which is causing the narrowing and its attached loop of skin is picked up on the forceps and demonstrated by pulling it away from the vaginal wall. In **12** the scissors are used to remove the raised hoop of tissue cutting sufficiently deeply to include the ring of fibrous tissue but not so deeply as to endanger the underlying structures.

13 Constriction ring removed from vaginal wall

The constricted tissue consisting of a fibrous circular band with overlying skin has been removed completely and a raw hoop or area of vaginal wall results. The fibrous tissue has been excised so that the previously narrowed area is now quite soft and pliable. If the skin edges were sutured together around the vagina at this stage the result would seem satisfactory but there would be a danger of further fibrosis developing under the suture line and it is therefore necessary to further widen the narrowed area. The small arrows indicate the raw area from which the constriction has been excised.

14

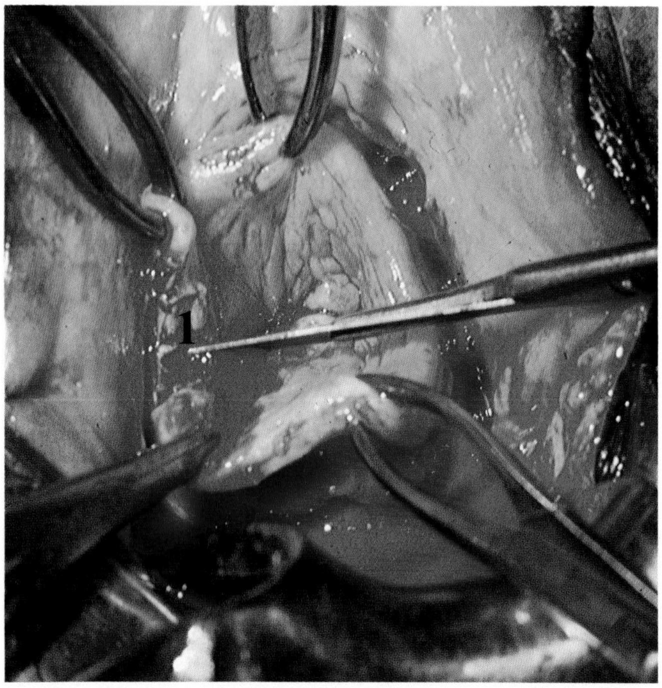

15

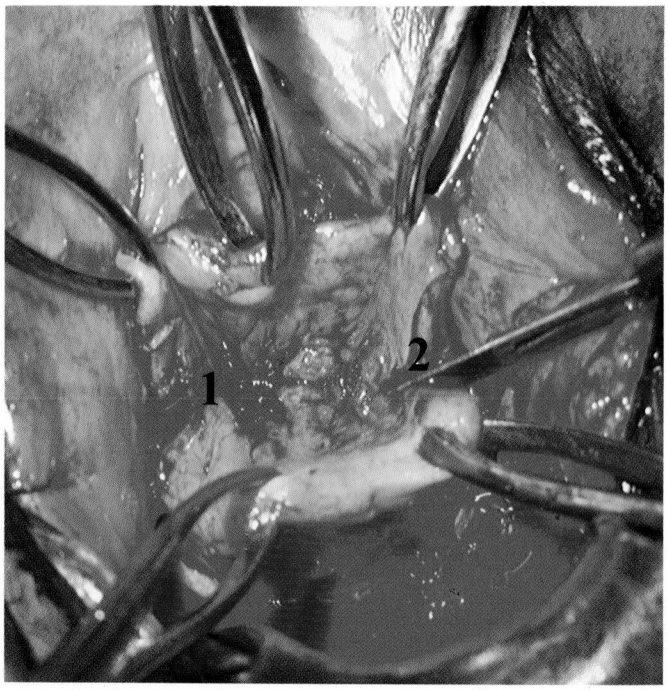

16

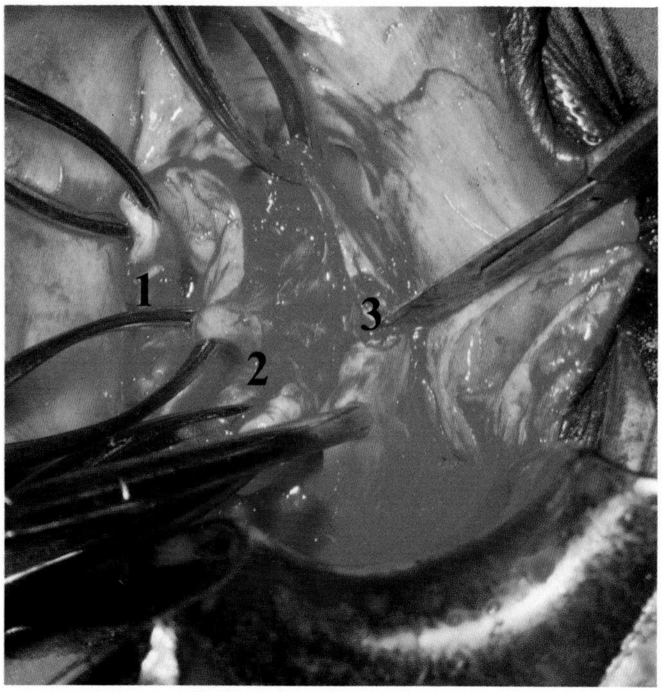

17

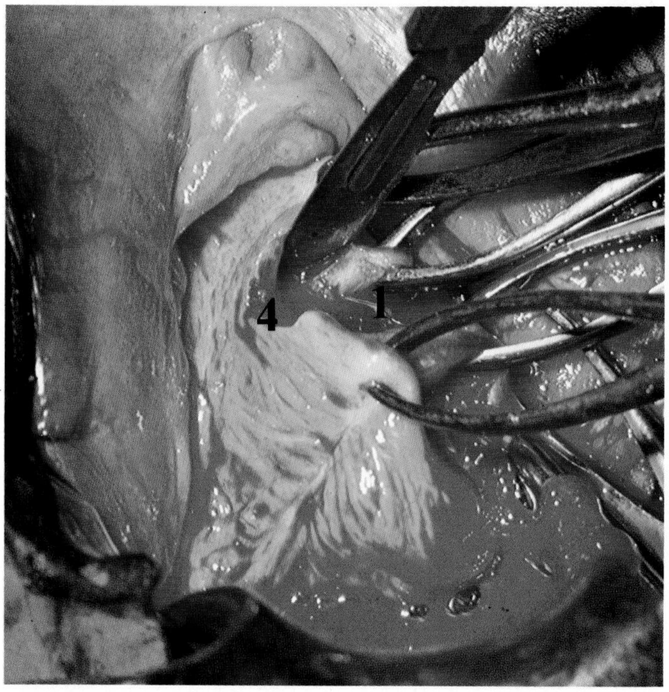

14–17 Outlining upper and lower skin flaps

To gain increased width it is necessary to form two upper and two lower skin flaps which, by being undercut, become mobile at their free edges. This is achieved by splitting both upper and lower skin edges vertically at their most lateral points as shown in the photographs.

In **14** the right upper edge is incised to a depth of 1.5 cm, in **15** the left upper edge is incised, in **16** the left lower and in **17** the right lower. In all cases the length of the incision is 1.5 cm. There are now four flaps, two upper and two lower, ready to be undercut. The numbers on the photographs correspond to those on **2** and **3**.

18

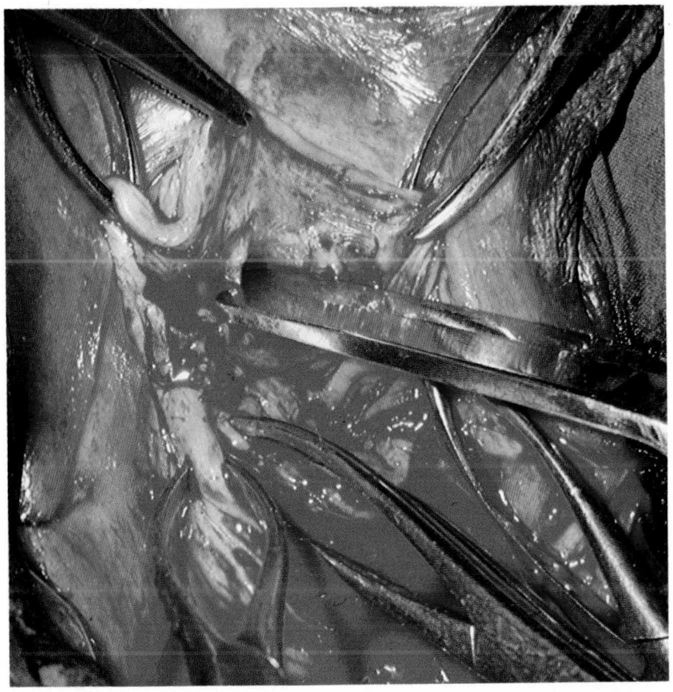

19

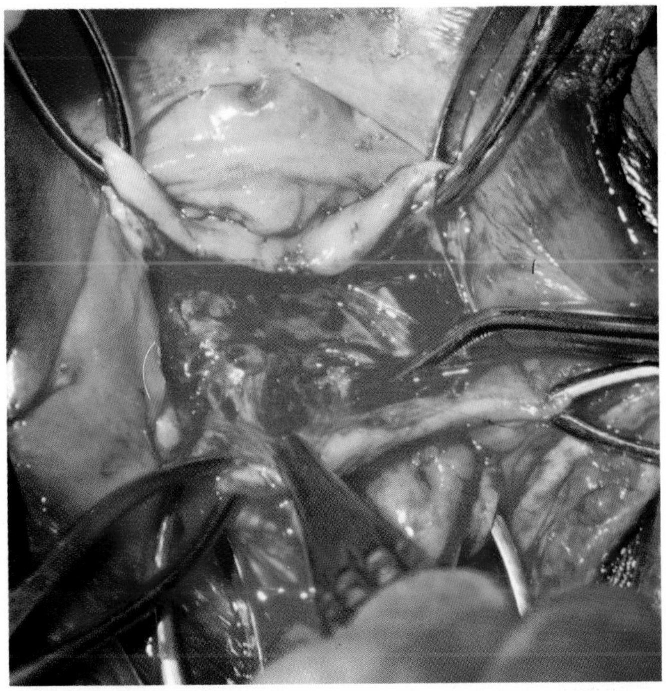

20

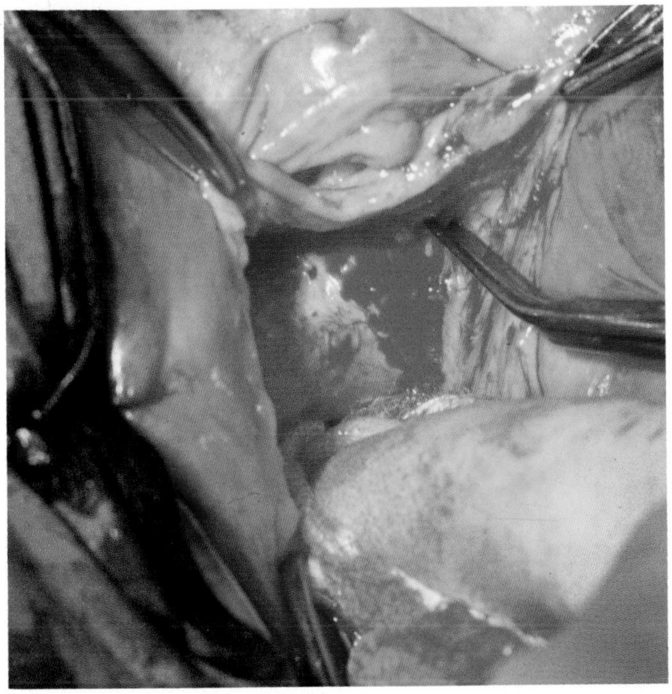

21

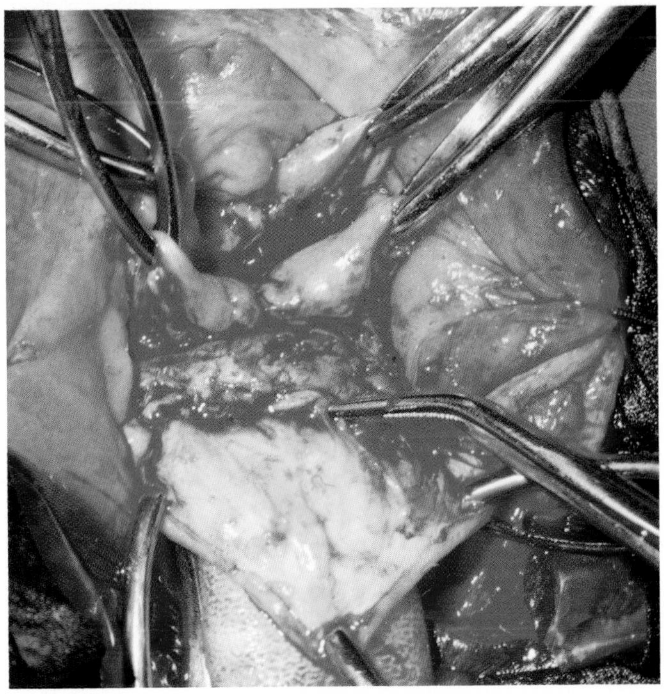

18–21 Undercutting upper and lower skin flaps

Steadying the flaps with Littlewood's forceps and Bonney's dissecting forceps the scissors are used to undercut the various flaps. Near the edge it is necessary to cut through the adherent tissues but a plane of cleavage is soon found and the skin is easily stripped off. In **18** the lower anterior flap is being freed and in **19** the upper is being dealt with similarly. In this photograph the flap is being undercut at the 5 o'clock position using the fine cleft-palate scissors. In **20** the upper posterior flap is being raised and in **21** the lower posterior flap is being well stripped back. The thick loose posterior wall skin is very elastic and ideal for covering a defect. This is used to advantage in the operation. The areas undercut correspond to those in **2**.

22

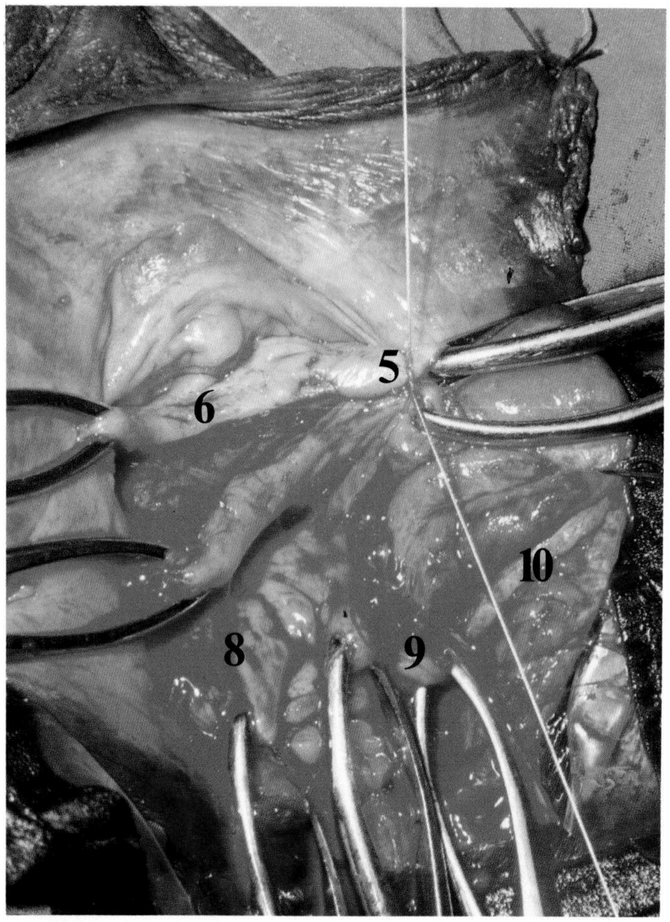

23

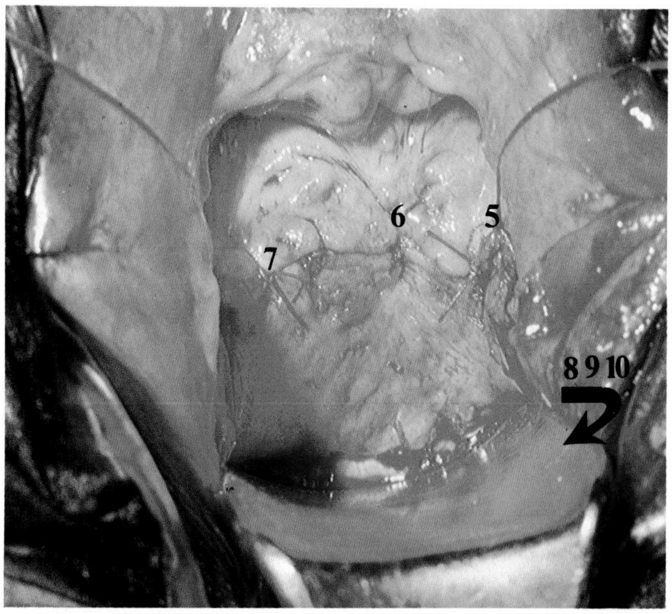

22 and 23 Approximation of upper and lower skin flaps (i)
The upper anterior and posterior skin flaps are now stitched to the respective lower ones and this recovers the vagina with skin except at the lateral angles as will be seen later. In **22** the lateral ends of the two anterior flaps are held by Littlewood's forceps and the closure of the gap is being commenced on the patient's left side where the first suture is being placed. In **23** the closed anterior wall is shown. The lateral stitches have been left long as holders and four stitches have been placed between them. The stitches numbered 5, 6 and 7 correspond to the same numbers in **3**. In **22** the Auvard speculum has been removed to show the posterior wall incision awaiting suture. The approximate position of these sutures is shown by the numbers 8, 9 and 10 in **22**.

24

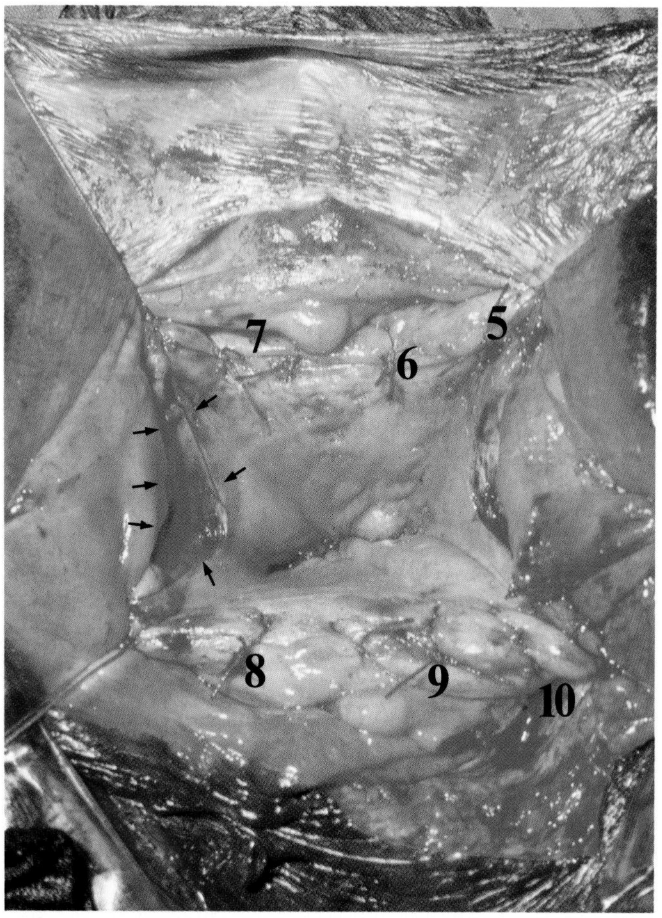

24 Approximation of upper and lower skin flaps (ii)
In this illustration the posterior wall has been closed in the same way as the anterior one and the Auvard speculum has been removed to show how the whole vagina is opened out and the narrowing dispelled. As already mentioned the lateral angles are still open and appear as a raw area. The previous rhomboid shape is now more crescentic because of the pull outwards of the uncut sutures (see diagram). The vault of the vagina is now accessible and clearly seen with the recently closed transverse suture line of the recently performed abdominal hysterectomy. The numbered sutures are all seen in place. The posterior stitches cannot be shown on **3**, because the anterior wall has already been closed.

25

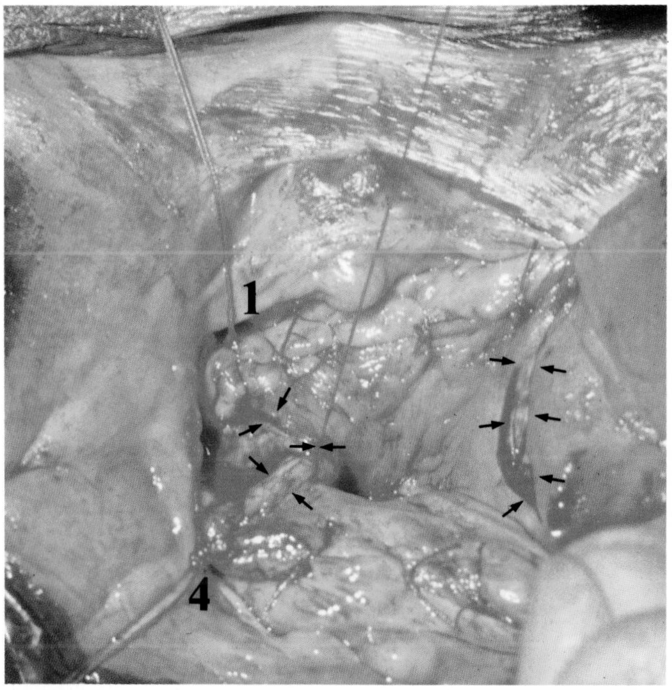

27

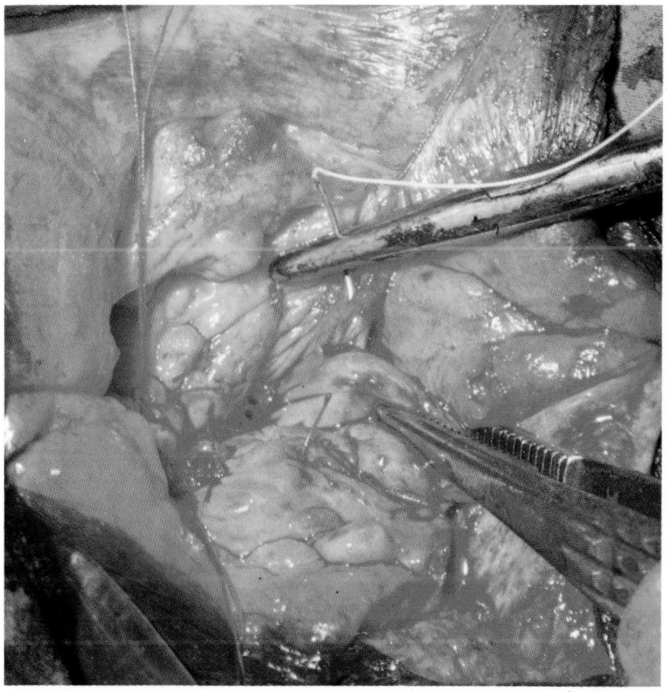

26

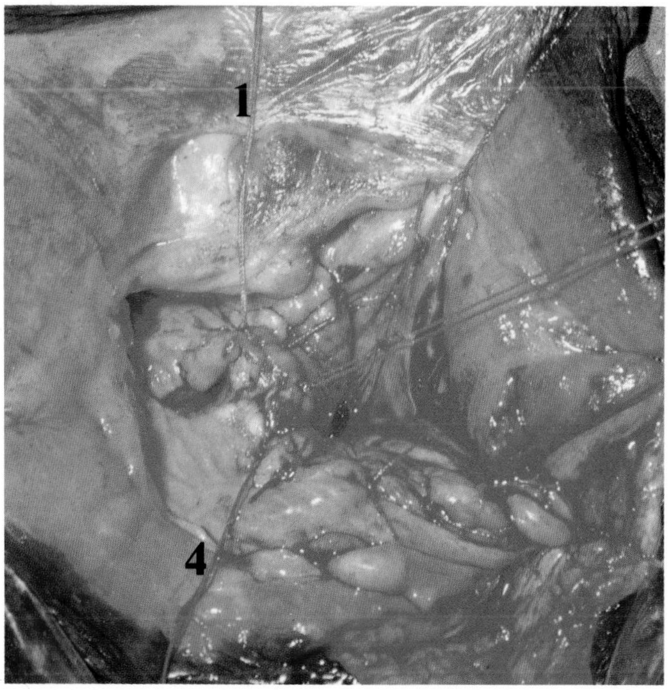

28

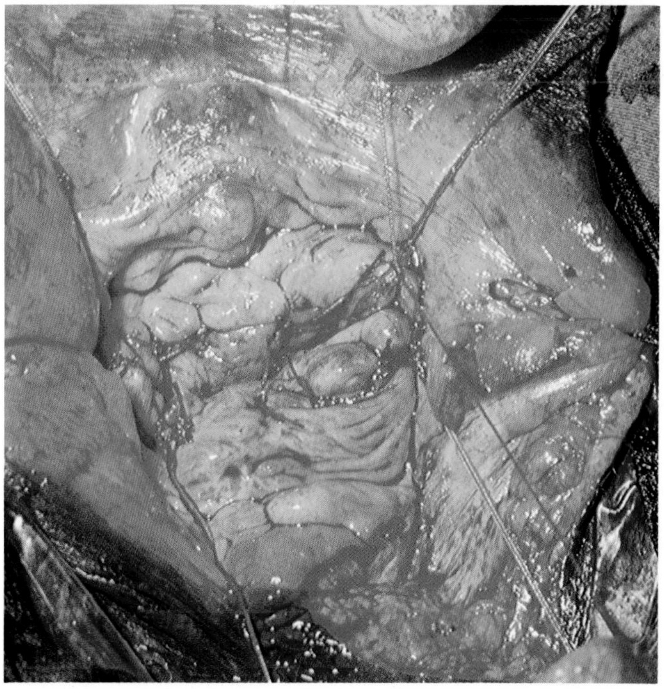

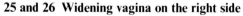

25 and 26 Widening vagina on the right side

The rhomboid or crescentic-shaped area between the two holding sutures (1 and 4) results from the vertical incisions of the two skin flaps laterally and the gap is now closed by horizontal sutures which increase the width at the expense of some length laterally. This results in slight puckering of the vaginal wall but this is quite temporary. In **25** a central stitch has just been placed to flatten the rhomboid or crescent to a more or less straight horizontal line but which actually appears to curve inwards in the illustration. In **26** the final stitch is ready to be cut. In both illustrations it will be seen that the raw crescentic area on the patient's left side is still open. The small arrows on **24** and **25** show where the stitches must be placed to flatten the rhomboid area on the right side.

27 and 28 Widening vagina on left side

The same procedure is carried out on the left side. In **27** the mid-points of each skin edge of the rhomboid or crescent are being approximated and in **28** the final suture is being tied.

29

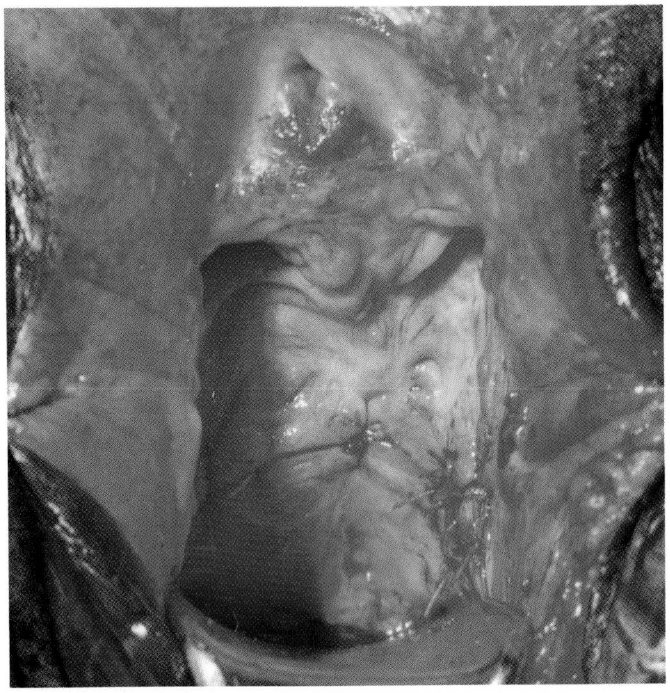

30

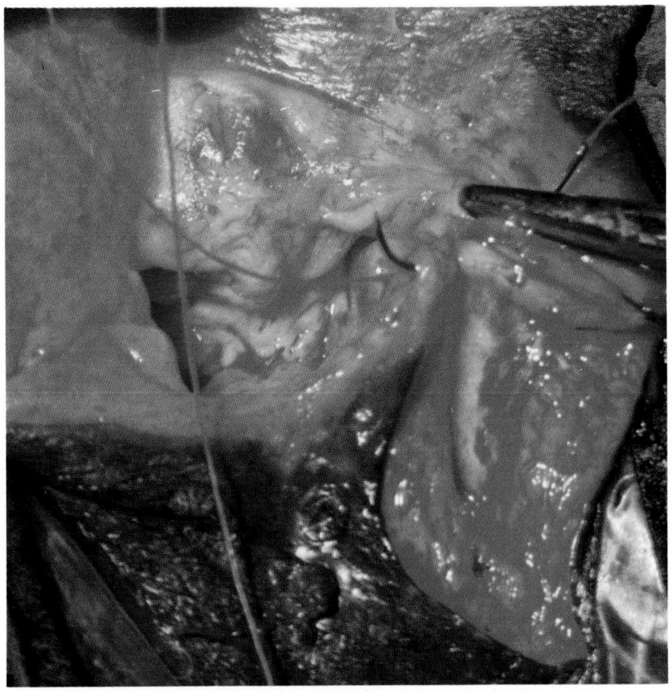

31

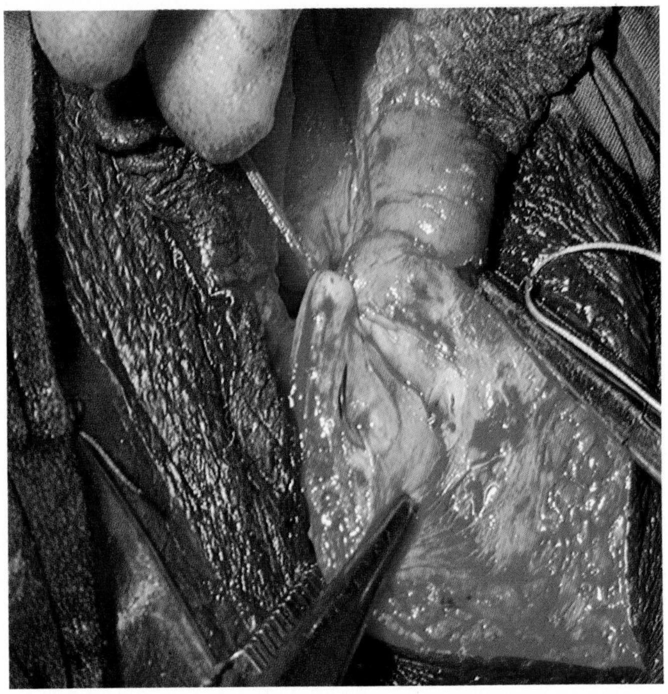

32

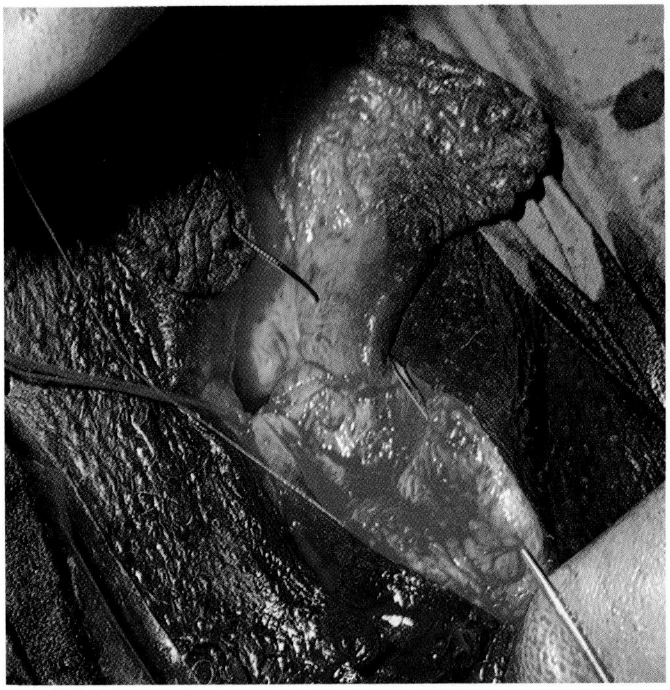

29–32 General appearance of upper vagina post-operatively and closure of episiotomy

The stay sutures have been cut and the posterior vaginal wall retracted to show the anterior suture line and the vault generally. The line of the lateral horizontal suturing is seen on the left but only the cut ends of stitches are visible on the right. There is now plenty of room at the vault and the flaps are healthy and without tension. The episiotomy is still open and is closed in three stages:

In **30** the posterior vaginal skin layer is about to be closed with a continuous suture. In **31** the first stitch in the levator muscle is being placed. In **32** a subcutaneous suture is closing the skin.

12: Repair of vesico-vaginal fistula

Vesico-vaginal fistulae fall into one of three groups according to their aetiology. They may result from three types of trauma, i.e. surgical, radiotherapy or obstetrical. Patients in the first group generally present with a bladder base defect of about 2 cm, but it may be considerably larger. There is always the possibility that a ureter may be involved in such cases and before attempting closure of the fistula this must be excluded. The post-radiation fistulae are notoriously difficult because of their large size and because the tissues have an impaired blood supply. Fistulae resulting from combined obstetrical obstruction and neglect are not seen in Britain, but are common in certain countries of the developing world. They are often large and tend to involve the urethra but the patients are young with healthy tissues which have a good blood supply.

The following photographs illustrate the three main types.

1

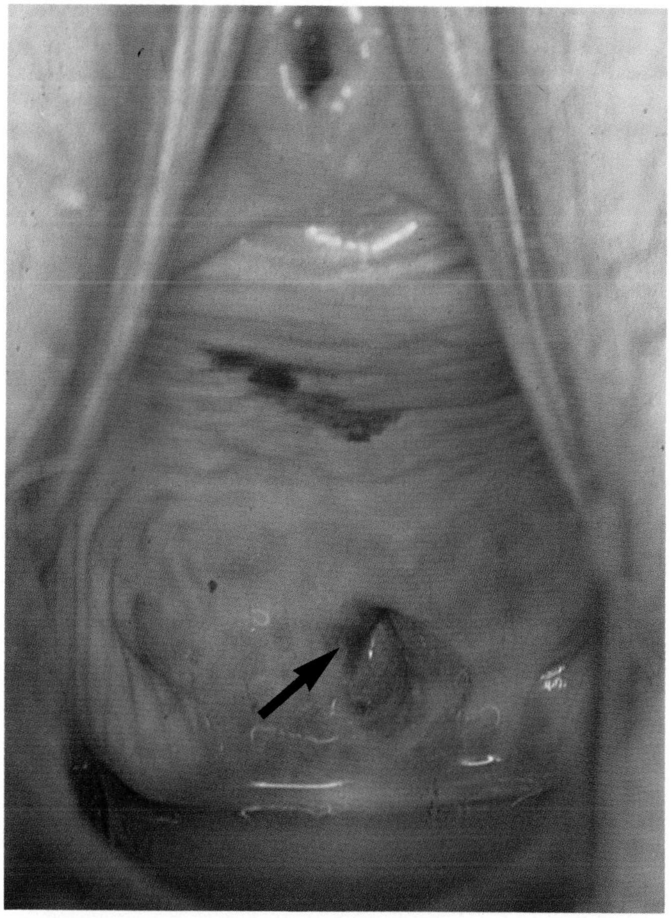

2

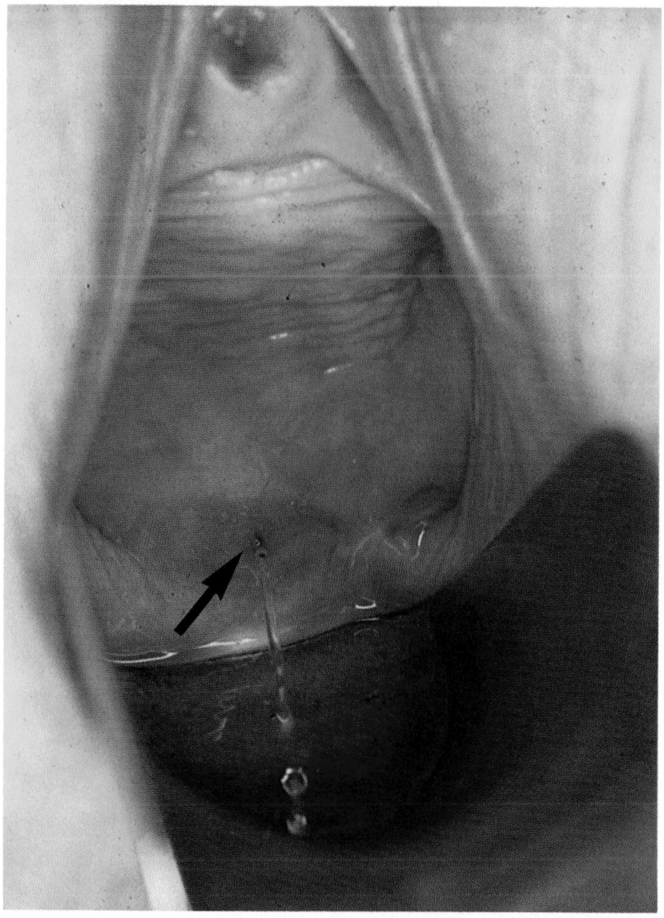

1 Fistula resulting from surgical trauma (i)

This figure shows a bladder fistula which followed a Wertheim hysterectomy for cervical carcinoma. The more usual injury resulting from that operation is a ureteric fistula due to necrosis following impaired blood supply to the ureter. One presumes that the bladder wall was actually damaged or opened during the operation in this case. The fistula is not unduly large and provided the ureters are intact should not present undue technical difficulty in closure. On the other hand the patient had pre-operative radiotherapy and that must devitalise the tissues to some extent.

2 Fistula resulting from surgical trauma (ii)

This figure shows a post-hysterectomy fistula of the bladder base and is of no great size. A stream of urine is seen escaping through the narrow opening when the bladder is compressed. It is likely that the bladder base was opened when it was reflected off the cervix at operation. If the ureters are not involved such defects can be closed by a standard double layer closure technique which will be described below. As mentioned in the introduction above it is essential to establish certain facts such as the size and position of the fistula as well as its relation to the ureters and their function, before attempting closure.

3

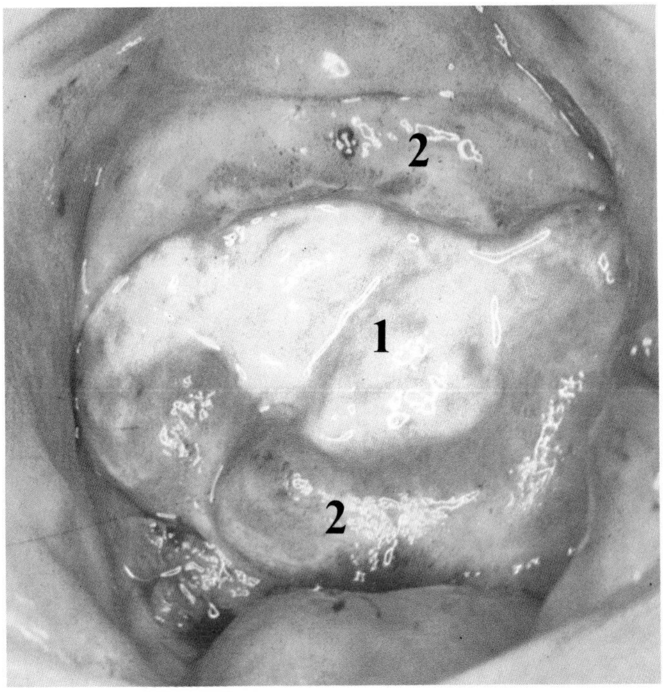

3 Fistula resulting from radiotherapy burn (i)

This photograph shows the effects of a severe radiotherapy burn. Sloughing of the bladder base (1) is occurring over a large area and a huge fistula is inevitable within a few days of the photograph being taken. The skin surrounding the slough (2) is severely affected by radiation and cannot be expected to heal well. It will be a considerable time before any form of closure can be contemplated.

4

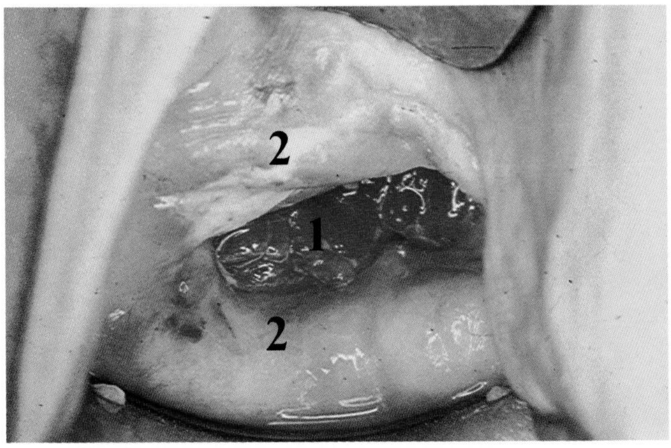

4 Fistula resulting from radiotherapy burn (ii)

The same patient when seen several weeks later has an extensive post-radiation fistula which is quite clean and the bladder mucosa seen in the centre of the picture (1) looks reasonably healthy. The surrounding skin, however, is atrophic and telangiectatic (2) and there is obviously tissue distortion. On palpation there is dense fibrosis around the fistula and the whole bladder base is fixed and inelastic. Closure will obviously be difficult and while it may be possible to saucerize and make a single layer closure with silver wire, colpocleisis is much more likely to be required.

5

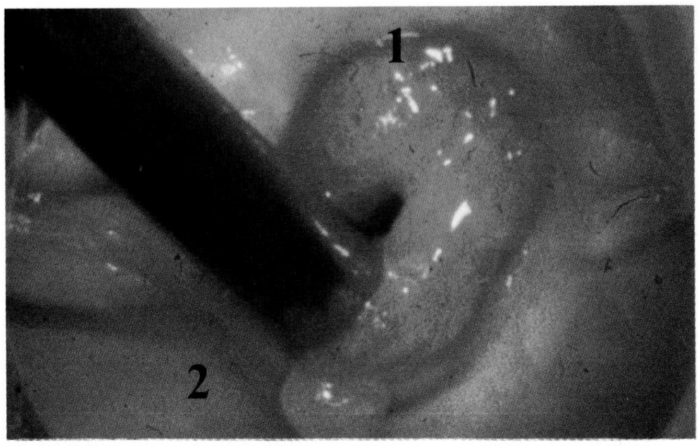

5 Fistula resulting from obstructed labour (i)

This figure shows a large oblique fistula extending from the urethrovesical junction (1) to the anterior aspect of the vaginal vault (2) and the bladder mucosa is everted through the opening. This opening is being demonstrated by a dilator and the defect is seen to be large.

Because of its aetiology there is little likelihood of ureters being involved but the possibility of one or both obtruding on the area of closure has to be taken into account in planning the operation. The main problem, however, is the size of the defect. If the layers of the repaired structures are satisfactorily approximated the tissues will heal in such patients: the important point is to effect closure with minimal scarring or distortion in view of possible future childbearing.

6

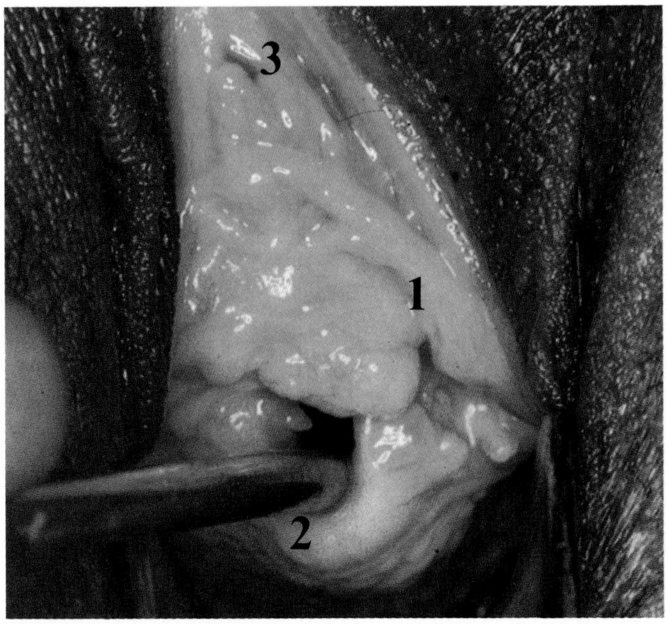

6 Fistula resulting from obstructed labour (ii)

This figure shows a fistula in a 13-year-old Indian girl and illustrates the type of lesion which is all too common in developing countries. It resembles **5** in that it extends from urethrovesical junction (1) to the vault of the vagina (2) and is wide. The urethral orifice is marked (3). As one would have expected the ureters were not involved and the tissues had a good blood supply. It was possible to close the fistula successfully by a double-layer technique as described below.

The techniques of closing vesico-vaginal fistulae

Closure of fistulae may be effected abdominally or vaginally, or by a joint approach from above and below. The urologist generally prefers the first and the gynaecologist the second but in complicated cases the interests of the patient are probably best served by a joint approach. Provided the ureters are not involved the operation should perhaps be done vaginally, the provisos being determined by cystoscopy and pyelography, and the case always assessed on an individual basis.

7

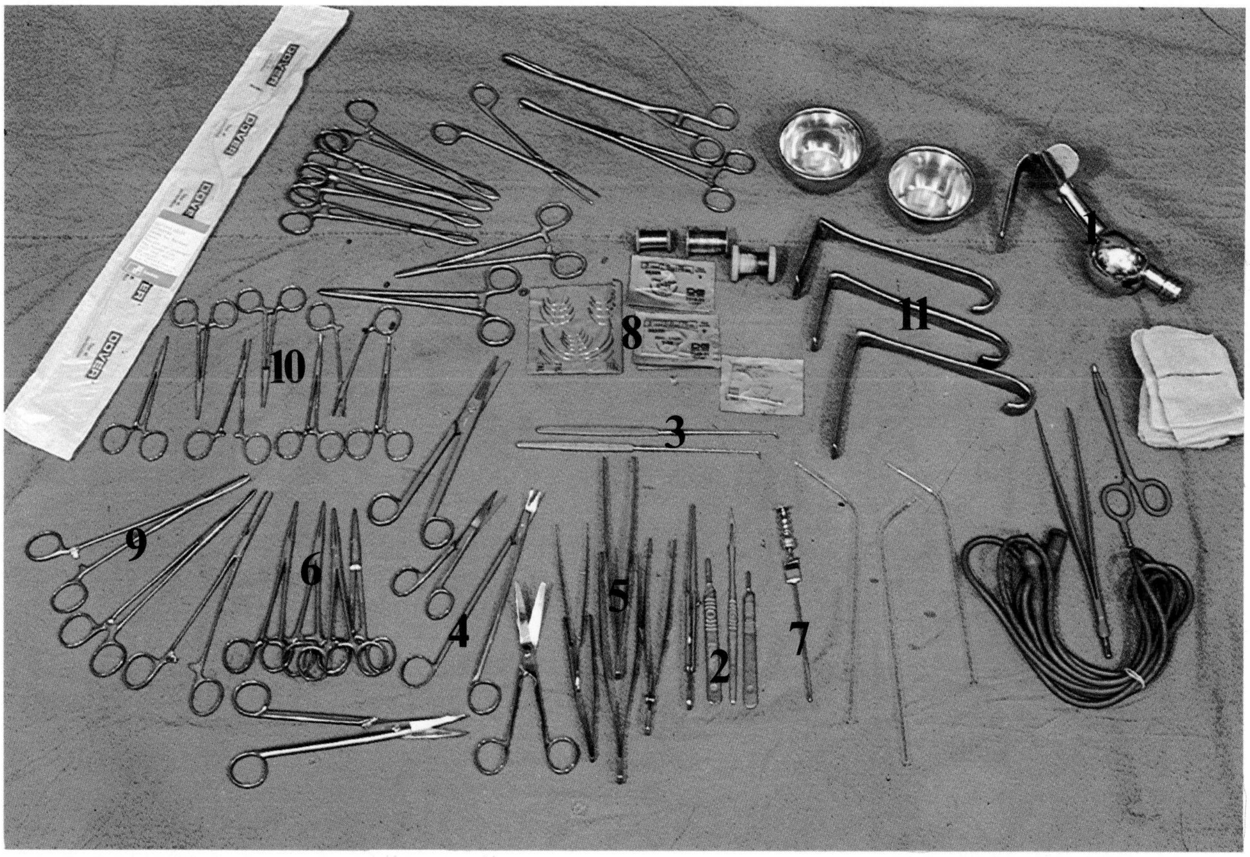

7 Special instruments required

It is both frustrating and dangerous to attempt this kind of surgery without appropriate instruments. In addition to the usual vaginal instrument tray (as shown on page 42), special items shown in this photograph should be available. These include:

1 Single-ended speculum
2 Small-bladed scalpel
3 Right-angled hooks (2)
4 Cleft-palate scissors
5 Fine-toothed dissecting forceps (2)
6 Mosquito forceps
7 Fine sucker
8 Assorted needles, sutures and fine silver wire
9 Allis's tissue forceps
10 Fine artery forceps
11 Vaginal retractors

Essential steps in double layer fistula closure

The essential steps in double layer, and also in single layer, fistula closure are shown in the succeeding drawings and the legend describes each step. The structures have been kept lifelike while at the same time employing the advantages of diagrams in simplifying the procedures as far as possible.

8

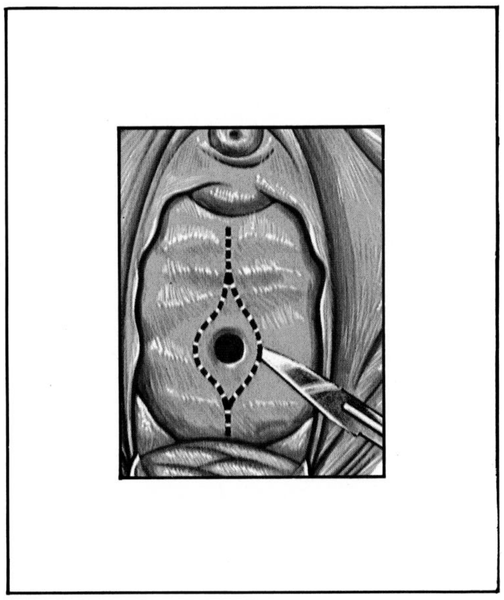

9

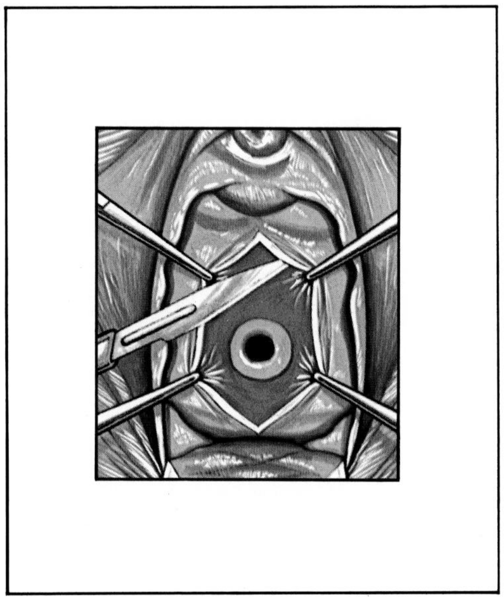

10

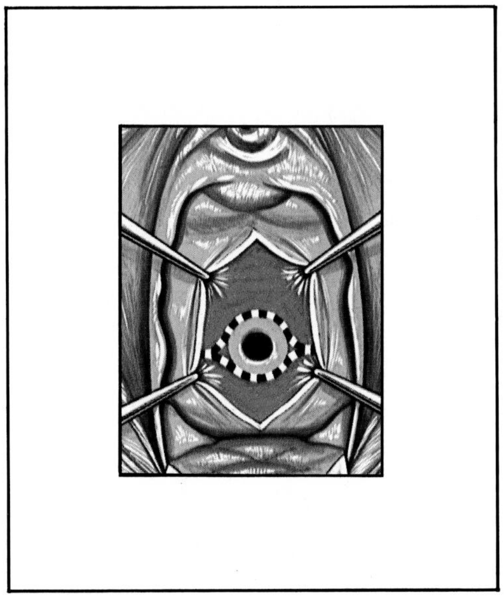

A vertical or oblique incision through skin only, diverges to encircle the area of the fistula which lies at its centre. Its course is shown by the dotted line in figure **8**. The vaginal skin flaps are dissected back from the incision line and from the isolated fistula using the small scalpel and the right angled hooks.

To aid fixation and access during dissection some surgeons prefer to insert a Foley balloon catheter into the bladder through the fistula, the assistant maintaining traction on it during dissection. Stay sutures are also sometimes helpful in maintaining the position of the skin closure. The appearance is now as in figure **9**.

The fibrous avascular edges of the fistula have to be excised and this is done transversely or as nearly at right angles to the skin incision as possible, using the cleft palate scissors. The line is indicated by dots in figure **10**.

11

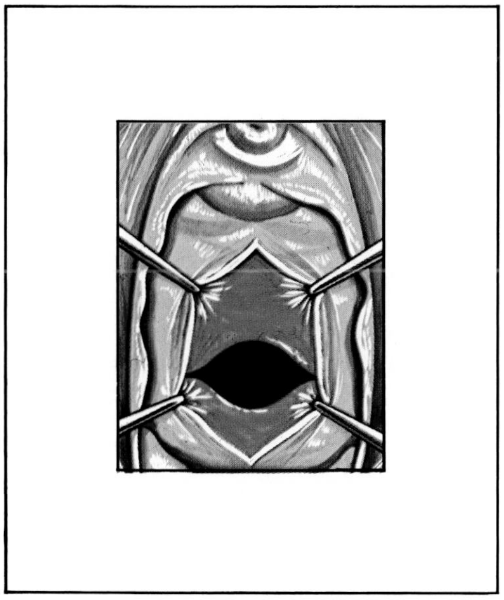

12

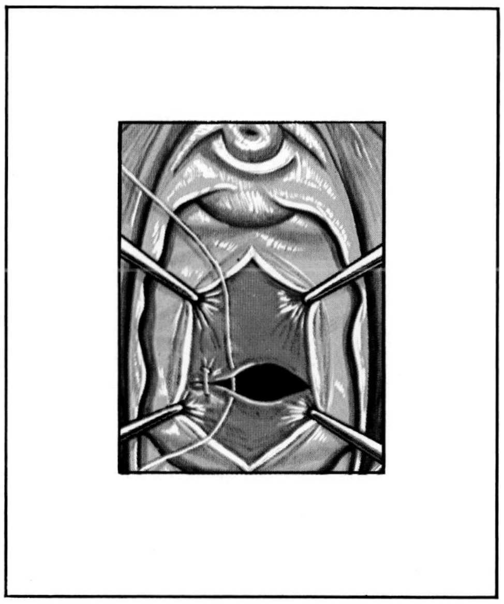

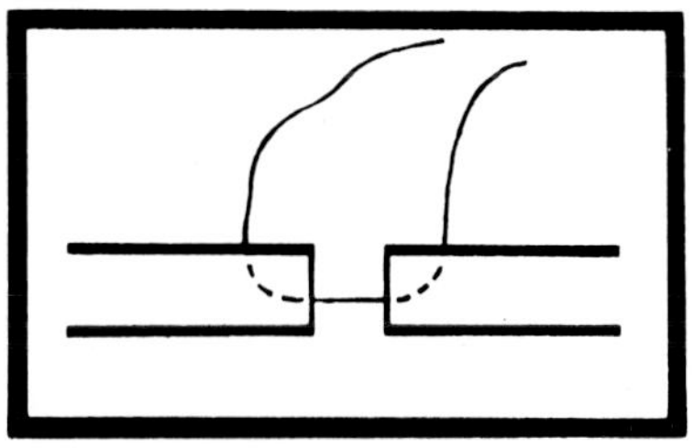

The transverse opening in the bladder with its freshened edges is shown in figure **11**. Transverse closure of the bladder wall by No. 000 plain catgut is shown in progress in figure **12**. The inset diagram shows how the stitches are placed to avoid their obtruding into the bladder.

13

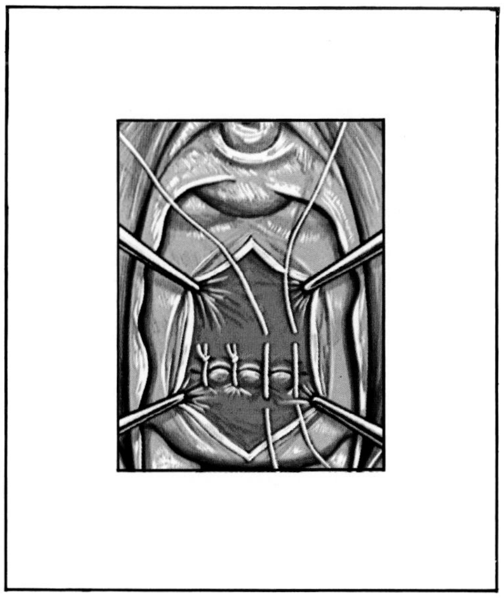

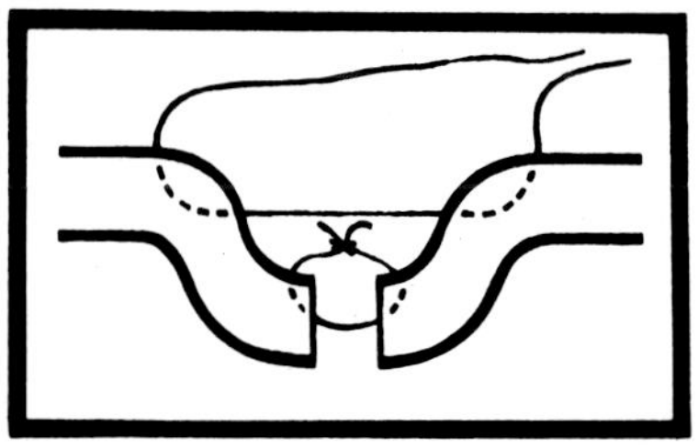

A second inverting layer of bladder sutures is placed over the first as shown in figure **13** and the area of tissue picked up is shown in the inset. With the bladder wall repaired the skin edges are held taut and ready for closure at right angles to the bladder incision as shown in figure **14**. Vertical mattress sutures are used to close the skin of the vaginal wall and the inset shows how each is placed.

14

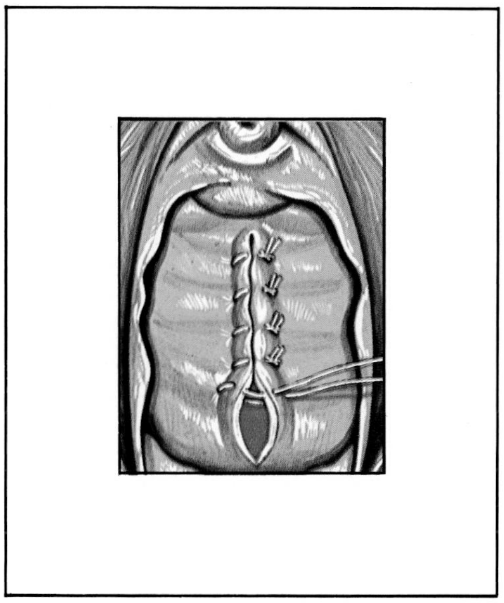

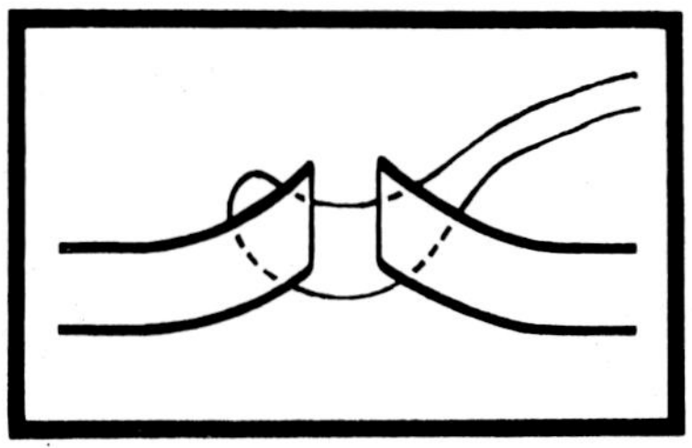

Essential steps in silver wire or nylon single layer closure of fistula

This method is only used where the two layers, namely the bladder wall and the vaginal skin, are not separable, as for example in the presence of gross fibrosis following radiotherapy. It is also the safest method where there is doubt about the viability of the tissues around the fistula. This again is usually where radiotherapy has caused the defect. The main objection is that the saucerisation entails the sacrifice of vaginal skin which brings its own disadvantages.

The area of the fistula is excised in such a way as to saucerise the wound and produce an elliptical defect which can be approximated without tension. The line of the incision depends on the shape of the fistula and the dotted line would be the appropriate one for the fistula shown in figure **15**. The incision is through the whole thickness of joint vaginal and bladder walls and approaches close to the fistula edge on the bladder mucosa, but is well slanted outwards on the skin edge to give a good wide saucerisation as shown in figure **16**. The inset shows the angle of incision through the tissues and the result achieved.

The ends of the ellipse are held taut by sutures (1 and 2 in figure **17**) to bring the freshened edges into correct alignment and a series of silver wire (or nylon) sutures are placed in position before starting to tie them; starting from each end in turn. The wound is shown with stitches *in situ* and ready for closure in figure **17** and the inset indicates the line of each stitch. Before tying each stitch and if the skin is healthy and sufficiently mobile the needle is taken through the skin edges to form vertical mattress sutures. The closed incision is shown in figure **18** with an inset to demonstrate the vertical mattress stitch.

15

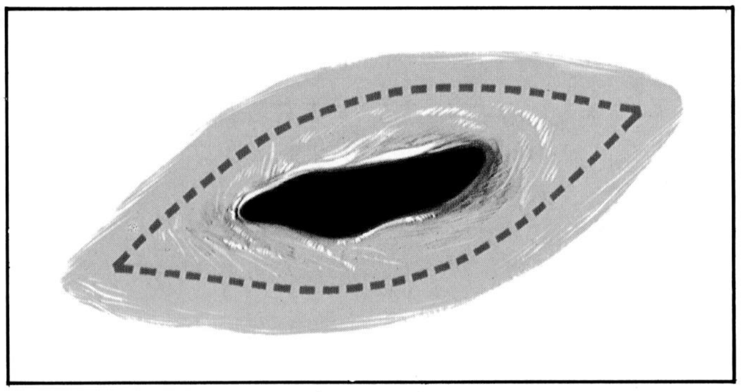

16

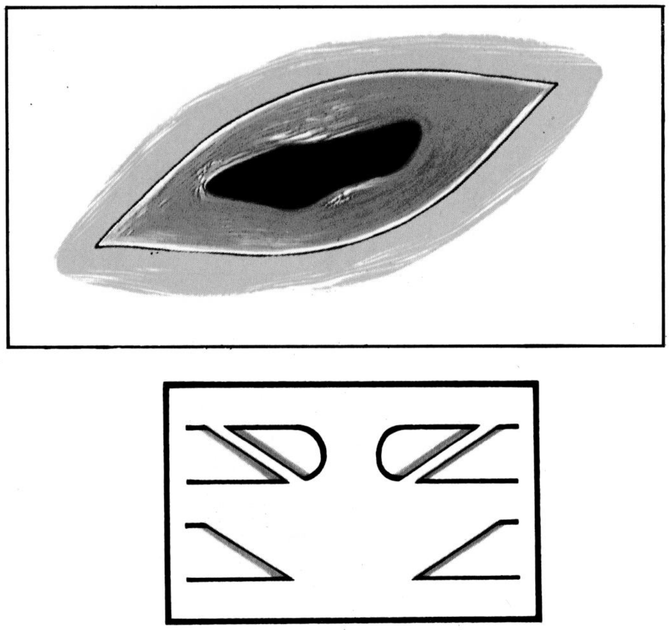

17

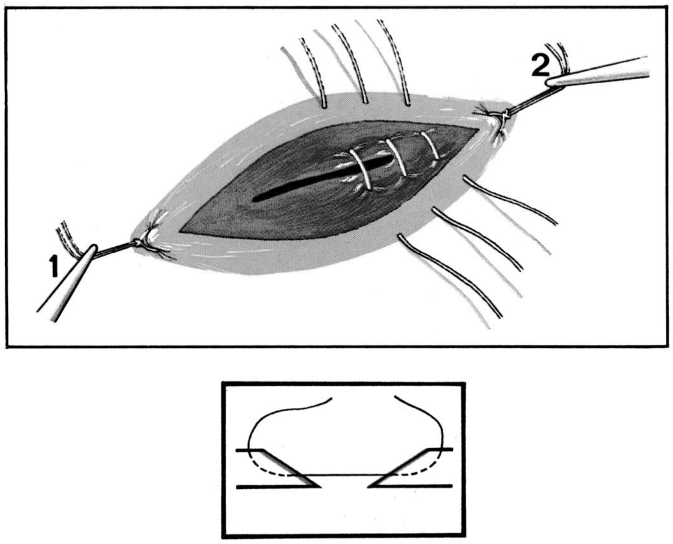

18

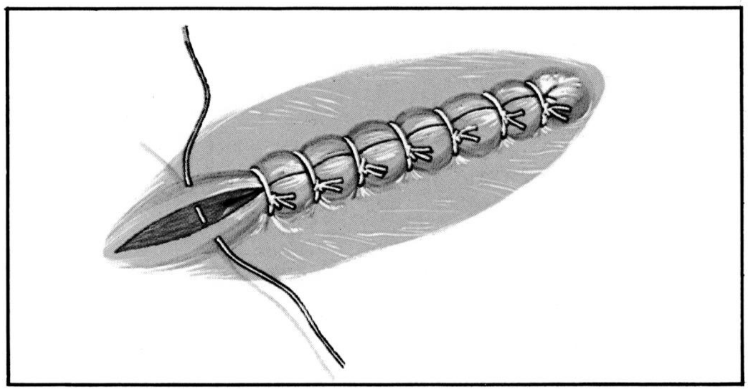

Acknowledgement

Figures **1** to **6** are from the collection of the University of Sheffield, Department of Obstetrics and Gynaecology, and were photographed by the late Professor C. S. Russell.

Suggested reading

1 Te Linde, R. W. & Mattingly, R. F. 'Operative Gynaecology', p. 584–623. Lippincott & Co., Philadelphia, 1970.
2 Moir, J. C. 'The Vesico-vaginal Fistula'. Oxford University Press, Oxford, 1967.
3 Russell, C. S. in 'Operative Surgery: Gynaecology & Obstetrics' **13,** p. 100–114, ed. Roberts, D. W. T., 2nd ed. Butterworths, London, 1977.

Index

Contents of further volumes in the Gynaecological Surgery series

Volume 2: Abdominal Operations For Benign Conditions

1 **Surgical Anatomy and Instruments**

2 **Opening and Closing of Abdomen**
Lower abdominal transverse incision
Midline (subumbilical) incision

3 ***Abdominal Hysterectomy***
Basic technique
Conditions demanding modification of basic hysterectomy technique:
Broad ligament fibroid
Cervical fibroid
Pelvic endometriosis
Chronic pelvic inflammatory disease (including hysterectomy for frozen pelvis)
Accompanying vaginal vault prolapse
Supravaginal (subtotal) hysterectomy
Removal of residual cervix

4 ***Myomectomy***

5 **Tubo-Ovarian Surgery**
Ovarian cystectomy
Salpingo-oophorectomy
Tubal ligation

6 **Endometriosis**
Conservative pelvic surgery, including ventrosuspension

7 ***Operation for Acute Pelvic Inflammatory Disease***

8 ***Appendicectomy***

9 **Laparoscopy**
Basic technique
Sterilisation procedures

10 ***Cysto-urethropexy*** *(Marshall–Marchetti–Krantz procedure)*

11 ***Ligation of Internal Iliac Artery***

12 ***Drainage of Abdominal Wound Haematoma***

13 ***Abdominal Closure of Pelvic Fistulae***
Vesico-vaginal fistula
Recto-vaginal fistula

Volume 3: Operations For Malignant Disease

1 **Instruments and Surgical Anatomy**

2 **Carcinoma of Vulva**
Biopsy of the vulva
Local vulvectomy
Radical vulvectomy
Radical vulvectomy with pelvic lymphadenectomy
Local excision of recurrent vulval carcinoma

3 **Cervical Carcinoma**
Preclinical Carcinoma
Colposcopy and cervical biopsy
Local destructive techniques:
Electrodiathermy
Cryosurgery
CO_2 laser
Cone biopsy
Abdominal hysterectomy with removal of vaginal cuff
Clinical Carcinoma
Examination, staging and biopsy
Radical hysterectomy with pelvic lymphadenectomy (Wertheim's Hysterectomy)

4 **Uterine Carcinoma**
Diagnostic dilatation and curettage
Extended hysterectomy
Radical hysterectomy and partial vaginectomy with pelvic node biopsy

5 **Ovarian Carcinoma**
Surgical clearance of pelvic growth (total hysterectomy and salpingo-oophorectomy)
Extensive surgical removal of abdomino-pelvic growth

6 ***Surgical Management of Recurrent Pelvic Malignancy***
(following failed radio-therapy)

7 **Radiotherapeutic Techniques**
Insertion of intrauterine and intravaginal radiation sources
External irradiation sources
Lymphography

Volume 4: Surgery Of Vulva And Lower Genital Tract

1 **Instruments and Surgical Anatomy**

2 **Urethral Operations**
Excision of caruncle
Excision of prolapsed urethra
Excision of para-urethral cyst

3 **Surgery of Bartholin Duct/Gland**
Excision of gland
Marsupialisation of cyst abscess

4 **Surgery of Vaginal Introitus**
Fenton's operation
Vaginoplasty with full thickness labial graft

5 **Surgery for Absent or Shortened Vagina**
Vulvo vaginoplasty (Williams operation)

6 **Surgery for Woolfian Duct Remnants**
Excision of paravaginal cyst
Marsupialisation of paravaginal cyst

7 **Treatment of Vulva Condylomata**
Excision diathermy
Cryosurgery

8 ***Surgery of Imperforate Hymen***

9 ***Haemorrhoidectomy***

10 ***Closure of Recto-Vaginal Fistula***

Volume 5: Infertility Surgery

1 **Instruments and Developmental Anatomy**

2 **Preliminary Investigations**
Hysterosalpingography
Intrauterine aspiration curettage (Vabra)
Laparoscopy

3 **Cervical Operations**
Trachelorraphy
Cervical cerclage (Shirodkar operation)

4 **Utero-Vaginal Operations for Congenital Malformations**
Division of vaginal septum
Uteroplasty (Strassman's operation)

5 **Tubo-Ovarian Operations**
Salpingolysis
Salpingostomy
Salpingostomy with prostheses
Implantation of Fallopian tube
Fallopian tubal reanastomosis
Conservative surgery of pelvic endometriosis

6 **Microsurgical Techniques in Infertility Surgery**
Implantation and reanastomosis of Fallopian tubes

Volume 6: Surgery Of Conditions Complicating Pregnancy

1 **Instruments and Surgical Anatomy in Pregnancy**

2 **Evacuation of Uterus**
Incomplete miscarriage
Hydatidiform mole

3 **Termination of Pregnancy**
During first trimester (suction curettage)
Under local anaesthetic (Karman cannula)
During second trimester (intra and extra amniotic drug instillation)

4 ***Abdominal Hysterotomy***

5 ***Cervical Cerclage*** *(Shirodkar operation)*

6 ***Ovarian Cyst in Pregnancy***

7 ***Appendicectomy in Pregnancy***

8 **Ectopic Pregnancy Surgery**
For complete tubal rupture (salpingectomy)
For intratubal haematocele (tubal conservation)
For abdominal pregnancy

9 ***Caesarean Section*** *(Lower Segment)*

10 ***Surgical Management of Uterine Choriocarcinoma***
(gestational trophoblastic disease)